DISABILITY
SPORT and RECREATION
RESOURCES

Third Edition

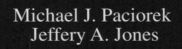

Michael J. Paciorek
Jeffery A. Jones

Disability Sport and Recreation Resources

3rd Edition

Michael J. Paciorek
Jeffery A. Jones

COOPER

Publishing
Group

Library of Congress Cataloging in Publication Data:

Paciorek, Michael J., 1953-
Jones, Jeffery A., 1956-

Disability Sport and Recreation Resources, 3rd Edition

Publisher: I. L. Cooper

Library of Congress Catalog Card Number: 2001086212
ISBN: 1-884125-75-1

Printed in the United States of America. Published by Cooper Publishing Group, LLC, P.O. Box 1129, Traverse City, MI 49685

10 9 8 7 6 5 4 3 2 1

Acknowledgements

Over the course of the last two years many people have graciously assisted us with the compilation of information and in lending their expertise. A book as comprehensive as this could never be the product of just two people. To the extent that we have succeeded in putting together a useful, informative, readable book, we owe them profound gratitude. To the extent we have failed, the shortcomings are ours alone. We would first like to recognize all of the students at Eastern Michigan University who helped to gather and research valuable resources. You are great students and will make even better educators.

Andy Ames, Jim Barnes, Jennifer Baughman, Hassen Berry, Dena Berstein, Angie Black, Melanie Bolton, Michael Bright, Ronda Brodsky, Julie Brouwer, Chandra Brown, Elizabeth Brown, Tom Carney, Scott Casebolt, Mary Colburn, Rob Conley, Michael Daily, Patrick Daugherty, Adrian Dean, Russ Dekker, T.J. Delamielleure, Lawrence DeWolf, Garrick Elston, Hugh Felt, Shaney Froysland, Chuck Fuller, William Grove, Rodericka Greaves, Tyice Griffin, Frank Haliburda, Patrick Hansen, Tim Hense, Melissa Hopson, Michael Huber, Erik Johnson, Seth Kenny, Danny Knipper, John Kramer, Andy Irvine, Mike Jackson, Jennifer Langston, Kevin Leszczynski, Carrie Lindsey, Mel Long, Matt Lumetta, Russ McKenzie, Kristy Meek, Molly Menard, Matt Merrill, Mary Frances Milke, Kim Morrow, Andy Osterholm, Laura Pasden, Stacy Peterson, Jamie Piasecki, Lisa Pinto, Erica Rahm, Jennifer Reid, Chris Robertson, Tracy Rynkiewicz, Darcy Schrieber, Becky Smith, Janet Smith, Jim Squibbs, Renee Staley, Kate Steele, Jennifer Tedesco, James Thiede, David Thompson, Jody Thompson, Ron Thornton, Brian VanDerziel, Todd Vokal, Susan Waldrop, Amy Zanetti, Brian Zawislak.

The inclusion of many wonderful photographs and illustrations were due to the efforts of a number of people. Our deep appreciation for providing photographs and illustrations goes to Chris Jordan of the Rehabilitation Institute of Chicago and the staffs at Special Olympics Michigan, and the United States Association for Blind Athletes (USABA). Extra special gratitude is extended to Valerie Miller of PVA Publications, specifically *Sports 'n Spokes*; and to Bob Radocy of Therapeutic Recreation Systems (TRS).

Gathering information from the many individual organizations associated with this book was, by far, the most rewarding aspect of this book. Our deep appreciation goes out to all the DSO's and NGB's who responded to our many requests for information.

There always seemed to be technical questions that had to be answered. In that regard we received much help. Some of the people that must be recognized are Lynn Rourke for her excellent review of the Archery Chapter, Patricia McCowan (CAN President), Jonathan Newman (BORP), Tim Shurtleff (Organization Effectiveness Consulting Practice), and Tommie Storm (AASSP). Clerical support from our staff at Eastern Michigan University especially Jennifer Rieger and Yulanda Woods was outstanding. Thanks to Fred Andres, Department Head at EMU for his understanding about the copying situation and for the support of the entire EMU administrative staff. Thanks to our good friend Erik Pedersen for taking the load off during critical times. Special thanks goes to Pearl Ragalie of the RIC Center for Health and Fitness. Thanks to Editors Butch and Joanne Cooper for your patience with us.

To all athletes who participate under the auspices of one or more of the organizations listed in this book, our deepest appreciation. You have motivated us to bring together the many resources listed here in the hope that others will follow in your footsteps. You are great athletes and this book is for you.

Although this book is dedicated to our families, their efforts must also be acknowledged here. They provided constant encouragement through many long days and nights. Without their support, this book would not have been completed. Deepest thanks are extended to our wives, Marybeth Jones and Karen Menke Paciorek for their support and love. To our children, Clark and Clay Paciorek, and Kristyn and Benjamin Jones, thank you for your support and respite from this long task. You brought smiles to our faces and encouragement to continue. To Loretta Paciorek, mother of the co-author, I know you were watching down over us and leading us to good sources. To Loretta Watkins, mother-in-law to Jeff Jones, thanks for the years of wisdom and support.

DEDICATION

For our spouses Marybeth Jones and Karen Menke Paciorek, and our children, Kristyn and Benjamin Jones, and Clark and Clay Paciorek. Without your continual support and encouragement, this project would never have been completed. Thank you for being there always.

"Having a physical disability is not the same as being disabled. Failing to make that distinction, we leave out the most important ingredient in human achievement, the desire in each of us to strive for the best we can be. Everyone lives in an age of opportunities and technological advances and yet, our most marvelous and moving experiences are still those victories of will and spirit against almost seemingly insurmountable odds."

Jean-Michael Cousteau
Freedom in Depth
Handicapped Scuba Association, 1985

Cover photo credits:

Soccer Player:	Eli A. Wolft, Washington, D.C.	
	1996 Atlanta Paralympic Games	
	Photographer: Jeffery Jones, Chicago, IL	

Cyclist:	Kyle Weber, Stroudsburg, PA	
	1996 Cycling in the Rocky Mountains	
	Photographer: John Weiland	
		2075 South Wright St.,
		Lakewood, CO 80228
	Phone:	(303) 986-8960

Skier:	Sandy Dokat, Chicago, IL	
	2001 U.S. Disabled Alpine Nationals	
	Photographer: Marshall Tate, Crystal Image Photography	
		Big Sky, MT
	Phone:	(406) 995-2426
		Bigsky photos.com

Contents

Preface

The high profile case of professional golfer Casey Martin illustrates the point that people with disabilities will not sit idly on the sidelines watching others participate in physical activity. Casey Martin has a rare circulatory disorder, which makes walking very painful. In 1998 Martin sued the PGA Tour for the right to use a golf cart during competition (it should be noted that the PGA Tour and the PGA of America are separate entities). Martin won the initial case and it was appealed by the Tour. The PGA Tour felt that by allowing Martin to use a cart it would change the nature of the competition, in a sense giving him an unfair advantage. It seems inconceivable that anyone who has a degenerative condition in their leg causing severe pain every time they move could have an unfair advantage in a sporting event. In March of 2000 the federal appeals court upheld the appellate courts ruling allowing Martin to ride. Yet, this issue is far from over. The day after the Martin ruling, another case heard in the Midwest involving a club-pro and the USGA on exactly the same issue and argument, was won by the USGA. These two rulings on the same argument has set-up the possibility of further litigation.

The ascent to the summit of Mt. Everest by Tom Whittaker in 1998, the first successful attempt by a person with a disability (single leg amputee) to climb the world's tallest mountain, was a terrific athletic accomplishment and provided great evidence that people with disabilities desire to participate in adventure activities. Mark Wellman's (a climber with spinal cord injury) two ascents of El Capitan 10 years apart, also were well-documented in the media and brought much attention about the capabilities of individuals with disabilities in tackling even the most challenging adventure activities.

This book is dedicated to those with the spirit of Casey Martin, Tom Whittaker, and Mark Wellman and the hundreds of thousands of children, teenagers and adults with disabilities throughout the world who are active in sports and recreation (Figure 1).

Known as the "Bible of Disability Sport", the 3rd Edition of *Disability Sport and Recreation Resources* includes a title change from *Sports and Recreation for the Disabled*. This book is the most complete guide to disability sports available and includes up to date information on almost four dozen sports and recreation activities that are accessible to individuals with disabilities, including people who are blind or deaf or who have amputations, cerebral palsy, spinal cord injuries, dwarfism, cognitive challenges or other physical disabilities (Figure 2).

There has been unprecedented growth in disability sports since the first edition of this book was published in 1989 as well as an increased knowledge of the benefits of physical activity. The book was developed under the premise that participation in athletic and recreational activity is the right of every individual, and is an integral part of leading a meaningful and balanced life. As Americans become increasingly sedentary and obese, we have seen an increase in the numbers of people acquiring coronary heart disease and diabetes. Individuals with disabilities are at great risk for complications from secondary conditions as a result of their inactivity. The Surgeon General's Report of 1996 identified physical inactivity as a major cause of death to Americans—cardio-

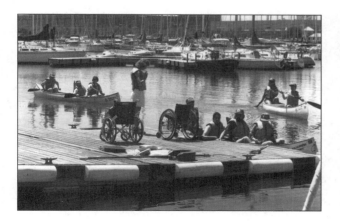

Figure 1. Wilderness Inquiry conducting a Learn to Canoe workshop in Chicago. (Courtesy of Oscar Izquierdo and Rehabilitation Institute of Chicago's Wirtz Sports Program)

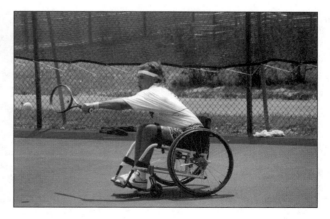

Figure 2. USA Tennis, the national governing body (NGB) for tennis, now coordinates wheelchair tennis nationwide. (Courtesy of Specialized Sports Unlimited)

vascular disease. The benefits of even moderate amounts of physical activity have been shown to significantly reduce the chances of many diseases in addition to improving mental health. National initiatives and goals such as Healthy People 2010 have identified the reduction of obesity and increase in physical activity as national priorities.

The central theme of this book is introducing ways in which individuals with disabilities can access sport and recreational activities from which they have been traditionally excluded. Chapters are organized alphabetically and start with All-Terrain Vehicles and end with Wrestling. In between is information on team and individual sports, competitive and recreational activities. The reader will soon realize that no sports are off-limits to a person with a disability.

The book is written for people with disabilities who refuse to have limits placed on their selection of physical activities. Physical education teachers, adapted physical education teachers, physical therapists, occupational therapists, recreation therapists, sports medicine professionals, physicians and health-care personnel, parents and anyone involved in assisting people with disabilities to achieve their maximum potential through physical activity will find this book to be an invaluable resource. It provides an excellent supplement to an adapted physical education or therapeutic recreation class, where time may not be available to discuss modification of activities in-depth. It should serve as the primary text in classes dealing specifically with disability sport and recreation.

The motivation for this book comes from the authors' feeling that sports and recreation are meant for all individuals and not just elite athletes. It is the right of all people to have access to opportunities for physical activity. The compilation of information for this edition took two years to complete. When the 2nd Edition of this book was published in 1994, there were no internet resources. The addition of the internet has brought access to information into our homes. Making contact with hundreds of resource individuals made it evident that the scope of sports and recreation for individuals with disabilities has grown tremendously. There are opportunities being presented by thousands of unselfish individuals dedicated by their love of physical activity and the understanding of its power. Certainly without their help, this text would not have been possible

PURPOSE OF THE BOOK

Disability Sport and Recreation Resources takes a cross-disability view of sporting and recreational opportunities for individuals with disabilities. The framework of this text features seven key cross-disability multisport organizations. Each of these organizations provides services in more than one sport to a target population based specifically on disability or groups of disabilities. The United States Olympic Committee officially recognizes these organizations as Disabled Sports organizations (DSOs). These DSOs include the following: Disabled Sports USA (DSUSA), the Dwarf Athletic Association of America (DAAA), Special Olympics, Inc. (SOI), the United States Association for Blind Athletes (USABA), the United States Cerebral Palsy Athletic Association (USCPAA), the United States Deaf Sports Federation (USDSF), and Wheelchair Sports USA (WSUSA). Some of these organizations have undergone name changes since the 2nd edition of this book. Disabled Sports USA was formerly National Handicapped Sports (NHS), the United States Deaf Sports Federation was formerly the American Athletic Association of the Deaf (AAAD) and Wheelchair Sports USA was formerly the National Wheelchair Athletic Association (NWAA). These name changes were a result of reorganization of some of these groups or done to better identify the organization's mission. Each of these organizations is discussed in greater detail further in the text. In addition to these seven multisport organizations, more than 200 national, regional and local organizations and programs provide sports and recreation opportunities for individuals with disabilities and are referenced within thee pages. The text is designed to provide resource information on almost four dozen competitive and recreational sports activities for individuals who have a wide range of abilities.

CHAPTER ORGANIZATION

Each chapter is organized specifically to provide the most current information available, and to allow individuals to access relevant information.

National Governing Bodies (NGB)

Where applicable, the national and international nondisabled National Governing Bodies (NGBs) are listed. Space limitations do not allow the inclusion of all the rules of each sport. In most cases specific information on rules can be received by contacting the nondisabled NGB or by accessing their web site. With an emphasis on inclusion, most of the competitions offered in disability sport is conducted under nondisabled NGB rules, usually only with slight modifications. Each of the nondisabled NGBs provides information to promote the growth and enjoyment of their sport. Many nondisabled NGBs have established committees or subgroups to address participation by individuals with disabilities.

Disability Sport National Governing Body

In many cases, NGBs exist for sports or activities open to individuals with disabilities. They function in much the same capacity as nondisabled NGBs, to oversee the development and conduct of their sports. Where applicable, names and addresses have been provided. Some may find it surprising that some sports, such as wheelchair tennis, are not listed as official sports of Wheelchair Sports USA. Wheelchair Sports does not offer tennis as an official sport. Wheelchair tennis is offered as part of the programming of USA Tennis. Other sports such as wheelchair bowling, equestrian and scuba, have specific national organizations which provide governance over the sport.

Official Sport Listing

For competitive events, the disabled sports organizations that offer the activity as an official or demonstration sport are identified. Do not assume that a sport is not possible for a person with a disability just because it is not offered as an official or demonstration sport. Organizations continue to expand their offerings as interest demands. As mentioned previously, some sports are offered through organizations other than the multisport disability sport organizations.

Primary Disability

In most cases, participation in any of the activities is not restricted by disability. In other cases however, activities have been developed for specific disabilities such as goalball and showdown for people who are blind, blowdarts for people who use power wheelchairs, and quad rugby for individuals with quadriplegia. We have attempted to match disabilities with the most suitable activities.

Sports Overview

A brief description provides general information and rationale for offering this activity to individuals with disabilities. Discussion throughout the book will focus on how activities are similar to and different from nondisabled sports. Descriptions of program offerings by the seven major disability sport organizations is included, as well as references to more than 200 other sports and recreation organizations. A quick reference, sport-by-sport listing of major organizations can be found in the appendix.

Historical Overview

A new feature of this book includes a brief historical overview of the sport and inclusion by people with disabilities. In some cases a detailed historical accounting of participation by people with disabilities is included, while in other cases very little information exists. It is hoped that this will spark an interest in historians to document participation by people with disabilities in the various sports. It is evident that further historical documentation is needed.

Adapted Equipment/Modified Rules

Although in most cases, individuals with disabilities will be able to enjoy physical activities with little, if any, equipment or rule modifications, a thorough review of the literature has discovered many unique sources and types of equipment that will allow a person with a disability to access sport and recreation opportunities. As with participation in all physical activities, there is an element of risk and potential for injury. It is up to the individual to assess the risks involved and participate in each activity within safe guidelines. It should be noted that the authors have not used these adaptive devices and it is the responsibility of the user to be a smart consumer by analyzing how the equipment would meet individual needs and if it is safe for use.

Equipment Suppliers and Manufacturers

It is of little use to be aware of an equipment adaptation but not know where to obtain one. This book lists over 250 equipment suppliers and manufacturers that market adaptive equipment for people with disabilities. This in itself should provide a valuable resource to therapists, professionals, athletes with disabilities, coaches and others with an interest in this area. Many local athletic supply stores can provide all the equipment that anyone will need for participation. Listing of a supplier or manufacturer in this book does not constitute an endorsement by the authors, but is provided as reference information only.

Additional Resources and Internet Resources

It has never been easier in the history of the world to access information related to disability sport. This section provides a variety of references to enable the person with a disability to access sports and recreation opportunities. It includes more than 200 sports and recreation associations and resources (many that cater only to athletes with disabilities), contact people, addresses, means to access the outdoors, training information, and videotapes geared to those with disabilities. An added and valuable feature includes new information on hundreds of electronic resources, such as website and email addresses for international and national disability and non-disability sport organizations. It should be understood that electronic resources have a tendency to change frequently. To minimize this, the authors have included only those sites that appear to be the most stable. The authors have conducted an extensive and time-consuming review of websites for each of the sports over the past two years. The majority of these major websites provide additional links to other resources and local programs. The 2nd edition of this book provided addresses for many individual programs such as all of the Special Olympics, Disabled Sports USA and Wheelchair Sports USA affiliated programs. The addresses and contacts for these programs had a history of frequent change making the information obsolete. The 3rd edition of the book does not include such information. This information is more easily accessed by using the website for each of these organizations. In many cases they provide direct links to these affiliated program websites. As long as websites are kept current, information will be easily accessed.

The sole purpose of this book is to provide the most detailed information available on how individuals with disabilities can access sports and recreation opportunities. It is not intended to be a coffee-table book, but is designed to be used on a daily basis. This book was organized to be user-friendly with information at your fingertips. We hope this book will be used by people with and without disabilities, will provide an insight into sports programs for people with disabilities, and encourage you to seek additional information. We wish to remind everyone that there is little a person with a disability cannot do if they have the desire, determination, motivation, and opportunity. Stay active, stay healthy, and have fun.

Introduction

It is well-documented that athletic competition has been an important component of human existence for thousands of years. Organized athletic competition for individuals with physical disabilities traces its beginnings to the Stoke Mandeville Hospital in England where Sir Ludwig Guttman used sport in his rehabilitation of injured World War II veterans. It was only a little more than 30 years ago when Eunice Kennedy Shriver believed enough in the power of physical activity to start Special Olympics for individuals with cognitive disabilities. In the past three decades, sports participation has become increasingly possible for individuals with developmental disabilities, cerebral palsy, dwarfism, visual impairments, and les autres conditions. The importance and benefits of athletic competition for athletes with disabilities is just as keen as it is for nondisabled athletes if not greater .

Athletes with disabilities participate in sport and recreation for the same reasons as nondisabled individuals. Physical and health benefits have been well documented. In the past, limited opportunities for athletic activity forced many individuals with disabilities to lead sedentary lives, resulting in the accumulation of health risk factors. This sedentary life is not limited to individuals with disabilities however. The Surgeon General, citing with alarm in 1996, that physical inactivity is one of the key factors in the leading cause of death in this country, cardiovascular disease, called for increased physical activity by all Americans. As people become better educated about the benefits of physical activity it is hoped that physical activity will become a normal part of everyone's lives. Individuals with disabilities are seeking out programs in greater numbers to maintain appropriate levels of fitness through physical activity to reduce these health risk factors.

The psychological benefits of physical activity are also well documented. Individuals who are physically active and physically fit are less likely to suffer depression and anxiety. If an individual finds that sports participation is still possible despite a congenital or acquired disability, then self-motivation often leads to other accomplishments. Issues of family, independent living, employment, and community participation are frequently addressed with a renewed perspective.

Individuals with disabilities have overcome many discriminatory barriers in recent years. The American's with Disabilities Act (1990) addresses many aspects of equal access including access to recreation programs. As a direct result of this act, facilities are being built that are accessible for all Americans. Golf course designers have turned many golf courses into accessible venues by experimenting with special grasses that will allow carts to be driven right into the green. Most road races now welcome individuals with disabilities and many have special race categories for athletes who use wheelchairs. Colleges and universities are slowly expanding athletic scholarships to include athletes with disabilities. The perception of the general public towards individuals with disabilities is changing dramatically as visibility in sports increases. Athletes with disabilities are now seen on television sponsored by major corporations. For instance, a powerful commercial features wheelchair racer Deanna Sodoma for Northwest Airlines. "If I can't get my wheelchair to the starting line", says Sodoma, "I can't win the race. I depend on Northwest Airlines". As the general public becomes accustomed to seeing people with disabilities participating on an equal basis, perceptions can be formed or altered. Our society assumes that people who are successful in sports, are successful in other aspects of life as well.

Sports and recreation opportunities for individuals with disabilities is receiving increased attention in universities, public schools, rehabilitation centers and recreation programs. Most professional physical education and recreation training programs within universities now offer at least one course in adapted physical education or sport for individuals with disabilities. Those that do not must alter their curricula to include such information. Many universities are also offering health-related physical activity courses for their students with disabilities.

Although organized sports for individuals with physical disabilities had its beginnings in a rehabilitation setting, it has only been within the last decade or so that programs of high quality are being offered in rehabilitation settings. Some examples of high quality programs that have emerged include the Wirtz Sports Program and Center for Health and Fitness at the Rehabilitation Institute of Chicago (Figure 1), the Shepherd Spinal Cord Center in Atlanta, the recreation program at the Roosevelt Rehabilitation Center in Warm Springs, Georgia, the Craig Rehabilitation Hospital in Denver and the adaptive sport program at the Charlotte Institute of Rehabilitation in North Carolina to name but a few. Additional rehabilitation centers are sending their staff to special seminars and workshops to help them to develop sports programs. Many rehabilitation centers offer community-based programs that serve a cross-disability population who have completed therapy at their centers, in addition to other individuals with disabilities who are general members of the community.

This book is dedicated to all athletes and educators who promote healthy and active living for all individuals. The success stories of individuals and organizations who have triumphed offer clear testimony that individuals with disabilities will no longer be content to sit on the sidelines (Figure 2). Participation in physical activity leading to healthy living is a right of all individuals, and opportunities must continue to be developed by professionals in the field. Although much has been accomplished in recent years, the challenges of equal access, funding, representation, public education, and appropriate classification systems still remain. These challenges may never be completely solved, but through the work of dedicated individuals, they can be minimized.

Public Recognition

Effective public recognition of sports and recreation programs for individuals with disabilities can serve two major purposes: public education and revenue generation.

Public Education: Promoting the abilities of individuals with disabilities in sports and recreation pursuits changes public attitudes. Sport is a very powerful medium that accentuates ability and normalization. Higher visibility of sports programs also increases participation by individuals with disabilities. Many people are still unsure about what programs are open and how to access them. Parents, teachers, and therapists must be informed about the programs available. Athletes with disabilities such as Jean Driscoll, Scot Hollonbeck, Tim Willis, Linda Mastandrea, Ann Cody-Morris, Tony Volpentest, David Larson, Brad Parks, Dennis Ohler, Trisha Zorn (Figure 3a and 3b), and many others have become public role models and spokespersons for the disability sports movement. Children with disabilities can now look up to these athletes as examples of what might be possible.

Revenue Generation: The marketing of Disabled Sports USA, the United States Disabled Athletes Fund, and Special Olympics at all program levels is testimony to what can be accomplished through effective public education. It is important to generate greater name recognition for all of the disability sport organizations. Organizations that are successful revenue generators have effective management teams from the national to local levels who work together to promote programs and generate funds. This great public recognition supports fundraising ventures that will help programming at all levels.

Although media attention has been inadequate nationally, especially during the 1996 Paralympic games, there have been some successes. Two journals worth mentioning include *Palaestra*, dedicated to providing professionals with information on adapted physical education, recreation and sport, and *Sports 'n Spokes*, dedicated primarily to sports and recreation for individuals who use wheelchairs. Both have filled a void and have provided timely and educational information. Inclusion of articles in other journals and magazines through the work of many professionals is proof that sports for people with disabilities is a viable area for study and research.

Increased Emphasis on Research

Increases in the numbers of programs and athletes with disabilities participating have boosted the quantity and quality of related research. Studies on athletes with disabilities are published in a variety of professional jour-

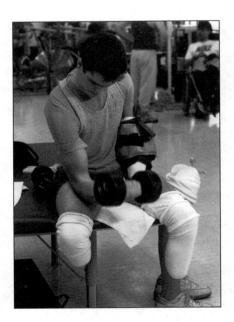

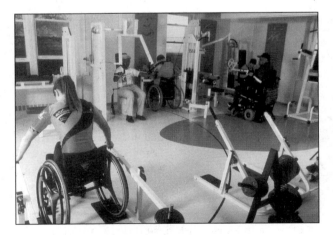

Figure 1. An increasing number of rehabilitation centers are offering strength and conditioning programs as part of outpatient or sports and recreation programming. (Courtesy of Oscar Izquierdo and Rehabilitation Institute of Chicago's Wirtz Sports Program)

Figure 2. Less than two years after an accident resulting in the loss of three extremities, B.J. Miller competed on the U.S. Sitting Volleyball Team at the Paralympic Games in Barcelona. (Courtesy of Oscar Izquierdo and Rehabilitation Institute of Chicago's Wirtz Sports Program)

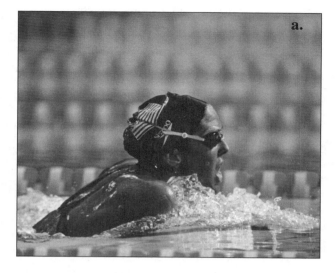

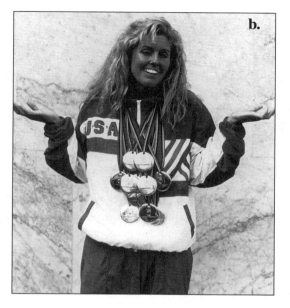

Figure 3 a-b. Trisha Zorn is the most successful visually impaired swimmer in history, winning 12 medals at the 1992 Paralympic Games in Barcelona, Spain. (Courtesy of USABA)

nals. *The Adapted Physical Activity Quarterly (APAQ)* is dedicated to individuals who have disabilities and presents the latest research in sports and physical activity. University exercise science labs must become more open to athletes with disabilities. Research needs to be conducted in all areas and the results disseminated to coaches and practitioners.

Inclusion with Nondisabled Athletics

An issue facing leaders in the sports movement for individuals with disabilities is the degree to which competition should include both the disabled and the nondisabled (Figure 4). Most national and international events for nondisabled athletes have been troubled by excessive numbers of participants. Although demonstration events for athletes with disabilities (wheelchair racers and skiers) have been a part of the Olympic Games since 1984, and the United States Olympic Festival since 1985, the cost of the Olympic Games is already prohibitive. There has been talk of imposing further limits on participation for nondisabled athletes but the idea of increasing disabled athlete participation in the Olympic Games is being vigorously discussed. In the next few decades a handful of events for athletes with disabilities may become official Olympic events; however, the merger of the Olympic and Paralympic games into a single competition does not appear to be feasible. Joint Olympic and Paralympic committees working cooperatively as in Seoul, Barcelona, Nagano, Sydney, and Salt Lake City will continue as decreed by the International Olympic Committee (IOC).

Athletes with disabilities compete with nondisabled athletes in sports in which disability is not a factor and in demonstration events at specific competitions. The United States Association of Blind Athletes (USABA) and Special Olympics have developed mechanisms to specifically address this issue. Athletes with visual impairments have routinely trained with sighted athletes especially in track and cycling events. Sighted guides in running and sighted pilots in cycling have been used for many years. The Special Olympics Unified Sports Program takes athletes with and without cognitive impairments and places them on the same team for integrated competition. Very specific rules ensure fairness for all athletes. This logical approach addresses the intent of such legislation as the Individuals with Disabilities Education Act (IDEA) and the Americans with Disabilities Act of 1990 (ADA).

Classification Issues

Classification systems are vital to competitions for athletes with disabilities. The various classification systems are discussed within the description of each disabled sports organization. Classification allows for equitable competition and helps to ensure that training and skill are the determining factors in winning and losing, and not the type or level of disability. The challenge continuing to face leaders in multi-disability competitions is the great number of classification categories which produces an organizational nightmare. A low number of entrants may diminish the quality of competition or force cancellations, confusing spectators and athletes alike. The integrated classification system utilized since the Paralympic Games in Barcelona has been met with mixed results. Although the intent to streamline the games is sincere, serious challenges have surfaced that need to be addressed.

While some sports are well suited to an integrated classification system (archery, shooting, and table tennis), others are not. Organizers of the Paralympic games have recognized that blind swimmers would be at a significant advantage compared with athletes who had physical disabilities. Blind swimmers are thus allowed to swim in their own category utilizing the traditional classification system for the blind. However, athletes with cerebral palsy and spinal cord injuries are at a distinct disadvantage compared to amputee swimmers. Athletes with cerebral palsy and spinal cord-injured swimmers find it difficult to win Paralympic swimming medals and even to make it to the finals, although their level of training is as advanced as ever. In this case, disability rather than training is the determining factor in their failure to succeed, undermining the very purpose of classification. Due to this inequitable classification system, fewer and fewer athletes with cerebral palsy and athletes with higher level spinal cord injuries are participating in Paralympic Games (Figure 5). We must address the management issues of these games, review the current integrated classification system, and revise it to ensure that all athletes have an equal opportunity for success based on ability, not disability.

Vertical Integration

In response to the passage of the Amateur Sports Act of 1998, there has been a greater emphasis on vertical integration. Vertical integration is the philosophy where National Governing Bodies takes greater responsibility for including elite athletes with disabilities into their programs as opposed to athletes participating in segregated programs. For instance, athletes with disabilities who are interested in cycling would now theoretically have programs available to them through USA Cycling. Many of the sport governing bodies have had programs representing athletes with disabilities in place for many years. In fact, USA Tennis has now taken complete control of Wheelchair Tennis programming as opposed to the old National Foundation of Wheelchair Tennis. Many NGBs have had modifications to their rules in their rulebooks for many years. The role of these NGBs and the role played by the disability sport organizations will be debated and refined during the next few years.

Grass Roots Programming

One potential outcome of vertical integration is that disability sport organizations may focus an even greater amount of their efforts to grass roots programs in local communities. National programs are developed for one major reason: to serve athletes in the local regions at the grass roots level to ensure maximum participation. Although the development of elite athletes is important and much attention is focused on national and international competitions, disabled sports make the most significant contributions in communities where the majority of participants may never qualify for international competition. Sports involve much more than the winning of gold medals. Their lasting value is in participation itself. All too often, national sport programs focus too heavily on the upper level athlete and neglect the majority of the athletes. The development of local programs needs more attention. All disabled sport organizations should adopt a

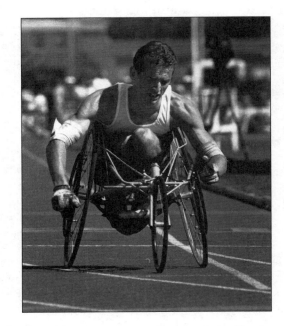

Figure 5. Although supporters of integrated classification consider the wheelchair to be the equalizing factor, the physiological difference among disabilities makes developing an equitable classification system very difficult. (Photo by Oscar Izquierdo)

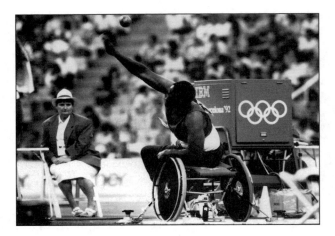

Figure 4. Inclusion of events for athletes with disabilities into the Olympic Games will be one of a number of priorities for disabled sports in the 1990's. (Photo by Oscar Izquierdo)

management team approach or a similar system. Within each local program a management team should include individuals with a variety of backgrounds. Management teams typically recruit volunteers who serve on committees for fund raising, public education, training, parents, sports competition, finance, medical, and other activities as needed. This cooperative team approach can be coordinated by a volunteer who ensures that priorities are established and goals accomplished. Job requirements should be spelled out clearly. The success of this system has been tremendous in Special Olympic programming. The national disability sports program should develop materials similar to SOI to direct volunteers. The characteristic that distinguishes the Special Olympics volunteers from volunteers in many other programs is evidence of adequate guidance.

Respect for the Entire Disability Sport Movement

Leaders in disability sport have worked tirelessly against the prejudices and biases of a society that has not been completely educated about the potential of athletes and individuals with disabilities. Athletes and individuals with disabilities want to be accepted and recognized for their abilities and for their accomplishments. No special treatment is ever asked of the able bodied community, only equal access and equal opportunity. The perception in much of the able bodied community for many years is that disability sport is not really sport at all and that much skill is not needed. These perceptions are slowly changing and society is beginning to realize the excitement of disability sport competition.

It is important to realize that each of the disability sport organizations is different in their programming and organizational structures and sometimes in their philosophy. For instance athletes who are deaf and who compete within the USA Deaf Sports Federation choose to not compete in the Paralympic Games. They choose to compete within their own international game structure, The World Games for the Deaf (WGD). Among the Deaf community there is overwhelming support for separate Games. Deaf people do not consider themselves disabled, particularly in physical ability. Rather, they consider themselves to be part of a cultural and linguistic minority. The Deaf athlete is physically able-bodied and able to compete without significant restrictions, with the exception of communication barriers. The purpose of the deaf games is to bring people together. Leaders in deaf sport believe this would be lost if deaf athletes competed in the Paralympic Games. Although some leaders within disability sport may view this as being counterproductive, it is important to respect this viewpoint from the oldest disability sport organization.

Likewise there has been criticism of the Special Olympic program from athletes involved in programs for the physically disabled. Athletes with physical disabilities have long since complained that they have not received the respect from the able-bodied community that they deserve, however some have done the same thing to athletes with cognitive challenges and to athletes with severe physical disabilities such as cerebral palsy. A perception exists at the highest level of disability sports that athletes involved in Special Olympics are not really athletes and that the program is more recreational than competitive. This perception is not only wrong in most cases, but it is potentially damaging to the disability sports movement. Athletes with disabilities have long fought for equal opportunity and status among the able-bodied sports world. For athletes with physical disabilities to criticize athletes with cognitive disabilities is hypocritical. The classification system in Special Olympic competition is somewhat different from other disability sport organizations, but it is similar in that it allows athletes with varying levels of functional ability to participate on an equal basis against people with similar abilities. We need to celebrate the fact that there are opportunities to participate in physical activity and not spend needless energy criticizing one another. If we cannot respect one another, how can we ask respect from others?

Much has been accomplished during the past few years in promoting programs for individuals with disabilities. All future challenges can be met by utilizing the greatest resource at our disposal, the talents and dedication of concerned people, with and without disabilities, who believe in the value of physical activity.

Disability Sport Organizations

Disabled Sports USA
451 Hungerford Dr., Suite 100
Rockville, MD 20805
(301) 217-9838
(301) 217-0968 (fax)
Email: information@dsusa.org
Website: http://www.dsusa.org/

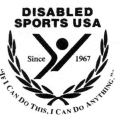

MISSION

The mission of Disabled Sports USA (DS/USA) is to provide the opportunity for individuals with physical disabilities to gain confidence and dignity through participation in sports, recreation and physical education programs, from preschool through college, and through elite sport levels. Initially involved primarily in winter sports activities, DS/USA chapters now promote year-round recreational activities and various levels of competitive sport (Figure 1).

FOUNDATION

Disabled Sports USA is a cross-disability sports program that has undergone a number of name changes as the organization has evolved. Originally known as the National Amputee Skiers Association, Disabled Sports USA was founded in 1967 by disabled Vietnam veterans. In 1972, due to the addition of other programs, the groups name was changed to the National Inconvenienced Sportsmen's Association. In 1976 the organization changed its name to the National Handicapped Sports and Recreation Association. In 1991, the program assumed responsibility for programming for athletes with amputees when the United States Amputee Athletic Association (USAAA) was dissolved. The name was shortened to National Handicapped Sports in 1992 and renamed Disabled Sports USA in 1994.

ELIGIBILITY

Individuals eligible for Disabled Sports USA general programming are those with physical disabilities including amputations (Figure 2), paraplegia, quadriplegia, cerebral palsy, head injury, multiple sclerosis, muscular dystrophy, spina bifida, stroke and visual impairments.

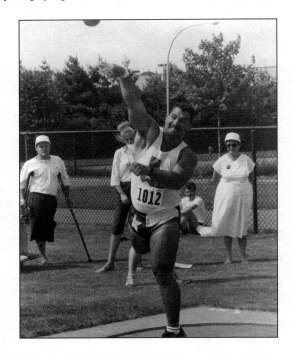

DS/USA-2. Since 1991, Disabled Sports USA has been responsible for the development of sports opportunities for athletes with amputations. (Courtesy of Specialized Sports Unlimited)

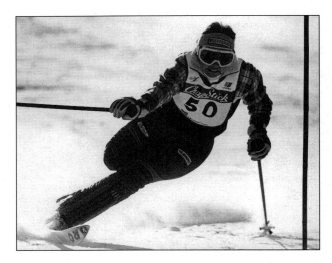

DS/USA-1. Disabled Sports USA is the disabled Sports NGB for skiing. (Courtesy of Disabled Sports USA)

SPORTS OFFERED AND COMPETITIONS

DS/USA sanctions and conducts winter and summer competitions in eleven sports, including archery, athletics (track and field), lawn bowling, cycling, powerlifting, sailing, skiing (alpine and nordic), swimming, table tennis, volleyball (standing and sitting). Training camps for novice and elite athletes are held in these sports. DS/USA also coordinates the US Disabled Volleyball (standing and sitting) teams.

UNIQUE PROGRAMS AND INITIATIVES

Adapted Fitness Instructor Workshops

A series of Adapted Fitness Instructor workshops (AFI) are held yearly at locations across the United States. The AFI program instructs adapted physical educators, occupational, physical and recreation therapists, fitness and health care professionals in adaptations of exercises for people with physical disabilities. The program provides training in strength training, adapted strength training, conditioning, aerobic and flexibility exercises through a combination of lecture and practical sessions. The training and certification of professionals assures that fitness, recreation, sport and physical education programs include people with disabilities.

"Learn To" Programs, Peer Support, Educational Materials

Disabled Sports USA offers a series of "Learn To" programs for their members in a variety of summer and winter recreation and sports activities in addition to their winter and summer competition programs for serious athletes.

Peer support is provided for families through a series of nationwide family-training workshops, while the production of videotapes and instruction manuals provides educational information for members as well as the general public.

CLASSIFICATION SYSTEM

Classification in Disabled Sports USA-sponsored events is in accordance with functional ability (consult DS/USA rules for specific information), and in many cases, according to adapted equipment used. National ski championships are divided into classifications by age and gender. Classification for summer athletes with amputations is based on the following nine classes.

Abbreviations:

AK = above or through the knee joint
BK = below knee, but through or above talocrural joint
AE = above or through elbow joint
BE = below elbow, but through or above wrist joint

Classification Code:

Class A1 = Double AK
Class A2 = Single AK
Class A3 = Double BK
Class A4 = Single BK
Class A5 = Double AE
Class A6 = Single AE
Class A7 = Double BE
Class A8 = Single BE
Class A9 = Combined lower and upper limb amputations

LOCAL, NATIONAL, INTERNATIONAL AFFILIATIONS

DS/USA is one of the seven disabled sports organizations recognized as a member of the United States Olympic Committee. It is a Paralympic Affiliated Sports Organization.

DS/USA has more than 80 community-based chapters (see website) in more than 30 states, providing year-round sports, recreation and social activities for people with disabilities. Each program offers its own schedule of programming.

Disabled Sports USA is represented internationally through the International Sports Organization for the Disabled (ISOD).

MOTTO

If I can do this, I can do anything.

Dwarf Athletic Association of America
418 Willow Way
Lewisville, TX 75077
(972) 317-8299
(972) 966-0184 (fax)
Email: daaa@flash.net
Website: http://www.daaa.org/

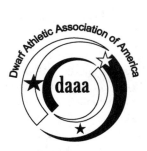

MISSION

The mission of the Dwarf Athletic Association of America (DAAA) is to develop, promote, and provide quality amateur athletic opportunities for dwarf athletes in the United States and to encourage people with dwarfism to participate in sports regardless of their level of skills.

FOUNDATION

The Dwarf Athletic Association of America was established in 1985 after 25 short-statured (dwarf) athletes participated successfully at the 1985 National Cerebral Palsy/Les Autres Games in East Lansing, Michigan. At that time in the development of sports for individuals with disabilities, the need was apparent for a formal organization of the les autres sports movement, of which the dwarfs were included.

With no organizational structure in place to handle the needs of a multi-disability sports organization, the dwarfs took an independent role and incorporated as the DAAA, using the parent organization, The Little People of America (LPA), on which to draw immediate membership. As a national organization with an established regional chapter network and an annual conference, the LPA also provided an immediate format for a yearly national sports competition (Figure 1). The first competition was held in Dearborn, Michigan in 1986.

ELIGIBILITY

DAAA is open to members who are dwarfs (4'10") due to chondrodystrophy or related causes.

SPORTS OFFERED AND COMPETITIONS

Clinics, developmental events, and formal competitions are offered at local, regional and national levels. DAAA offers programs for children through elite athletes. DAAA athletes compete in the following events: athletics (track & field), basketball, boccia, power lifting, swimming, skiing (alpine), table tennis, volleyball, badminton, and soccer, and equestrian events.

UNIQUE PROGRAMS AND INITIATIVES

DAAA offers youth events (ages 8-15) emphasizing the achieving of personal best. For children seven and under, DAAA offers special "Futures Team" non-competitive sports programs where everyone is a "Winner".

CLASSIFICATION SYSTEM

For the National Dwarf Games, athletes compete under age, gender, and functional ability classifications.

LOCAL, NATIONAL, INTERNATIONAL AFFILIATIONS

DAAA is one of the seven disabled sports organizations recognized as a member of the United States Olympic Committee. It is a Paralympic Affiliated Sports Organization.

Since the condition of dwarfism is considered a les autres disability in sport, the DAAA is represented inter-

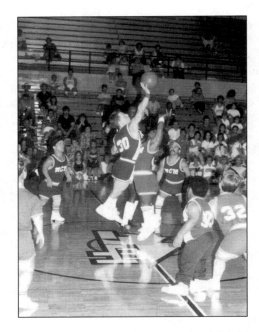

DAAA-1. Basketball competition at a national DAAA event. (Courtesy of DAAA)

nationally through the International Sports Organization for the Disabled (ISOD). ISOD recognizes only one national organization per country. At the time DAAA was established, the United States already had one ISOD member, Disabled Sports USA. This fact requires Disabled Sports USA to act as the official international link between DAAA and ISOD. Athletes compete internationally in the Paralympic Summer and Winter Games.

Dwarf World Games are held under the auspices of the International Dwarf Athletic Federation (IDAF). The IDAF was established in 1996 to promote and develop international sport for dwarfs throughout the world and to hold Dwarf World Games every four years. The first World Dwarf Games were conducted in Chicago in July of 1993. This event was the first international competition for dwarf athletes using their own classification system.

Special Olympics
1325 G Street, NW, Suite 500
Washington, DC 20005-3104
(202) 628-3630
(202) 824-0200 (fax)
Email: SOImail@aol.com
Website: http://www.specialolympics.org

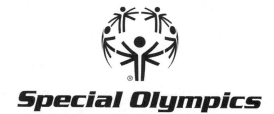

MISSION

Special Olympics provides year-round sports training and athletic competition in a variety of Olympic-type sports for individuals with mental retardation by giving them continuing opportunities to develop physical fitness, demonstrate courage, experience joy and participate in a sharing of gifts, skills and friendship with their families, other Special Olympics athletes and the community.

FOUNDATION

Special Olympics was founded in 1968 by Eunice Kennedy Shriver with the first games being held for 1,000 athletes from 26 States and Canada at Chicago's Soldier Field, with competition in track and field, swimming and floor hockey. Special Olympics has experienced unprecedented growth and now serves over 1 million athletes worldwide with programs in all 50 states and over 160 countries. Special Olympic World Summer Games now routinely include over 7,000 athletes from over 143 countries, while World Winter Games include 2,000 athletes from 73 countries.

ELIGIBILITY

Special Olympics competition is open to individuals who are at least 8 years of age and identified by an agency or professional as having one of the following conditions: mental retardation, cognitive delays as measured by formal assessment, or significant learning and vocational problems due to cognitive delay that require or have required specially-designed instruction.

SPORTS OFFERED AND COMPETITIONS

Special Olympics provides year-round training and competition in 26 sports. Training programs for each of these sports (and the Motor Activities Training Program) are outlined in Sports Skills Guides providing a developmental approach to teaching and coaching each sport. Training and competition are offered at various levels including athlete demonstrations, minimeet, local league, local tournament, city tournament, county area, district, section, state, provincial, national, regional, and World Winter and Summer Games. More than 15,000 games, meets, and tournaments in both summer and winter sports are held worldwide each year. World Games for selected representatives of all programs are held every two years, alternating between summer and winter. Official summer sports offered include aquatics, athletics, basketball, bowling, cycling, equestrian, football (soccer), golf, gymnastics (artistic and rhythmic), powerlifting, roller skating, softball, tennis, and volleyball. Official winter sports offered include Alpine skiing, cross country skiing, figure skating, floor hockey, and speed skating. Nationally popular sports offered include badminton, bocce, sailing, snowboarding, snowshoeing, table tennis, and team handball.

UNIQUE PROGRAMS AND INITIATIVES
Mega-Cities Program

Special Olympics has recognized that the opportunity to participate in Special Olympics has been limited for a large segment of the population living in the major urban communities of the United States and around the world. Since 1989, the Mega-Cities program has provided grant money to provide sports training and competition for athletes with mental retardation living in major urban communities throughout the world. The Special Olympics Mega-Cities program coordinates Special Olympics training and competition in schools, community recreation programs, group homes, and institutions in 11 large metropolitan areas.

Unified Sports™

Many of the Disabled Sports Organizations actively encourage and facilitate inclusive opportunities of training and competition within the expanded community. The Special Olympics Unified Sports™ program brings persons without mental retardation together on the same team with persons with mental retardation of comparable age and athletic ability. Founded in 1987, Unified Sports™ fosters the integration of persons with mental retardation into school and community sports programs. Special Olympics now offers Unified Sports™ in all 25 summer and winter sports.

Motor Activities Training Program (MATP)

The Motor Activities Training Program was developed for athletes with severe disabilities. MATP trains participants in seven basic motor skills designed to relate to specific skills. While the goal of MATP is not necessarily to prepare persons with severe disabilities to participate in sports, many may gain the skills required to compete in certain Special Olympics sports. MATP trains participants in aquatics, dexterity-athletics, electric wheelchair-athletics, manual wheelchair-athletics, kicking (soccer), and striking (softball).

CLASSIFICATION SYSTEM

Athletes are divided into competition divisions based upon their ability, age, and gender. Competition divisions are structured so that athletes compete against other athletes of similar ability in equitable divisions. In team sports competition, Skills Assessment Tests scores (submitted with registration) and a classification round of games are used to determine competitive divisions. A classification round involves teams competing in a short version of the official team sport. Special Olympics believes that competition among those of equal abilities is the best way to test its athletes' skills, measure their progress, and inspire them to grow (Figure 1). By assigning athletes to divisions commensurate with their ability, Special Olympics gives every athlete a reasonable chance to win. Athletes from all divisions may advance to Chapter, National, and World Games. Age

groupings used for individual sports are 8 to 11, 12 to 15, 16 to 21, 22 to 29, and 30 and older. Age groupings used for team sports are 15 and younger, 16 to 21, and 22 and older. Additional age groupings may be established if there are a sufficient number of competitors in older age groups.

LOCAL, NATIONAL, INTERNATIONAL AFFILIATIONS

There are accredited Special Olympics programs in more than 145 countries. Special Olympic Programs are established in all 50 states, the District of Columbia, Guam, the Virgin Islands, and American Samoa. Over 25,000 communities in the United States have Special Olympic Programs headed by local area directors. Many public schools include Special Olympics through their physical education programs and many provide extracurricular and interscholastic sports to their students with mental retardation.

Special Olympics is one of the seven disabled sports organizations recognized as a member of the United States Olympic Committee.

Special Olympics is represented internationally through Special Olympics, Inc. Athletes compete internationally in the Special Olympics Summer and Winter Games. The first Special Olympics International Games to be held outside of the United States took place in Salzburg and Schladming, Austria in 1993.

MOTTO

Let me win. But if I cannot win, let me be brave in the attempt.

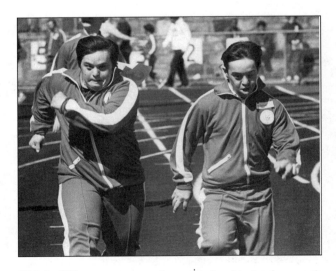

SOI-1. SOI state games track meet is head-to-head competition. (Courtesy of Michigan Special Olympics)

United States Association of Blind Athletes
33 N. Institute Street
Colorado Springs, CO 80903
(719) 630-0422
(719) 630-0616 (fax)
Email: usaba@usa.net
Website: http://www.usaba.org

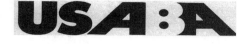

MISSION

The mission of the United States Association of Blind Athletes (USABA) is to change the attitudes of the general population about the abilities of the blind and visually impaired. Since its founding in 1976, the USABA has reached over 100,000 blind individuals. During that time, the organization has emerged as more than just a world-class trainer of blind athletes, it has become a vocal champion of the abilities of America's legally blind residents.

In addition to providing world-class coaching and training, the USABA reaches into hundreds of communities across America, helping thousands of blind and disabled youth discover their own unlimited potential - in school, sports, the community and the achievement of their own personal dreams.

Where many blind and visually impaired individuals have heard enough about their limitation; USABA gives them the tools to experience the reality of success without limits (Figure 1).

FOUNDATION

At the 1976 Olympiad for the Disabled in Toronto, Canada, the United States was represented by 27 men and women who were blind, who brought home nine medals. After such success, a group of national leaders, educators and coaches of the blind met in Kansas City in November 1976 to discuss the formation of an organization to promote and sponsor competition for blind athletes.

ELIGIBILITY

Any individual regardless of ability is eligible to join in the capacity of a volunteer or coach. Competition is designed for visually impaired and blind athletes.

SPORTS OFFERED AND COMPETITIONS

USABA has an active membership of 3,000 blind and visually impaired athletes (within three visual classifications, see following) in nine sports—alpine and nordic skiing, goalball, judo, powerlifting, swimming, tandem cycling, track and field and wrestling. USABA and its

athletes have accomplished membership in the U.S. Olympic Committee and have won dozens of world and Paralympic records. USABA has been a leader in the move to inclusion as it was one of the first organizations to routinely include athletes with and without sight at their competitions. Opportunities for sighted athletes are available as sighted guides for track (Figure 2) and as sighted pilots in tandem cycle racing.

CLASSIFICATION SYSTEM

During competition, all legally blind athletes are classified according to visual acuity into one of the following three USABA visual classifications. Athletes generally compete against others of the same class, but competition among classes occur in such sports as goalball.

Class B1-Possessing no light perception in either eye up to light perception, but inability to recognize the shape of a hand at any distance or in any direction.

Class B2-From ability to recognize the shape of a hand up to visual acuity of 20/600 and/or a visual field of less than 5 degrees in the best eye with the best practical eye correction.

Class B3-From visual acuity above 20/600 and up to visual acuity of 20/200 and/or a visual field of less than 20 degrees and more than 5 degrees in the best eye with the best practical eye correction.

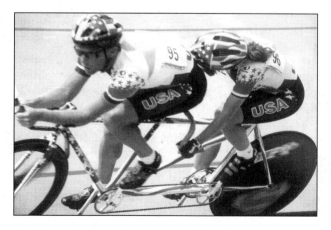

USABA-1. Tandem cycling has developed into a very competitive sport for USABA. (Courtesy of USABA)

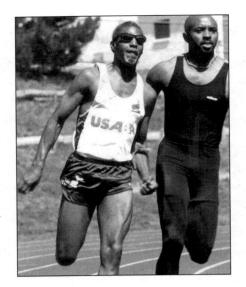

USABA-2. A sighted guide with a blind track runner. (Courtesy of USABA)

LOCAL, NATIONAL, INTERNATIONAL AFFILIATIONS

The United States Association of Blind Athletes is represented internationally through the International Blind Sports Association (IBSA) and participates in the Paralympic Games. IBSA was founded in Paris in 1981 and is a fully fledged member of the International Paralympic Committee. The purpose of IBSA is to develop and promote the concept of sport for people who are blind or have visual impairments throughout the world.

MOTTO

If I can do this, I can do anything.

United States Cerebral Palsy Athletic Association
25 West Independence Way
Kingston, RI 02881
(401) 792-7130
(401) 792-7132 (fax)
Email: uscpaa@mail.bbsnet.com
Website: http://www.uscpaa.org

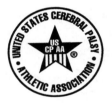

MISSION

The mission of the United States Cerebral Palsy Athletic Association is to provide both individualized sports training and competitive opportunities for athletes with cerebral palsy (CP), or other similar disabilities, such as traumatic brain injuries (TBI) or strokes. The guiding philosophy, equal opportunity for all, is personified in USCPAA's eight level classification system (Figure 1). This system, based on the functional level of the athlete, provides a fair and equitable starting point for competitions. Assisting athletes to discover and recognize their abilities is a primary goal.

FOUNDATION

The dream of developing a sports organization for individuals with cerebral palsy was realized in 1978 with the founding of the National Association of Sport for Cerebral Palsy (NASCP), as a departmental program of the United Cerebral Palsy Association, Inc. (UCPA). In the Fall of 1985 officials and program leaders decided that an organizational structure separate from UCPA's day-to-day operation was needed to facilitate the growth of cerebral palsy sports. The United States Cerebral Palsy Athletic Association (USCPAA) was established in November 1986, as the disabled sports organization for individuals with cerebral palsy. Originally based in Westland, Michigan, USCPAA headquarters has moved from Dallas, Texas, to Newport, Rhode Island to it's current home at the University of Rhode Island in Kingston.

NATIONAL ALLIANCE FOR DISABILITY SPORT (NADS)

USCPAA recently changed their corporate name to the National Alliance for Disability Sport (NADS). The National Alliance for Disability Sport will be an umbrella organization that will include USCPAA. Athletes with cerebral palsy will still be members of USCPAA. USCPAA will remain the member organization of NADS responsible for the oversight of sports opportunities for athletes with cerebral palsy.

The purpose of USCPAA's corporate name change was the need for USCPAA to identify additional athlete recruitment sources. Specifically targeted for recruitment will be athletes with head injuries and stroke survivors who traditionally have not identified themselves with the U.S. Cerebral Palsy Athletic Association. USCPAA's restructuring and name change to National Alliance for Disability Sports, establishes an organizational structure similar to that of Wheelchair Sports, USA and the USA Deaf Sports Federation, which includes member groups as part of their overall organization's structure.

For the purpose of this text, all references will be to USCPAA. Readers should note, however, that in all sports mentioned opportunities are available to individuals with similar conditions including head injuries and strokes.

ELIGIBILITY

USCPAA competitions are open to individuals with cerebral palsy (CP), traumatic brain injuries (TBI), and stroke survivors (cerebrovascular accident). Because loss of motor function, commonly seen as a residual effect of strokes and head injuries, manifests itself in a similar manner to that of congenitally acquired CP, individuals disabled by strokes and head injuries are eligible to participate.

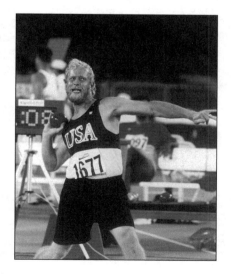

USCPAA-1. Tom Becke, world class field competitor. (Courtesy Rehabilitation Institute of Chicago's Wirtz Sports Program)

SPORTS OFFERED AND COMPETITIONS

USCPAA offers local, national, and international training and competitive opportunities in the following sports: athletics (track and field), boccia, bowling, cross country, cycling, equestrian, powerlifting, soccer, indoor wheelchair soccer, swimming, table tennis and target shooting. Many regional programs also offer slalom and archery. Basketball is a developing sport at the national level

CLASSIFICATION

Classification for competition in cerebral palsy sports is a much more complex process than it is in other disabled sports organizations. Objective criteria used by other disabled sports organizations (loss of sight or hearing, level of spinal cord injury, or number and location of amputation) are not applicable. A more subjective process using a series of functional tests is used to classify athletes in one of eight categories ranging from severe to minimal dysfunction (4 wheelchair categories and 4 ambulatory classes)

This classification system is used in all individual sports, including athletics (track and field), swimming, cycling and cross-country - where athletes compete only against athletes with their same classification. In the remaining sports, athletes are grouped in divisions according to classification. An extensive description of the classification system can be found in the USCPAA Classification/Rule Manual. A brief explanation of the eight classes include:

Class 1: Severe involvement in all four limbs. Limited trunk control. Unable to grasp a softball. Poor functional strength in upper extremities, often necessitating the use of a power wheelchair for independence.

Class 2: Severe to moderate quadriplegic (all four limbs involved), normally able to propel a wheelchair very slowly with arms or by pushing with feet. Poor functional strength and severe control problems in the upper extremities.

Class 3: Moderate quadriplegic, fair functional strength and moderate control problems in upper extremities and torso. Propels wheelchair independently.

Class 4: Lower limbs have moderate to severe involvement. Good functional strength and minimal control problem in upper extremities and torso. Uses wheelchair.

Class 5: Good functional strength and minimal control problems in upper extremities. May walk with or without assistive devices for ambulatory support.

Class 6: Moderate to severe quadriplegic. Ambulates without walking aids. Less coordination. Balance problems when running or throwing. Has greater upper extremity involvement.

Class 7: Moderate to minimal hemiplegic (one side of the body involved). Good functional ability in non-affected side. Walks/runs with noted limp.

Class 8: Minimally affected. May have minimal coordination problems. Able to run and jump freely. Has good balance.

Local, National, International Affiliations

Already, in over 40 states across the United States, USCPAA is a resource that member athletes can turn to for help in coordinating their training. Headquartered on the campus of the University of Rhode Island, USCPAA strives to enable its athletes to compete at their peak on local, regional, national, and international levels (Figures 2 and 3).

USCPAA is one of the seven disabled sports organizations recognized as a member of the United States Olympic Committee. It is a Paralympic Affiliated Sports Organization.

USCPAA is represented internationally through the Cerebral Palsy International Sports and Recreation Association (CP-ISRA).

MOTTO

Sports by ability, not disability.

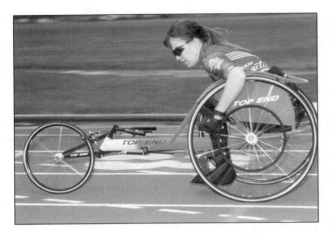

USCPAA-2. Linda Mastandrea, 5 time world record holder and 1996 Paralympic Games gold and silver medallist. (Courtesy Rehabilitation Institute of Chicago's Wirtz Sports Program)

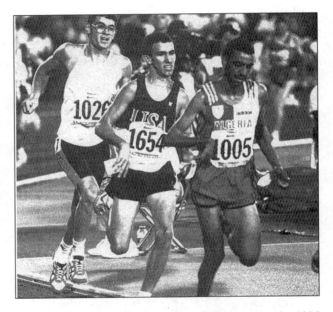

USCPAA-3. Class 7 Cerebral Palsy 1500 meters at the 1996 Atlanta Paralympic Games. (Courtesy of Specialized Sports Unlimited)

USA Deaf Sports Federation
3607 Washington Blvd., Suite 4
Ogden, UT 84403-1737
(801) 393-7916 Office (TTY: use state relay service)
(801) 393-2263 (fax)
Email: usadsf@aol.com
Website: http://www.usadsf.org

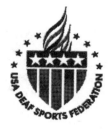

MISSION

The mission of the USA Deaf Sports Federation (USADSF) is to provide year-round training and athletic competition in a variety of sports at the state, regional, national, and international level for developing and elite athletes, and to assist athletes in developing physical fitness, sportsmanship, and self-esteem. The USA Deaf Sports Federation believes that through recreational opportunities, sports training, and competition, deaf and hard of hearing people can benefit physically, mentally, socially, and spiritually in an environment of equality, mutual respect, and acceptance.

FOUNDATION

Established as the American Athletic Union of the Deaf (AAUD) in 1945 by Art Kruger, after the Akron Club of the Deaf sponsored their first national basketball tournament, the USA Deaf Sports Federation is one of the oldest sports organizations for people with disabilities in the country. The name was soon changed to the American Athletic Association of the Deaf (AAAD), until it was renamed as the USA Deaf Sports Federation in 1997. Its purpose was to foster and regulate uniform rules of competition and provide social outlets for deaf members and their friends; serve as a parent organization for regional sports organizations; conduct annual athletic competitions; and assist in the participation of United States teams in international competition. Today, the USADSF provides programming to thousands of individuals who are deaf or hearing impaired through 18 national sport organizations.

SPORTS OFFERED AND COMPETITIONS

USA Deaf Sports Federation sanctions and conducts winter and summer competitions through its 18 National Sports Organizations offering programming in aquatics, athletics, badminton, baseball, basketball, bowling, cycling, flag football, golf, hockey, skiing/snowboarding, soccer, softball, table tennis, team handball, tennis, volleyball and wrestling.

UNIQUE PROGRAMS AND INITIATIVES

Mini Deaf Sports Festival

Participation in deaf sports has always been a cultural as well as an athletic experience. The involvement of youth in deaf culture is an important component of USADSF programming, accomplished to a great degree by participation in the Annual Mini Deaf Sports Festival. The festival has taken place every year since 1983. Starting with only seven people, it has grown to include hundreds of participants. It is the only event of its kind in the United States, and is specifically designed for deaf children ages 6-18. For further information contact:

Timothy Owens
(502) 634-3359
(502) 776-3913 (fax)
Email: timo01@aol.com

ELIGIBILITY

In deaf sports there is no need for a sport classification system similar to those used by organizations for people with disabilities. Since deafness is a communication barrier and not a physically disabling condition, only those deaf and hard-of-hearing individuals with a hearing loss of 55dB or greater in the better ear are eligible for full participation. The use of hearing aids is prohibited in competitions. Members of the US Team must be American citizens.

LOCAL, NATIONAL, INTERNATIONAL AFFILIATIONS

USA Deaf Sports Federation's international representative is the Comite International des Sports des Sourds (International Committee for Silent Sports). The CISS is a recognized member of the International Paralympic Committee (IPC). Although CISS is a member of the IPC, Deaf athletes do not compete in the Paralympic Games. Athletes participate in international competition at the Summer and Winter World Games for the Deaf held every four years, recognized by the IPC as the equivalent of the Paralympic Games. Among the Deaf community there is overwhelming support for separate Games. People who are deaf do not consider themselves disabled, particularly in physical ability. Rather, people who are deaf are considered to be part of a cultural and linguistic minority. The deaf athlete is physically able-bodied and able to compete without significant restrictions, with the exception of communication barriers. These barriers may be evident when deaf athletes compete in hearing competitions or competitions with athletes who have physical disabilities. The deaf athlete invariably experiences social isolation and exclusion. By participating in separate games such as the World Games for the Deaf, Deaf athletes can usually communicate with other Deaf athletes, regardless of which country they may be representing. In the Deaf Games, athletes are able to compete and interact with others freely and without sign language interpreters, except where hearing officials are involved. Deaf sports are regarded as a means to maintain a unique cultural identity and opportunity to exchange culturally relevant information. Sports attract individuals who are deaf into athletic activity and deaf athletes gain exposure to cultural activities of the deaf community.

Wheelchair Sports, USA
3395 E. Fountain Blvd., L-1
Colorado Springs, CO 80910
(719) 574-1150
(719) 574-9840 (fax)
Email: wsusa@aol.com
Website: http://www.wsusa.org/

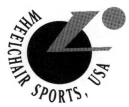

MISSION

The mission of Wheelchair Sports, USA, is to provide athletic experiences for athletes with physical disabilities paralleling those of the able-bodied, from novice through elite levels.

FOUNDATION

The beginnings of Wheelchair Sports USA can be traced back to the mid-1940s as thousands of permanently disabled veterans returned from World War II with their love of sport intact. Sir Ludwig Guttman is credited with being the founding father of wheelchair sports, as well as the Paralympic Games, when he utilized athletic competition and participation as part of the rehabilitation program at Stoke Mandeville Hospital in England. Dr. Guttman was one of the first individuals to realize the tremendous benefit that sport participation can have on people with physical disabilities. Although the initial Stoke Mandeville Games only included a few dozen competitors, the idea of wheelchair sports was fully established, eventually leading to the Paralympic Games in 1960.

Wheelchair basketball was the preferred sport of many during the first few years after the war, however, athletes soon wanted to participate in more sports than just basketball (Figure 1). Initially known as the National Wheelchair Athletic Association when it was founded in 1956 by World War II veterans to meet the need for additional sport participation, the name was changed in 1994 to Wheelchair Sports USA.

Today, Wheelchair Sports, USA, represents over 4,500 athletes, coaches, officials and support staff and is organized geographically into fourteen regional associations, each responsible for developing local wheelchair sports programs and for conducting qualifying meets for the National Wheelchair Games.

ELIGIBILITY

Any individual is eligible to join Wheelchair Sports, USA in the capacity of a volunteer or coach. Competition is designed for those individuals with lower extremity impairments who use wheelchairs as their primary means of locomotion. Athletes must compete in wheelchairs for all events (except weightlifting). Competition is offered for juniors (18 and younger) and adults (19 and older). Disabilities served by WS/USA include post polio, spinal cord injured, spina bifida and amputees.

SPORTS OFFERED AND COMPETITIONS

Wheelchair Sports USA has structured itself into a wheelchair sports federation comprising various wheelchair sports governing bodies. Sports offered include, aquatics, archery, basketball, hand cycling, fencing, quad rugby, racquetball, shooting, sled hockey, table tennis, tennis, water skiing, and weightlifting. Sports are offered at local, regional, national, and international levels (Figure 2).

UNIQUE PROGRAMS

Youth Development Program

Wheelchair Sports, USA, has recognized the importance of developing programs for youth and has expanded its offerings to junior athletes which make up 30% of the total membership. Regional associations now conduct annual local competitions for youths aged five to eighteen. The WSUSA Junior National Championships, the organizations largest annual event, was first held in July 1984. This event provided the first national program of competitions for junior athletes.

CLASSIFICATION SYSTEM

Wheelchair Sports, USA utilizes a complex and sophisticated medical classification system to determine and athlete's level of muscular function, striving for fair competition among individuals with similar degrees of disability. The lower the number, the higher the degree of spinal cord lesion. The classification is anatomically based with IA, IB, and IC representing the quadriplegic classes with injuries in the cervical region. Class II in-

cludes athletes with injuries beginning in the high thoracic region, Class III in the middle thoracic region, and Class IV in the lower thoracic and lumbar region. Class V includes athletes who have power to ambulate (majority disabled through polio), and Class VI (used only for swimming) represents athletes with the least muscle weakness of all. Observation of trunk balance and performance of muscle strength tests are used for classifications.

LOCAL, NATIONAL, INTERNATIONAL AFFILIATIONS

WS/USA is one of the seven disabled sports organizations recognized as a member of the United States Olympic Committee. Wheelchair Sports USA is represented internationally by the Stoke Mandeville Wheelchair Sports Federation (SMWSF). It is a Paralympic Affiliated Sports Organization.

MOTTO

Dedicated to the Guidance and Growth of Wheelchair Sports.

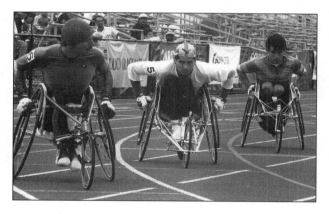

WS/USA-1. Track and road racing have become one of the most popular sports offered by Wheelchair Sports, USA. (Courtesy of Oscar Izquierdo and Rehabilitation Institute of Chicago)

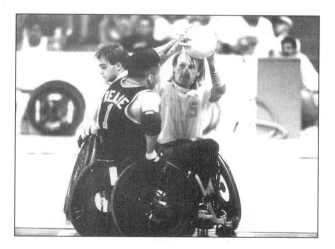

WS/USA-2. USA Quad Rugby won the gold medal in both the Atlanta and Sydney Paralympic Games. (Courtesy Rehabilitation Institute of Chicago's Wirtz Sports Program)

Chapter 1

All-Terrain Vehicles

SPORT OVERVIEW

Since the major idea behind this book is accessibility of sports and recreation opportunities, it is only appropriate that the book begin with a chapter dealing specifically with accessibility. It is the hope of the authors that readers will be better prepared to participate in a variety of sports and recreation opportunities because of the information presented. In many cases, accessing a new opportunity will require the use of equipment. Outdoor activities may be accessible for some only with the use of "mobility-enhancing equipment" (Figure 1.1).

All-terrain vehicles (ATV's), or off-road vehicles as they are more commonly known, are discussed in this book for that reason. Off-road vehicles can allow individuals with disabilities independent access to outdoor activities such as hunting, fishing, camping and even hiking(Figures 1.2, 1.3, and 1.4). Some are large enough to carry equipment such as tents, fishing gear, hunting blinds and other outdoor equipment.

Several types of ATV's and off-road vehicles are described in this chapter. The purchase price of these vehicles vary greatly depending on whether the vehicle is motorized or not and what types of additional features are involved. Motorized vehicles come with a price range of $3,500-$6,500 while off-road wheelchairs are considerably less expensive. The purchase of a motorized ATV should be done with the same consideration given when purchasing a car. Service plans, reliability, and warranties should all be considered. Within the last few years more options have become available due to the increased demand for such equipment. We have not personally field tested these vehicles, nor is their mention considered to be an endorsement. Due to the variety of models and different reasons for use, individuals interested in ATV's should thoroughly investigate products prior to purchase. The use of motorized ATV's is potentially dangerous.

Each individual must determine their ability to use an ATV in a safe and responsible manner (see concerns below). ATV's and various off-road models are designed for out-of-the way, and accessibly challenging places. Caution should be exercised when using any type of off-road device.

Due to the potential dangers, no one under the age of 16 should operate a motorized ATV or an ATC (all-terrain cycle) (Figure 1.5). A helmet and gloves should be worn when in any off-road situation, and motorized vehicles should never be operated by a person under the influence of alcohol or drugs.

For the sports person considering purchase of a motorized ATV, the first step is to determine what the vehicle will be used for, where the vehicle will be used, and if use is allowed in a particular location. Although a hunter with a physical disability can access areas that were once inaccessible, many public hunting areas do not allow the use of ATV's, even by individuals with disabilities. It is advisable to check with the land manger and DNR when considering use on public lands.

PROBLEMS TO BE CONSIDERED WHEN USING ATV'S

In many cases, the use of a standard 4-wheel ATV will be sufficient for a person with a physical disability. Each individual should consider their own personal situation when looking for features or making modifications. The intended use is always a factor in purchasing an ATV. Will it be used for work, recreation, or both? Although most people regard ATV's as primarily recreational, they are used by many for non-recreational activities such as farming, yard work, and snow plowing (Figure 1.6). People with physical disabilities generally have 4 types of problems to consider when using an ATV.

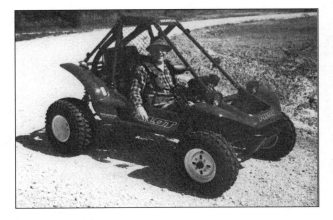

Figure 1.1. The jeep-like ATV with four or six wheels has many of the same features as a standard car. (Courtesy of *Disabled Outdoors*)

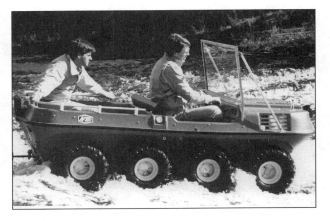

Figure 1.2. The eight-wheel Amphibious Argo Off-Road Vehicle provides a safe way to access outdoor recreation opportunities (Courtesy of Ontario Drive & Gear Ltd.)

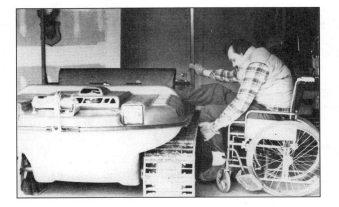

Figure 1.3. Most ATVs are at a height to allow easy transferring from a wheelchair. (Courtesy of *Sports 'n Spokes* 3/82:21)

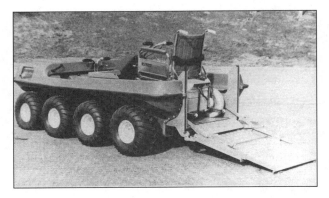

Figure 1.4. Certain models of ATVs are easily modified to include a wheelchair ramp.

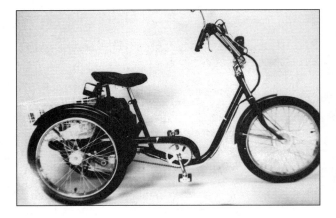

Figure 1.5. Other ATC models are designed for daily mobility: pedal, motor, or both. The Litening Trike offers exercise and economical transportation. (Courtesy Of Electric Mobility)

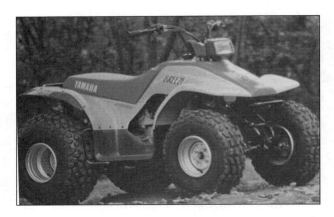

Figure 1.6. Four-wheel ATV by Yamaha.

1. Getting on and off the ATV may present a significant challenge for some individuals due to their physical disability. No one should use an ATV unless they have demonstrated the ability to safely transfer into and out of the vehicle.

2. The ability to maintain a stable sitting position when riding is also of concern. Individuals with balance problems may want to consider some type of custom support system such as a harness or backrest. API Outdoors offers their Ride-N-Rest back rest to ATV owners (see Equipment Suppliers at the end of the chapter). This device is adjustable and can adapt to almost any ATV for less than $50. Other types of seat or harness modifications should be accomplished by your local ATV dealer.

3. Contact with a heated surface by a person with a disability who has reduced skin sensation can be of concern. Serious burns can occur very quickly even with the use of heavy pants and boots. The rider should take extra precautions to ensure they are not in contact with any heated surface.

4. Shifting of gears for some models may be of concern but alternatives exist to solve this problem. Some models use shiftless (automatic) gears. Just put the vehicle in gear and let the machine do the rest (Figure 1.7 a and b). The Electrix Shift by Cycle Country is an excellent option. Check with your local ATV dealer for other models using automatic shifters. For ATV's without automatic transmissions, the solution is adapting the shift gear. A simple shift lever can be attached to the foot shifter that will allow the rider to change gears with his or her left hand. For the cost of about $20, API offers a device, called the Speed Stick Shifter, that works very well. The Speed Stick Shifter quickly attaches to most any ATV. Electric shifters are also a viable solution to this problem. Shifting is accomplished by simply the push of a button.. Shifting is accomplished by a small electric motor. Even with electric shifters installed on your ATV, gears can still be shifting manually.

EQUIPMENT

Motorized ATV's

Motorized ATV's come in a variety of styles from single person to multi-person designs. Single person designs such as the Tramper, and ones designed by Tomco Conversions, are designed to cover rough ground, mud and grass with little difficulty. The Tomco Conversion model can be used in either electric or gasoline modes.

The 6-wheel multi-person ATV, such as ones provided by BC Wheels and 6wheeldrive.com, is designed for the serious outdoors person who may be traveling longer distances and packing more equipment. This type of vehicle is designed for all types of rugged terrain and is good for extended trips into the wilderness.

The Freedom Children's Electric Wheelchair, designed by Tibby's of Vancouver Island, allows children with disabilities to explore the wilderness with friends and family. It is a three-wheeled, single-seat vehicle that is joystick operated, allowing children independent exploration of their natural environment. For added safety, a remote shut-off switch was added to the Freedom. This is an extremely versatile and environmentally sensitive vehicle, well suited to the needs of children exploring the wilderness. Information on this vehicle can be accessed by contacting the British Columbia Mobilities Opportunities Society (see equipment suppliers at the end of the chapter).

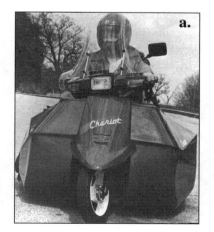
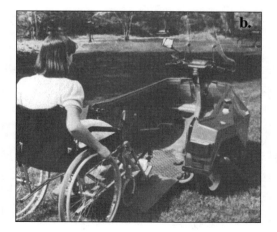

Figure 1.7 a and b. The Chariot is a three-wheeled, street-legal vehicle that provides a smooth ride to 35 mph. (Courtesy of Cottle Industries, Inc.)

Manual Off-Road and Beach Vehicles and Wheelchairs

A variety of manual off-road "mountain chairs" have been introduced to the market place over the past few years and provide functional outdoor use. Manual ATV's fall into two categories; dependent manual ATV's and independent manual ATV's. Dependent manual ATV's may require the assistance of a another individual to provide the locomotion (pushing/pulling). Most of these models are designed to be used in sand and water when at the beach, or to be pushed through snow or mud (Figures 1.8, 1.9, 1.10, and 1.11). Access to Recreation and other dealers offers 2 models, the Landeez All-Terrain and the Seeker Wheelchair. The Landeez with its soft plastic pneumatic tires rolls easily over snow, sand, and gravel. Beach wheelchairs have become very popular. With the many suppliers now routinely providing a wide assortment of beach wheelchairs, access to sandy terrain is no longer an obstacle.

The second type of independent manual ATV's are basically all-terrain wheelchairs built specifically for rough outdoor terrain (Figures 1.12, 1.13, 1.14, and 1.15). These wheelchairs boast larger front and rear tires similar to what is found on a typical mountain bike.

They allow the individual to wheel over gravel, sand, and rough terrain. Eagle Sports Chairs and Majors Medical Supply are examples of 2 companies that offer excellent products in this area. The Kili-Kart by Disability Options (Figure 16a and b) is a unique all-terrain wheelchair that has been tested in at Mt. Kilamanjaro and in Alaska. The rugged cart travels over rough terrain, logs, rock and ice. The Kili-Kart is designed to withstand harsh condi-

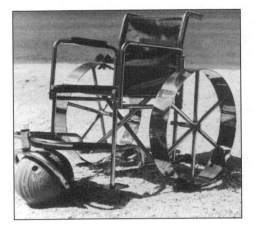

Figure 1.8. The Beachmaster Aquatic Wheelchair is designed to be wheeled over sand and into the water. (Courtesy of Access to Recreation and Beach Wheels, Inc.)

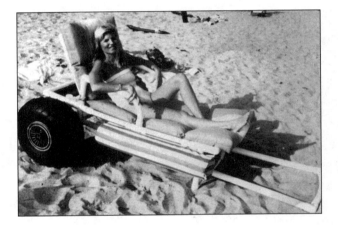

Figure 1.9. The Sand-Rik is another type of manual beach unit that provides mobility in the sand and water. (Courtesy of Access to Recreation)

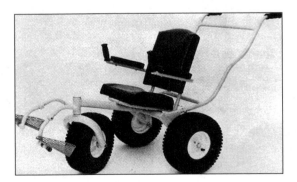

Figure 1.10. The Adventurer is designed for various off-road situations. (Courtesy of Westport Mobility Products)

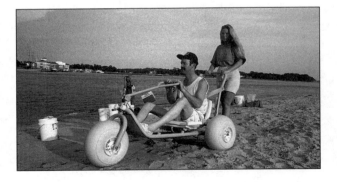

Figure 1.11. The Sport Wheeler allows independent steering by the seated person while the vehicle is being pushed from the rear. (Courtesy of Roleez Wheel System)

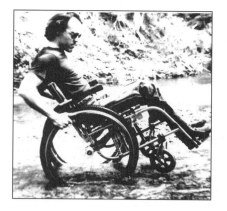

Figure 1.12. The Iron Horse—the industry's first suspensioned wheelchair is functional in on-and off-road situation. (Courtesy of Iron Horse Productions, Inc.)

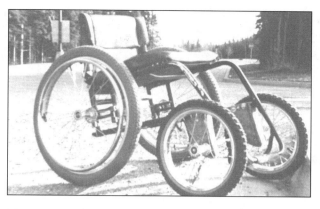

Figure 1.13. The Mountain Chair front end attachment.

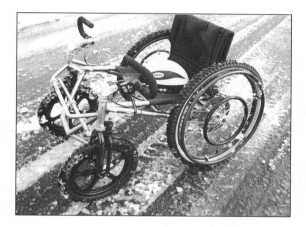

Figure 1.14. The All-Terrain Chair by Enduro Wheelchairs.

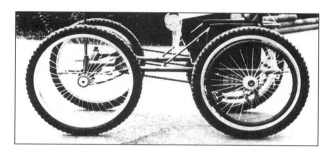

Figure 1.15. The Sure Foot is promoted as the perfect backpacking and camping wheelchair. (Courtesy of Access to Recreation)

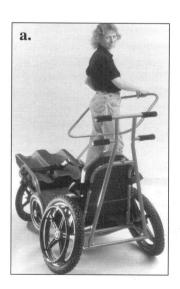

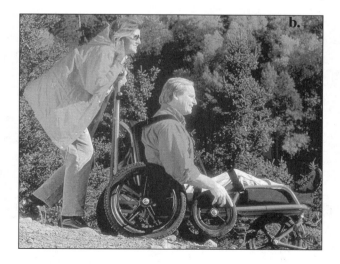

Figure 1.16 a and b. The Kili Kart is specially designed to travel over uneven ground to enable individuals with physical disabilities and their family and friends to enjoy outdoor activities. (Courtesy of Disability Options, Inc.)

tions, yet it is lightweight and durable. The entire cart is just 50 pounds and folds down for easy transport or storage. It features a stable, three-wheel design with low center of gravity. Push and tow bars enable friends and family to assist.

EQUIPMENT SUPPLIERS

For the individual with a disability who wishes to fish, most equipment suppliers and retailers will be suitable. Many new online companies offer an extensive line of equipment. The following are some representative companies.

Backrests

API Outdoors
602 Kimbrough Blvd
Tallulah , LA 71282-5420
(318) 574-4903

Beach Wheelchairs

The list of companies supplying beach and aquatic wheelchairs is abundant. The list provided here is a representative sample only. Other companies should be explored by the reader.

AAA Medical Sales, Inc.
2095 West Hampden Avenue
Englewood CO 80110
(800) 525-8586
Email: aaamedical@aaamedical.com
Website: http://www.medmarket.com

Access to Recreation, Inc.
8 Sandra Court
Newbury Park CA 91320
(800) 634-4351
(805) 498-7535
(805) 498-8186 (fax)
Email: dkrebs@gte.net
Website: http://www.accesstr.com
ATR provides Off-road "mountain bike" wheels that easily attach to a wheelchair for a softer ride over unpaved surfaces

Accessible Structures, Inc.
1311 Greenwood Street
Titusville, FL 32780
Phone 321-268-0166
(888) 639-8090
(321) 268-0579
Email: asifla@aol.com
Website: http://www.accessibilityplus.com

Deming Designs Inc.
141 W. Pinestead Rd.
Pensacola, Fl 32503
(850) 478-5765
Email: kmdeming@aol.com
Website: http://www.beachwheelchair.com

Dmeonline
P.O. Box 2069
Tricities, WA 99302
Email: dmestuff@owt.com
Website: http://www.dmeonline.com

Hotshot Products (Electric Beach Wheelchair)
1920 Del Amo Blvd. #A
Torrance, CA 90501
(888) 663-5911
Email: blhotshot@hotshotproducts.org
Website: http://www.hotshotproducts.org

Innovative Products Unlimited (Land Roller)
4351 W. College Avenue
Suite 505
Appleton, WI 54914
(920) 738-9090
(800) 424-3369
(920) 738-9050 (fax)
Email: ipu@ipu.com
Website: http://www.ipu.com/

Interior Mediquip Ltd. (Steel Wheel Aquatic Chair)
3401 33rd Ave.
Vernon, B.C.
Canada V1T2P2
(800) 561-8998
(604) 542-1363
(604) 549-3002 (fax)
Website: http://www.intermedd.com

Natural Access
P.O. Box 2222
Princeton, NJ 08543-2222
(800) 411-7789
Email: natural@superlink.net
Website: http://www.beachwheelchair.net

Sportaid & Medaid
78 Baycreek Road
Loganville, GA 30052
(800) 743-7203
Website: http://www.sportaid.com

Surf Chair, Inc.
2052 South Peninsula Dr.

Daytona Beach, FL 32118
(904) 253-0986
(904) 767-5707

Electric Shifters

Cycle Country Accessories Corporation (Electrix Shift)
2188 Hwy.86
Milford, Iowa 51351
(800) 841-2222
Email: ccac@cyclecountry.com

Manual Off-road Wheelchairs
Disability Options, Inc.
P.O. Box 1967
Palmer, Alaska 99645
(907) 745-3900
(907) 746-6678 (fax)
Email: info@disabilityoptions.com
Website: http://www.disabilityoptions.com/

Eagle Sportschairs
2351 Parkwood Road
Snellville , GA 30039
(770) 972-0763
(770) 985-4885 (fax)
Email: bewing@harb.net
Website: http://www.eaglesportschairs.com

Majors Medical Supply (Terratrek All-Terrain)
211 Rock Hill Road
Bala Cynwyd, PA. 19004
(800) 625-6770
(800) 783-5825 (fax)
Email: majorsmedical@majorsmedical.com
Website: http://www.majorsmedical.com/terratrek.htm

Motorized Off-road Vehicles/Wheelchairs

Alternative Driving Solutions (Freedom Car ATV)
1298 Sawleaf St.
San Luis Obispo, CA 93401
(805) 783-7195
(805) 474-4859 (fax)
Website: http://www.gocortez.com/

Beamer Ltd. (Tramper)
Email: info@tramper.co.uk
Website: http://www.tramper.co.uk/

BC Wheels (Six-Wheeled All-Terrain Vehicles)
Hwy 22 PO Box 914
Wyocena, WI 53969
(800) 279-4335
Email: bobc@bcwheels.com
Website: http://www.bcwheels.com

Electric Mobility World Headquarters,
One Mobility Plaza
P.O. Box 156
Sewell, NJ 08080
(800) 662-4548 Ext. 7474
Website: http://www.electricmobility.com/

JP Conversions, Inc.
4017 Bluff St.
Torrance, CA 90505
(310) 375-8699

Ontario Drive-Gear Limited
P.O. Box 280 Bleams Rd.
New Hamburg, Ontario
Canada N08-2G0
(519) 662-2840
(519) 662-2421 (fax)
Website: http://www.argoatv.com

6wheeldrive.com
(877) 299-7627
Website: http://www.6wheeldrive.com

Recreatives Industries, Inc.
60 Depot St.
Buffalo, New York 14206
(800) 255-2511
(716) 855-1094 (fax)
Website: http://www.maxatvs.com/
The World's Largest Manufacturer of Six-Wheel Drive, Amphibious All-Terrain Vehicles

Tomco Conversions (All-Terrain Motorized Wheelchair and TARA All-Terrain Vehicle)
P.O. Box 30
Rte. #321
Wilcox, PA 15870
(888) 516-4814
(814) 929-5284 (fax)
Email: info@tomcoconversions.com
Website: http://www.tomcoconversions.com

Venture Products, Inc.
12657 Church Rd.
P.O. Box 148
Orrville, OH 44667
(330) 683-0025
(330) 683-0000 (fax)

ADDITIONAL RESOURCES AND WEBSITES

ATV Safety Institute
(800) 887-2887

Beach Wheels
Email: rwest51034@aol.com
Website: http://www.beachwheels.com
   BeachWheels Inc. is a non-profit organization dedicated to making beaches more accessible to persons with disabilities by planning and holding recreational and awareness events at the South Jersey Shore. Example for other communities.

British Columbia Mobilities Opportunities Society
Plaza of Nations
Box 27, Suite A-304
770 Pacific Boulevard South
Vancouver, BC V6B 5E7
(604) 688-6464
(604) 688-6463 (fax)
Email: bcmos@reachdisability.org
Website: http://www.reachdisability.org/bcmos/

Buckmasters Online
Website: http://buckmasters.rivals.com/
   Although primarily a site for hunting and fishing, Buckmasters Online offers information on various outdoor activities, including ATV use. A special section for the sports-person with a disability is included.

National Off-Highway Vehicle Conservation Council, Inc.
4718 S. Taylor Drive
Sheboygan, WI 53081
(800) 348-6487
(920) 458-3446 (fax)
Email: trailhead@nohvcc.org
Website: http://www.nohvcc.org/
   The National Off-Highway Vehicle Conservation Council (NOHVCC) is a publicly supported, education foundation organized for the sole purpose of promoting safe, responsible, family oriented off-highway recreational experiences. They are a forum for organizations and supporters of OHV recreation, including OHV manufacturers, related businesses, affiliated foundations, OHV dealers, clubs and enthusiasts, to become partners in creating a positive future for the sport.

Off-Road.com
Website: http://www.off-road.com/
A complete website for the off-road enthusiast.

Chapter 2

Archery

SPORT GOVERNING BODIES:
National: National Archery Association (NAA)
International: International Archery Federation (FITA)

Official Sport Of: _____DAAA   _____USABA   *__USCPAA
                                 __x__DS/USA   _____USADSF   __x__WS/USA
                                 _____SOI
*some regional competitions

DISABLED SPORTS ORGANIZATION:
National: NAA Wheelchair Archers USA
International: none

PRIMARY DISABILITY: All

SPORT OVERVIEW

The memory of the lighting of the torch at the 1992 Paralympic Games in Barcelona, Spain remains as one of the most thrilling opening ceremonies in any event in history as Antonio Rebollo, a Paralympic archer with polio shot a flaming arrow 100 feet into the air lighting the torch. Rebollo had matched the feat he had accomplished just 3 weeks earlier as he lit the flame to begin the Olympic Games. Rebollo remains the only person to light both the Olympic and Paralympic torch. The use of the arrow to light the torch was significant because archery is one of the most popular summer camp, recreational, and competitive activity for individuals with a variety of disabilities. The adapted equipment discussed in this section makes it possible for almost anyone to participate successfully. This chapter is dedicated to archery as a competitive or recreational activity. Information on the use of archery equipment in hunting can be found in the hunting chapter.

SPORT ORIGIN

The use of the bow and arrow dates back to prehistoric times and has been used throughout the centuries to gather food, as a weapon, and as means of competition. The official national governing body for archery is the National Archery Association (NAA) founded in 1879. Archery was one of the original events of the modern Olympic Games in 1900. The Federation Internationale de Tir a l'Arc (FITA), was founded in 1931 as the international governing body for the sport of archery. The organization implemented standardized rules for competition which allowed the first World Championship to be held that same year.

Archery for individuals with disabilities was one of the original sport activities offered at the Stoke Mandeville Hospital by Sir Ludwig Guttman. Archery opened the 1948 International Wheelchair Games and it has been a sport at every Paralympic Games since its inception at Rome in 1960. Events are held in both standing and wheelchair divisions. Athletes participate in individual and team events under the International Archery Federation's (FITA) Olympic round competition and scoring systems. Competitors shoot at a 122-centimeter target from a distance of 70 meters.

In the United States, Wheelchair Sports USA has regional and national competitions. Each disability sports organization uses a sport classification system specific to its disability group. In major international competitions such as the world championships and Paralympics, archery is offered on an integrated basis with all disability groups competing in two divisions; standing- or sitting in a wheelchair. Competitions for these organizations are conducted according to FITA rules with only minor variations.

Wheelchair Archery USA

Wheelchair Archery USA is a Federation of Wheelchair Sports USA. They work closely with the National Archery Association's disabled archers committee in promoting and sanctioning archery competitions for individuals with disabilities. Wheelchair archery in the United States recognizes men's and women junior (U-18), senior (U-50), and master's classes. There are five shooting divisions recognized by Wheelchair Archery-USA.

- AR1: This category is for individuals with quadriplegia. Archers shoot using a compound or recurve bow and mechanical releases, mouth release or finger release is allowed.
- AR2: This category is for paraplegics. They shoot while sitting in a wheelchair and use a recurve bow shooting at the same distances and using the same rules as the able-bodied archer.
- AR3: This category encompasses all disabilities. Athletes shoot while standing or sitting and include archers with amputations who may or may not use prosthetic devices or mechanical releases. It also includes those athletes with cerebral palsy who do need a wheelchair for functional mobility.
- Open Compound Bow: This division is open to any competitor wishing to shoot with a compound bow.
- Bowstand: This division is for those who have only functional control on one side of their body. These individuals use a stand to hold the bow for them and they may use a recurve or compound bow in addition to mechanical releases.

Paralympic Archery

The Paralympic program includes individual and team events, and the competition and scoring procedures are identical to those used in the Olympic Games. Archers shoot from 70 meters at a 122 cm target face, as in Olympic archery competition. Each of the categories identified above have the following classifications:

AR 1 (Quadriplegia)
AR 2 (Open class-Paraplegia)
AR 3 (Standing)

Archers provide their own equipment that must conform to current FITA Rules. Generally, the same equipment, accessories and sighting equipment allowed in Olympic competition, is allowed in archery competitions for individuals with disabilities. Certain allowances regarding mechanical release devices are made for the AR1 Class.

Wheelchair Archers: Wheelchair archers represent ISMWSF, ISOD, and CP-ISRA. Some general rules regarding competition by wheelchair archers is provided below. Technical rules may be found on the International Paralympic Committee (IPC) website, or through the National Archery Association (NAA).

- FITA rules are applicable for wheelchair competitions, except in cases when the archer, because of his/her disability, cannot shoot correctly.
- Archers who belong to class AR1/CP 4-5 may have mechanical aids, recurve or compound bows but the sighting aids must be according to current FITA rules.
- Competitors with upper limb disabilities may use a releasing aid in cases where the drawing is made with a prosthesis or an orthosis.
- Strapping is allowed in certain cases when a medical certificate given by the classification panel is available. No body support or strapping to the chair is allowed in the AR2 class.
- Only quadriplegics and archers with upper limb disability may use the bow tied or bandaged to the hand. They may also have the arm which subjects the bow in a sling, a splint or some other device may be bandaged to the bow arm.
- No part of the wheelchair may support the bow arm while shooting.
- An assistant may load AR1's arrows into the bow. The assistant may not give the archer any verbal or other assistance, especially regarding the spotting of arrows.

Standing Archers: Standing archers represent ISOD and CP-ISRA.

- FITA Rules are applicable except in cases when the archer, because of his/her disability, cannot shoot correctly.
- Competitors may choose to compete standing or sitting.
- A competitor with upper limb disabilities may use a releasing aid in cases where the drawing is made with a prosthesis or an orthosis.

Archery for Individuals with Visual Impairments

The United States Association for Blind Athletes (USABA) has organized developmental archery competitions for the blind. A unique aiming device called the "Sightless Sight System"(Figure 2.1), developed in 1974 and modified in 1989, has opened up opportunities for the visually impaired (Gray, 1990). Developed by an avid 30-year-old archer and radio sound systems repairman, who was blinded as a result of diabetes, the sighting system works on a principle of two different pitched sounds. One indicates alignment, the other elevation. Monitoring by earphones, the archer releases the arrow when both tones are heard simultaneously. Introduced to USABA in demonstration form in 1989, the system was first used in competition at USABA's 1990 national championships.

EQUIPMENT

In choosing or developing assistive devices, the focus should be on assisting the athlete to shoot rather than replacing skill with mechanical devices (Jones, 1988). A number of mechanical devices are available through the archery equipment suppliers listed at the end of this chapter.

Trigger Releases

Trigger releases and release cuffs assist the archer who has fine motor grasp difficulty and/or reduced muscle strength draw and release the bow string smoothly and efficiently. Releases are usually used by spinal cord-injured quadriplegics and individuals with cerebral palsy and various les autres disabilities who experience grasp problems (Figure 2.2 a and b). Releases are also widely used in hunting, for they allow a hunter to hold a bow at full draw for an extended period of time. The use of a trigger release in sanctioned competition is permitted only for individuals with spinal cord injuries and cerebral palsy quadriplegia. Interested persons should consult the appropriate rule book for specific information.

Wrist and Elbow Supports

Wrist and elbow supports provide additional support and stability to the wrist and elbow of the bow arm (Fig-

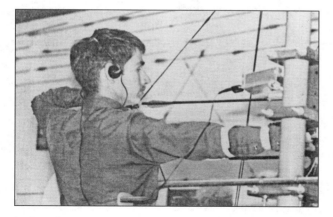

Figure 2.1. The Sightless Sight System developed by Al Lefebvre has made archery available to the visually impaired. Tones monitored through earphones indicate when the archer is on target. (Courtesy of *Disabled Outdoors*)

ure 2.3 a-e). Initially developed for use by spinal cord quadriplegics, supports are now being used by individuals with a variety of disabilities.

Both wrist and elbow supports are manufactured commercially as well as independently in rehabilitation engineering departments across the country.

Standing Supports

Standing supports allow wheelchair users to choose between shooting in a standing or a sitting position (Figure 2.4). The Courage Center of Golden Valley, MN has developed the Bowstand which holds the bow on a lightweight stand.

Bow Supports

A variety of custom-made bow supports provide adequate reinforcement and stabilization to the bow in cases where the archer is unable to grasp the bow, or lacks the strength to support its weight in a conventional manner (Figure 2.5 a and b). Drawing the bowstring and aiming, is still left to the participant in most cases. The Bow-Brace is one example of a commercially-made bow support.

Bow supports are not allowed in most sanctioned competitions but are permitted in limited use in United

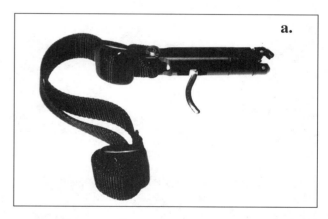

Figure 2.2 a and b. Two releases commonly used in archery. (Courtesy of True-Fire Corp.)

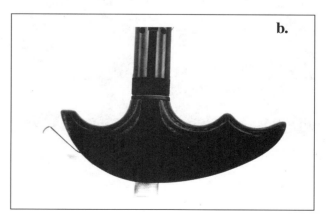

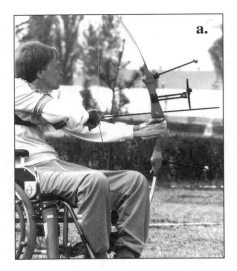

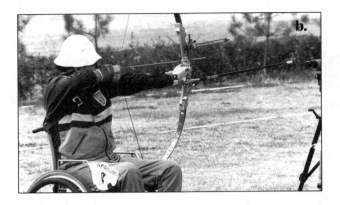

Figure 2.3 a-e. Archers with arm, wrist, and grasp difficulties use arm and wrist supports for additional stabilization. (Courtesy of Specialized Sports Unlimited, Lynn Rourke, and Michael Paciorek)

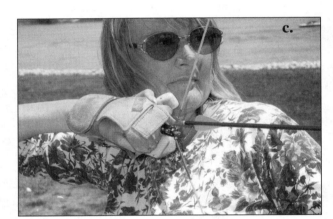

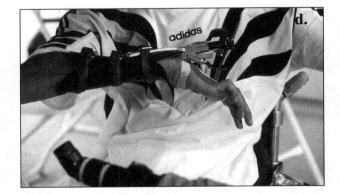

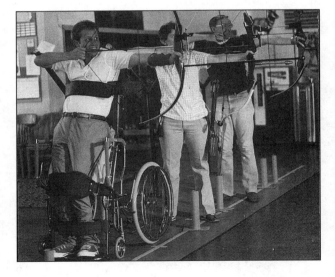

Figure 2.4. The Riser wheelchair provides a participant the option of shooting from a sitting or a standing position. (Courtesy of Imex Healthcare, Inc.)

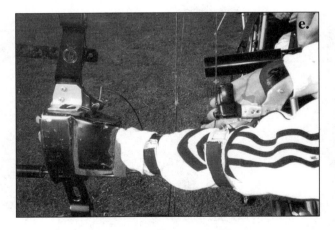

States Cerebral Palsy Athletic Association (USCPAA) regional competitions. The recreational shooter will benefit the most from the use of bow supports.

Crossbows

The use of crossbows has grown rapidly over the last few years (Figure 2.6). Crossbows allow individuals who do not have the strength to draw and hold the bowstring to participate. Assistance from another individual is usually required. Additional stability can be introduced by securing the cross bow to a bow support. Crossbows are now being widely used in hunting but are not sanctioned in Paralympic competition.

The National Crossbowmen (TNC) is an organization of people interested in promoting the crossbow. This organization promotes the use of crossbows for target shooting as well as hunting. Indoor and outdoor national championships are held leading to international championships.

TNC is a member of the International Armbrustschutzen Union (IAU) headquartered in Vaumarcus, Switzerland and is recognized internationally as the governing body of the Archery Crossbow shooting sport in the United States. TNC is also an affiliate of and a division within the National Archery Association of the United States (NAA). More information can be found on the NAA website.

Compound Bows

Many archers use compound bows to provide a lighter draw and maintain a bow poundage heavy enough to deliver an arrow accurately at longer distances. Compound bows are now allowed in Paralympic competition for the AR1 class (Figure 2.7). USCPAA competitions in the United States also allow the use of compound bows.

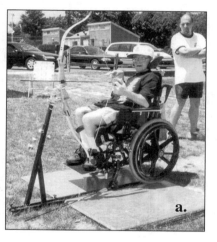

Figure 2.5 a and b. Bow supports have helped to increase the recreational value of archery in many local programs. Chairs serve as a suitable support for Class 2 athletes with cerebral palsy. (Courtesy of Human Kinetics)

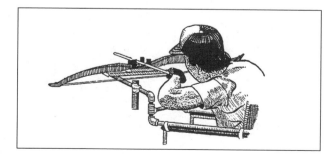

Figure 2.6. Crossbows allow successful participation by the more severely involved Individual. (Courtesy of Human Kinetics)

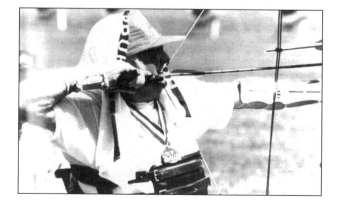

Figure 2.7. Compound bows work on a pulley system that provides a heavier poundage at an easier draw. (Courtesy of *Sports 'n Spokes* 10/91:27; Curt Beamer)

Mouth Pieces

Several types of mouth pieces have been used by individuals with various upper extremity hemiplegia impairments in order to draw the bowstrings with their mouths. Devices can be as simple as a piece of strapping or athletic tape looped around the bowstring and held between the archer's teeth (Figure 2.8 a-c), or as complicated as a trigger unit that is activated by a wired mouth piece.

Prosthetic Devices

Upper extremity amputees are faced with some unique challenges in archery. A review of the literature suggest the answers are quite simple. Radocy (1987) describes how a bow riser (handle) is modified to suit certain types of terminal devices by wrapping it with consecutive layers of rubber (Figure 2.9). Other simple devices include a home-made wooden apparatus to release the bowstring (Figure 2.10).

Standing Wheelchairs

Although most archers who require the use of a wheelchair participate in archery in a seated position, there are other options. With the development of standing wheelchairs, individuals interested in archery now have the option of shooting from a standing position.

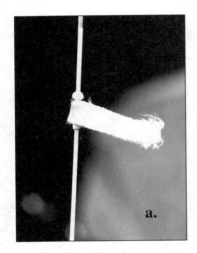

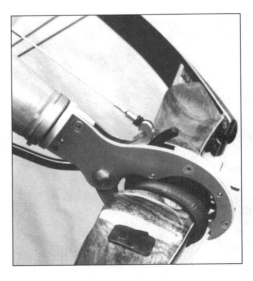

Figure 2.8 a-c. A strip of nylon cloth attached to the bowstring acts as a mouth piece, Allowing a hemiplegic archer to compete. (Courtesy of Specialized Sports Unlimited)

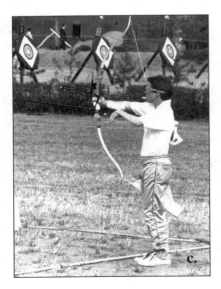

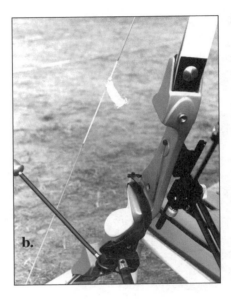

Figure 2.9. The use of several layers of rubber provides for a more secure grasp of the prosthetic terminal device. (Courtesy of TRS)

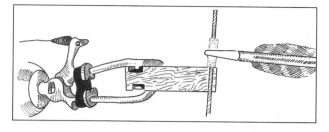

Figure 2.10. A home-made wooden device allows a smooth re-lease of the bowstring for the amputee archer.

EQUIPMENT SUPPLIERS

Archery equipment can be purchased through many athletic vendors. With the exception of grasp and release devices, little modification is needed for an individual with a disability to participate in archery. A sampling of archery equipment suppliers and online sites is listed below.

Hickory Creek Inc.
21595 Yankeetown Road
Saucier, MS 39574
(228) 832-2649
Website: http://www.drawloc.com

Hoyt USA
543 North Neil Armstrong Road
Salt Lake City, Utah 84116 USA

Lancaster Archery
2195-A Old Philadelphia Pike
Lancaster, Pa. 17602 U.S.A.
(800) 829-7408
(717) 394-7229
(717) 394-8635 (fax)
Email: las1@lasarchery.com
Website: http://www.lancasterarchery.com

"Sightless Sight System"
c/o Al Lefebvre
11 112 Wilmington Road
Lake Placid, NY 12946 OR
Colonel Earl Bass P.O. Box 22
Marvell, AK 72366

Bow Stand

Courage Center
3915 Golden Valley Road
Minneapolis, MN 55422
(763) 520-0520
(888) 8INTAKE

(763) 520-0577 (fax)
Email: jenim@courage.org
Website: http://www.courage.org/

Bow Support

The Bow Brace
20-9th Ave., NE
Glenwood, MN 56334
(320) 634-3660

Mechanical Releases

Tru-Fire Corporation
N7355 State Street
North Fond du Lac, WI 54937-1572
(920) 923-6866
(920) 923=4051 (fax)
Email: info@trufire.com
Website: http://www.trufire.com/

ADDITIONAL RESOURCES AND WEBSITES

Archers will find many websites related to their sport. Because this sport is accessible for those with and without disabilities, most participants will find the following sites satisfactory for gathering information.

International Archery Federation (FITA)
Avenue de Cour 135
1007 Lausanne, Switzerland
41-21-614-3050
41-21-614-3055 (fax)
Email: fita@worldcom.ch
Website: http://www.archery.org

National Archery Association
One Olympic Plaza
Colorado Springs, CO 80909-5778
(719) 578-4576
(719) 632-4733 (fax)
Email: info@usarchery.org
Website: http://www.USArchery.org

National Archery Assn.- Wheelchair Archers USA
Lyn Rourke
528 N. Bauman Street
Indianapolis, IN 46214
317-244-2377
Email: LMR1970@aol.com

National Field Archery Association
31407 Outer I-10
Redlands, CA 92372
(909) 794-2133

(800) 811-2331
(909) 794-8512 (fax)
Website: http://www.nfaa-archery.org/

Physically Challenged Bowhunters of America (PCBA)
Karen Vought
RD#1, Box 470
New Alexandria, PA 15670-9240
(724) 668-7439
Email: mkvought@westol.com
Website: http://www.bowhunting.net/pcba/

United Foundation For Disabled Archers (UFFDA)
Dan Hendricks
P.O. Box 250,
29th Ave
Glenwood, MN 65334
(320) 634-3660
Email: dhendricks@hunting.net
Website: http://www.hunting.net/uffda/
    Founded in 1994, The United Foundation For Disabled Archers promotes and provide a means to practice all forms of archery (target/hunitng) for any physically challenged person.

Other Equipment Websites

    The following online site provides a complete line of equipment for archery/bowhunting.
        http://www.archery.net/

VIDEOS

"The Incredible PCBA Story"
"Overcoming The Challenge, Adaptive Equipment Guide"
PCBA, Inc. Videos
RR 1 Box 470
New Alexandria, PA 15670-9240
The preceding videos are available for $15.00 each or 2/$25.00.

BIBLIOGRAPHY

Gray, N.L. (1990). Sightless archery. Disabled Outdoors 5(1):12-14.
Mugford, M. (1999). Bulls-Eye! Archery for Anyone. *Active Living* 8(3)49-52.
Radocy, B. (1987). Upper extremity prosthetics: Considerations and designs for sports and recreation. Clinical Prosthetics and Orthotics 11(3):131-153.
White, E. (1995) Making Archery a Sport for the Visually Impaired. *Strategies* 8(8)12-14.

Chapter 3

Basketball

SPORT OVERVIEW

Basketball is the oldest organized sport for individuals with disabilities. Since 1948 the National Wheelchair Basketball Association (NWBA) has set the pace for disability sports. Played with little or no rule adaptations by athletes from many disability groups, basketball continues to be one of the most exciting sports for players and spectators alike.

This chapter will discuss the programs offered by various disability sport organizations, as well as adapted equipment suggestions for developmental versions of the game. Two versions of basketball are popular within disability sport-ambulatory and wheelchair basketball.

AMBULATORY BASKETBALL

Four disability sport organizations offer ambulatory basketball competition. The Dwarf Athletic Association of America, Special Olympics, USA Deaf Sports Federation have offered basketball for many years while it is a new sport in the United States Cerebral Palsy Athletic Association. Rules for their programs are virtually identical to nondisabled rules.

Basketball has also been successfully played by peo-ple with upper and lower limb amputations (Figure 3.1). For upper extremity below the elbow amputees, the Super Sport prosthesis (Figure 3.2) by Therapeutic Recreation Systems can be an ideal solution. The device comes in different sizes and was specifically designed for use in recreational activities and ball sports.

Dwarf Basketball

The Dwarf Athletic Association of America follows the National Federation of State High School Basketball Rules with minor exceptions. Competition is offered in 5 vs. 5 and 3 vs. 3 (half court) in two divisions, open and junior. Separate classification systems are used for each division. Competition in the Junior Division is for players age 7-15 with the following classification system being used based on the age of the participant.

DAAA Junior Division Basketball Classification.

Age	Class/Points
7-9	1
12-	2
13-15	3

No team may have more than 12 points on the court at one time in 5v5 competition or 7 points for 3v3 junior competition. For instance; in a 5v5 situation a team may have 3 players on the court who are age 13-15 (total of 9 points), one 10-12 year player (2 points), and a player age 7-9 (1 point) for a total 12 points. Various combinations of players may be used but the total number of points on the court cannot exceed 12. A junior size ball is used in this division.

For the Open Division, classification is based on DAAA's Functional Classification System that assigns athletes to one of three classes for competition. Class 1 athletes are considered 1 point, class 2 athletes are considered 2 points and class 3 athletes are considered 3 points. Similar to the Junior Division, no team may have more than 12 points on the court at one time in 5 vs. 5 competition or 7 points for 3 vs. 3 competition. A regulation size women's ball is used in the Open Division.

Cerebral Palsy Basketball

The United States Cerebral Palsy Athletic Association first introduced basketball at its 1999 National Sports Festival. Similar to DAAA, USCPAA conducts competition under National Federation of State High School Basketball Rules. Co-ed competition is promoted and a point classification system is being developed.

Deaf Basketball

The first national deaf basketball tournament was held in April 1945. Recently, USA Deaf Basketball (USADB) and American Basketball Association of the Deaf (ABAD) merged in order to provide a comprehensive national basketball programs for deaf and hard of hearing people under the auspices of USA Deaf Sports Federation. There are no modifications from the traditional game.

Special Olympics Basketball

Basketball is offered as an official sport of Special Olympics (Figure 3.3). The game was first played at the inaugural games in Chicago in 1968. Currently the game is played by more than 69,000 Special Olympic athletes in over 40 countries, and in every U.S. State.

Special Olympics offer a variety of basketball official events in which athletes can participate, ranging from full team competition to individual skills competition.

The Official Special Olympics Sports Rules govern all Special Olympics basketball competitions. As an international sports organization, Special Olympics has created these rules based upon the Federation Internationale de Basketball (FIBA) and the National Federation of State High Schools Association (NFSHSA) Rules for Basketball. FIBA rules are employed in all international competitions; NFSHSA rules are employed in US competitions.

SOI offers competition in a variety of events, including Team Competition (5-on-5 Full Court), Half Court Team Competition (3-on-3), and Unified Sports® Competition (athletes with and without mental retardation competing together). The following events provide meaningful competition for athletes with lower ability: Individual Skills Contest (Target Pass, Ten Meter Dribble, and Spot Shot), Speed Dribble, and Team Skills Basketball. Specific rules may be found in the SOI Official Rule Boom.

A copy of the *Basketball Sports Skills Program Guide* is available for purchase through Special Olympics. This guide provides a developmental approach to teaching and coaching basketball. It is an excellent resource for physical education classes.

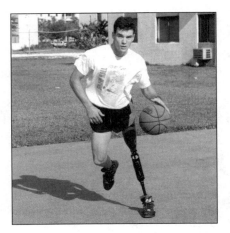

Figure 3.1. The use of the QSA Single Axis Knee and a quantum foot allows Doug Turner, an above-the-knee amputee, to enjoy basketball. (Courtesy of Hosmer Dorrance Corp.)

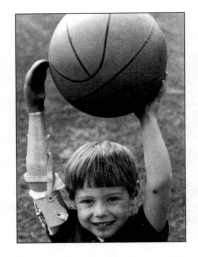

Figure 3.2. The Super Sport prothesis is specially designed for recreational activities such as ball sports. (Courtesy of TRS)

Wheelchair Basketball

Wheelchair basketball is physically and technically demanding and enjoys a high profile as a sport for people with disabilities (Figure 3.4). The sport is governed in the United States by the National Wheelchair Basketball Association (NWBA) and internationally by the International Wheelchair Basketball Federation (IWBF). The rules and player classification adopted by the NWBA is slightly different than the IWBF. The court size and basket height, are the same as ambulatory basketball. Any individual who, because of permanent severe leg disability or paralysis of the lower portion of the body, will benefit through participation in wheelchair basketball and who would be denied the opportunity to play basketball were it not for the wheelchair adaptation, is eligible.

Although the game of wheelchair basketball may look very different when first watched, the similarities with ambulatory basketball greatly outweigh the differences. However, the sport has its own unique style. Zone and man to man defenses are similar to the ambulatory game. Possessing a unique dribbling rule to accommodate the movement of players in wheelchairs, this high-intensity sport reveals its own system of attack. A three-guard offense is often used to increase speed and movement on the court. Wheelchair basketball's forwards or centers generally face and move towards the basket. The pick and roll is an effective offensive tactic.

The National Wheelchair Basketball Association (NWBA) is comprised of 181 basketball teams within twenty-two conferences. The NWBA was founded in 1948 (women's division in 1976), and today consists of men's, women's, intercollegiate, and youth teams throughout the United States of America and Canada. The NWBA is a member organization of Wheelchair Sports-USA.

The choice of a suitable sport wheelchair is critical to involvement in competitive leagues. Mobility is enhanced by the use of certain chairs. Appendix B lists many lightweight wheelchair manufacturers.

General Wheelchair Basketball Rules

Some unique rules of wheelchair basketball include the following:

- The wheelchair is considered to be part of the player, therefore, general rules of contact apply similar to the ambulatory game.
- The height of the seat may not exceed 21" from the floor.
- The height of the foot platform must be no more than 4.875" from the floor
- Seat cushions are permitted for medical reasons, however the thickness of the cushion allowed varies between classes.
- Players with the ball cannot push more than two strokes with one or two hands to advance without dribbling the basketball. However, a player may wheel the chair and dribble the ball simultaneously.
- More than two strokes of the wheel(s) without dribbling is a traveling violation.
- A player is out of bounds when any part of the chair touches the line.
- An offensive player cannot remain in the free throw lane for more than 4 seconds.
- There is a 30-second shot clock for offensive possessions.

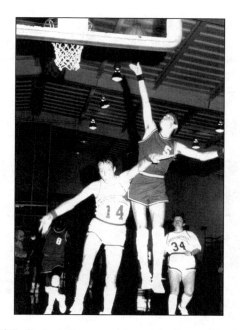

Figure 3.3. Basketball competition at the International Summer Special Olympic Games. (Courtesy of Special Olympics Michigan)

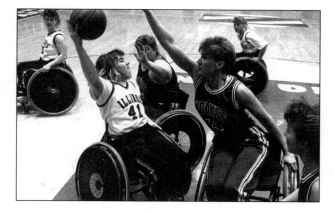

Figure 3.4. The National Wheelchair Basketball Association (NWBA) offers competition in four divisions: men, women, junior, and intercollegiate. (Courtesy of the Rehabilitation Institute of Chicago, Oscar Izquierdo, and Specialized Sports Unlimited)

Wheelchair Basketball Classification

Wheelchair basketball players are classified according to their level of functional ability. Muscle function related to the basketball skills of shooting, passing, rebounding, pushing and dribbling are evaluated. Athletes are given a point value or classification that is specific to basketball. This rating system is used to allow players with a variety of abilities and disabilities to compete together. The National Wheelchair Basketball Association uses a simple three-point system based on functional ability, with players being either class 1, 2, or 3. Teams are not allowed to have more than 12 points on the court at any one time. The classification system for international competition is more detailed using classes 1.0, 1.5, 2.0, 2.5, 3.0, 3.5, 4.0, and 4.5. Teams in international play are not allowed to have to have five players whose group point total is greater than 14 points on the court at the same time.

SPORT ORIGIN

Describing the 50+ years of wheelchair basketball is beyond the scope of this book. Readers interested in the complete history are encouraged to visit the website of the National Wheelchair Basketball Association. It is agreed that wheelchair basketball started in 1946 in Veterans Hospitals by a group of World War II veterans who were looking to maintain the active living they had experienced before sustaining spinal cord injuries. It quickly proved to be an extremely popular sport among wheelchair users and its growth spread to other countries. By 1948 there were six teams all representing VA Hospitals but soon the first non-veterans hospital team, the Kansas City Wheelchair Bulldozers began play. The organization experienced continual growth as interest increased and more teams were added. The National Wheelchair Basketball Association was formed to include players with disabilities other than spinal cord injured, such as amputee, polio and other orthopedic impairments.

In 1949, the University of Illinois under the guidance of Ted Nugent became the first college team to compete in the sport and formed the first National Wheelchair Basketball Tournament that continues to this day. Today over 150 teams in almost 2 dozen conferences vie for the title every year. The first women's team was also formed at the University of Illinois but because of lack of competition, they had to play able-bodied opponents from 1970-1974 until other organized women's teams emerged.

Wheelchair basketball, which has spread to every continent, is now an integral part of all regular international wheelchair games: The Pan American Games, the Commonwealth Games, the European Games, the Far Eastern as well as the South Pacific Games.

In 1977, the University of Illinois hosted the First Intercollegiate Wheelchair Basketball Tournament (NIWBT). The Southern Illinois University Squids winning the first title.

A significant reorganizing of wheelchair basketball occurred in the 1990's and has set the stage for continued growth and recognition of the sport entering the millennium. Internationally, wheelchair basketball was known as the Basketball Section of the International Stoke Mandeville Federation for 17 years until it was organized as the International Wheelchair Basketball Federation in 1990.

In the United States the Congress of USA Basketball voted to admit the NWBA as an active member in 1991, following eleven years as an Associate Member. The action represented a significant advance in the integration of the sport into the national governing body.

Adapted Basketball Games

A variety of modified versions of basketball with special equipment can be used for skill development. These range form a non-contact, non-running, and non-dribbling game called *Bankshot Basketball* to several games using lower and/or netted basketball rims that allow the ball to be returned to the wheelchair user by a ramp (Figure 3.5). Since there is no running, dribbling or jumping in *Bankshot Basketball*, the game relies on shooting skills. A series of shooting stations are set up, each with uniquely shaped angled, curved and brightly-colored backboards. For this reason it has been described a "mini-golf with a basketball". The players must score off the backboard from three different positions in order to move to the next station (see reference at the end of the chapter). Bankshot is non-aggressive and entirely inclusionary for ambulatory or wheelchair users. Each Bankshot requires a different banked shot to score. Some shots demand caroms off two backboards, some are ricochets and one diabolically maddening shot has three backboards and two rims. Players use a scorecard to track their score as they shoot increasingly difficult shots at each of the stations.

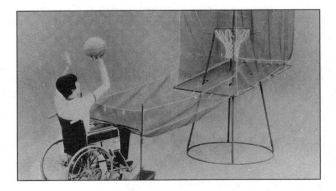

Figure 3.5. A netted basketball rim makes retrieving balls more efficient. (Courtesy of Access to Recreation)

The adapted game of *Twin Basketball* was developed in Japan for athletes with cervical level spinal cord injuries, with players divided into three classes based on functional ability. It is one of the few sports designed for individuals with quadriplegia and rules vary for each player based on functional ability. The game, played on a regulation basketball court, features both a high and low goal. Players with lower functional ability shoot at the lower goal (1.2m high) that is eye level to a seated player, while higher-level players shoot at the higher basket (3.05m high). A rubber playground ball is used to assist in grasping and shooting. See the reference following for a complete set of rules.

ADDITIONAL RESOURCES AND WEBSITES

Basketball and wheelchair basketball players will find many websites related to their sport. Because this sport is accessible for those with and without disabilities, most participants will find the following sites satisfactory for gathering information.

Bankshot Basketball
The Bankshot Organization
785 F Rockville Pike, PMB 504
Rockville, MD 20852
(800) 933-1040
(301)-309-0260
(301)-309-0263 (fax)
Email: info@bankshot.com
Website: http://www.bankshot.com

Canadian Wheelchair Basketball Association
1600 James Naismith Dr.
Gloucester, Ontario
K1B 5N4 Canada
(613) 841-1824
(613) 841-5151 (fax)
Email: cwba@cwba.ca
Website: http://www.cwba.ca

International Basketball Federation (FIBA)
P O Box 70 06 07, D-81306
MÜNCHEN, Germany
Tel:+49 89 7481 580 Fax:+49 89 7481 5833
Email: secretariat@office.fiba.com
Website: http://www.fiba.com

International Wheelchair Basketball Federation (IWBF)
Robert J Szyman, Secretary General

5142 Ville Maria Lane
Hazelwood, MO 63042–1646
(314) 209 9006
(314) 739 6688 (fax)
Email: iwbfsecgen@aol.com
Website: http://www.iwbf.org

National Wheelchair Basketball Association
Charlotte Institute of Rehabilitation
c/o Adaptive Sports/Adventures
1100 Blythe Blvd.
Charlotte, NC 28203
(704) 355-1064
(704) 466-4999 (fax)
Website: http://www.nwba.org

Special Olympics Director of Basketball
1325 G Street, N.W., Suite 500
Washington, DC 20005
(202) 628-3630
(202) 824-0200 (fax)
Email: SOImail@aol.com
Website: http://www.specialolympics.org

Twin Basketball
C/o Japan Wheelchair Basketball federation
207 ezondosharu 4-7-22
Minami Kudan Chiyodaku
Japan
10+03-3263-0381 (fax)

BIBLIOGRAPHY

Frogley, M. (1999). Part 1: University of Illinois Wheelchair Skills Workout. *Sports 'n Spokes*, 25(1), 46-47.

Frogley, M. (1999). Part II: University of Illinois Wheelchair Skills Workout. *Sports 'n Spokes*, 25(2), 57-58.

Official Special Olympics Summer Sports Rules (1996-1999). Special Olympics International: Washington, D.C.

Suyama, T., Nihei, R., Kimura, T., Tobimatsu, Y, Yano, H., and Mizukmi, M. (1998). Twin basketball for those with cervical cord injuries. *Palaestra*, 14(1), 20-24, 44-45.

Yilla, A.B., LaBar, R.H., and Dangelmaier, B.S. (1998). Setting up a wheelchair for basketball. *Sports 'n Spokes*, (24)2, 63-65.

Chapter 4

Beep Baseball

SPORT GOVERNING BODIES:

Official Sport Of: _____DAAA   _____USABA   _____USCPAA
_____DS/USA   _____USADSF   _____WS/USA
_____SOI

DISABLED SPORTS ORGANIZATION:
National: National Beep Baseball Association (NBBA)

PRIMARY DISABILITY: Blind and Visually Impaired

SPORT OVERVIEW

Beep Baseball (or beepball) is a modified game of softball developed for individuals who are blind or visually impaired. The object of the game is to bat a softball and to score more runs than your opponents. The games are six innings long with three outs in each inning. This is where the similarity to the traditional game of softball ends.

The Field

A large grassy area free of obstructions provides the best setting for a beep baseball field. The field is set up with a pitchers mound and only 2 bases (first and third). There is no second base in beep baseball. Bases are made of padded canvas or vinyl cylinders 48"-54" tall with speakers, placed one-hundred (100) feet down their respective lines and ten (10) feet off the foul line to prevent a runner from colliding with a defensive fielder. The bases contain sounding units that give off a buzzing sound when activated (Figure 4.1).

The Teams

Teams consist of six players on the field at any one time with each player having a number to identify a defensive position. For instance, the first baseman is one; right fielder-two; middle-three; left fielder-four; third baseman-five; and back fielder-six. One or two *sighted* spotters are positioned in the outfield, one on either side of the field (Figure 4.2). When the ball is hit, the spotter calls out the number indicating the direction the ball is traveling. This alerts the player in that position that the ball is approaching. When batting, each team has their own *sighted* pitcher and catcher. All players with the exception of spotters wear blindfolds making it an excellent activity for inclusion of people with and without visual impairments.

Playing the Game

Understanding the game is simple once you realize there are sighted people to guide players on each team. Each team has its own sighted pitcher and catcher. The catcher sets the target where the batter normally swings. The pitcher attempts to place the ball, which emits a beeping tone, on the hitter's bat while pitching from 20 feet away. The pitcher announces that the ball is tossed to alert the batter and fielders that the ball is in play. Prior to releasing the ball, the pitcher says "Ready." As the ball is released the pitcher says "Pitch" or "Ball." Each player is allowed four strikes and the fourth must be a clean miss, not a foul ball.

When the ball is hit, the base operator activates one of the bases and it becomes a race between the fielders and the runner. The runner does not know which base will be activated. The runner must identify which base (1st or 3rd) is activated and run to it before the ball is fielded by a defensive player (Figure 4.3). If the runner is safe, a point is scored. There is no running to other bases. A hit ball must travel at least forty (40) feet to be considered fair. If it does not reach the forty (40) foot line it is considered foul. A ball that travels one hundred eighty (180) feet in the air with the runner making it safely to the base, is scored as 2 runs.

A key to success in any baseball team is the effectiveness of their pitcher (Figure 4.4). Beep baseball is the only version of the game where it is very desirable to have a pitcher with a high ERA.

On defense, sighted spotters guide the players in determining the direction of the ball. Spotters can only call out numbers to indicate the general direction in which the ball is traveling. For safety reasons spotters can also call out warnings to prevent players from being hit with the ball or colliding with another player. Once the ball is picked up off the ground and is in the hand of the defense, the play is over. No throw is required and it is a rare occasion when a player catches the ball on the fly. When this does happen the inning is automatically over. A good defensive player learns to use the body and the

ground to trap or block the ball, then pick it up and display it for the umpires call.

Beep baseball is a game packed full of competitive action. Scrapes and bruises are a part of the game. New and improved training and coaching methods continue to be developed. New teams are being formed each year ensuring the success of this sport.

Official rules are available on the NBBA website or by writing Jeanette Bigger, Secretary, N.B.B.A., 2231 West First Street, Topeka, Kansas 66606.

SPORT ORIGIN

The founding of Beep baseball in 1964, is credited to Charly Fairbanks, an engineer with Mountain Bell Telephone who implanted a small beeping sound module into a regulation sized softball. The game was slow to catch on or to develop due to faulty equipment and lack of per-

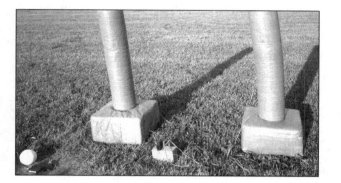

Figure 4.1. Official set of beep baseball bases. (Courtesy of Jeanette Bigger, NBBA)

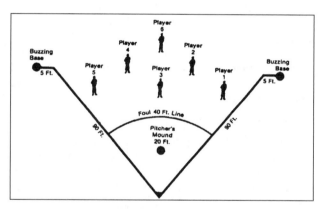

Figure 4.2. Beep baseball field diagram. (Courtesy of NBBA)

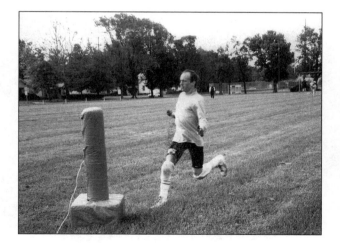

Figure 4.3. John Parker (Topeka GOFORS) running to the base. (Courtesy of Jeanette Bigger, NBBA)

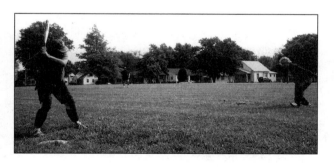

Figure 4.4. Joe Perez (Mid America Tornadoes) batting, Ed Valdez Pitching. (Courtesy of Jeanette Bigger, NBBA)

fected pitching styles. In the spring of 1975, the Minnesota Telephone Pioneers developed a newly designed 16-inch beep ball with an improved sound module designed to withstand the impact of being hit solidly. With a revision and standardizing of the rules, the game was ready to take off.

Since its primitive beginnings, beep baseball has become a very popular action-packed sport with more than 100 teams competing nationally. The game allows people with visual impairments to participate in a popular and demanding sport, enjoy physical activity, and obtain the same benefits offered to sighted baseball players. Although developed primarily for the visually impaired, anyone with an interest can play beep baseball. The game engages blind, visually impaired, and sighted individuals and encourages friendship among them. Games have even been played incorporating wheelchair softball and beep baseball rules, allowing individuals with various disabilities to compete.

The sport is governed by the National Beep Baseball Association (NBBA) and is not affiliated with the United States Association for Blind Athletes. The NBBA serves to promote the development of beep baseball throughout the United States and to elevate the ability of blind and visually impaired individuals to perform recreational and competitive athletics.

Telephone Pioneers of America

The influence of the Telephone Pioneers of America on the game has been great. The Telephone Pioneers of America is a non-profit organization of over 800,000 active and retired employee volunteers from sponsoring companies within the telecommunications industry in the United States, Canada and now Mexico. They are the world's largest industry-related community service organization, with a special focus on education. This organization helped introduce beep baseball making a form of the game of baseball accessible to people who were blind or visually impaired. The beep baseball was produced solely by the Pioneers with 25,000 beepballs having found their way to ballparks and sandlots in every state and province in the U.S. and Canada, as well as Europe, the Far East, South America and Australia. The Pioneers also devised a set of knee-high, cone shaped, rubber bases that contained electrically powered sounding units that emitted a high pitched whistle. That laid the foundation for the initial experimentation's with beep baseball. Various schools for the blind introduced this newest form of baseball for the unsighted.

EQUIPMENT

Equipment needed to play this game is similar to that needed for baseball or softball game with two notable exceptions, the bases and ball.

Bases

The bases are battery-powered and made of rubber or plastic. They stand at least four-feet high and emit a buzzing noise.

Ball/Bat

The ball is a 16-inch auditory beep baseball (Figure 4.5) and the bat must be an official approved softball bat.

Blindfolds

To enhance fairness, all players, regardless of vision, must wear blindfolds.

EQUIPMENT SUPPLIERS

Beep baseball equipment can be purchased by contacting the following individuals.

Bases:
Wyjo Council-Telephone Pioneers
Larry Tate
(816) 275-3062
@$175/set

Beep Baseballs:
Merrimack Valley Works Chapter #78
Telephone Pioneers of America
1600 Osgood Street
North Andover, MA 01845
(508) 960-2311
@ $25/ball

Pioneer Audio Ball Workroom
Connie Worsham
1332 Mickey Way Houston, TX 77055
@$18/ball

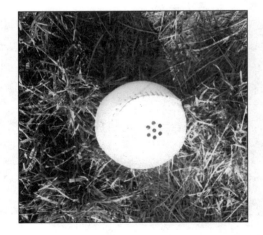

Figure 4.5. Official beep baseball. (Courtesy of Jeanette Bigger, NBBA)

F.H. Reid Beeper Ball Manufacturing
931 14th Street - Room 1400
Denver, CO 80202
(303) 624-8600
$30/ball
Blindfolds:
South Dakota Assoc. of Blind Athletes
Steve Bruggeman
800 West Ave.
North Sioux Falls, SD 57104
(800) 656-5441
@ $7.00 each

1-70 Council Pioneers
Jackie McBride
137 South Seventh
Salina, KS 67401
(913) 826-1188
@ $4.00 each

Repair of Beep Baseballs:
Merrimack Valley Works Telephone Pioneers - Chapter #78
Leo Pouliot 1600 Osgood Street
North Andover, MA 01845
(508) 960-2311
@ $10.00 per ball

ADDITIONAL RESOURCES AND WEBSITES

National Beep Baseball Association
Email: info@nbba.org

Website: http://www.nbba.org

Michael Garrett, NBBA President
4427 Knottynold
Houston, TX 77053

Jeanette Bigger
Secretary, NBBA
2231 West First Street,
Topeka, Kansas 66606

Chapter 5

Blowdarts

SPORT GOVERNING BODIES:
National:
International:

Official Sport Of: _____DAAA   _____USABA   _____USCPAA
                        _____DS/USA   _____USADSF   _____WS/USA
                        _____SOI

DISABLED SPORTS ORGANIZATION:
National:
International:

PRIMARY DISABILITY: High Level Spinal Cord Injured

SPORT OVERVIEW

In most adapted sports, an existing activity is modified or a new activity is developed when someone or some group is presented with a particular problem or challenge. This was the case with Andrew Batavia, a long-distance runner whose life was altered after a 1977 car accident left him a C2-3 spinal cord injured quadriplegic. He was faced with a situation that confronts thousands of high level quadriplegics: how to be an active participant in sports and recreation.

As a researcher for the National Rehabilitation Hospital in Washington, D.C., Batavia spent years investigating potential forms of non-passive entertainment for high-level quadriplegics. His research and practical testing of blowguns has led to the introduction of blowdarts as a viable athletic sport for quadriplegics.

Target shooting with a blowgun has all the recreational advantages of throwing darts at a target, yet it does not require any hand function by the user. Blowdarts gives the user a strong physical release and a real sense of control over the environment (Batavia, 1987). Batavia also notes the potential physical benefits since it requires physical exertion of the user's respiratory muscles, which is likely to increase respiratory capacity (1988). Although

not an official sport of any disability sports group, blowdarts has the potential to become an official sport as more people with high-level quadriplegia look for competitive opportunities (Figures 5.1 a and b).

Although a use exists for recreational use, it is important to realize that the blowgun has been, and is still used primarily as a weapon for hunting. It is the responsibility of the user to ascertain, and obey, all applicable local, state, federal and international laws in regard to the possession and use of blowguns.

BLOWGUN HISTORY

Although the history of blowdarts as a sport is very recent, the use of blowguns is perhaps the oldest of all known activities. Used specifically for survival, there is evidence of blowgun use over 40,000 years ago as a means of protection and hunting. The blowgun is still used for these purposes today. As a recreational or competitive activity, it can be assumed that informal contests among hunters have existed for thousands of years

Many scholars believe that blowguns appeared simultaneously in several parts of the world. Earliest evidence of blowguns appeared in parts of Africa and Asia. Blowguns are still used today by the Dyak tribe of headhunters

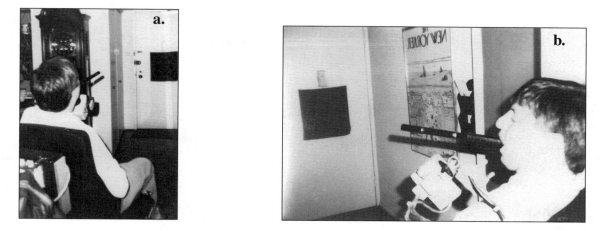

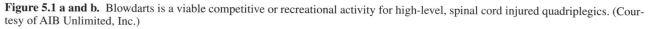

Figure 5.1 a and b. Blowdarts is a viable competitive or recreational activity for high-level, spinal cord injured quadriplegics. (Courtesy of AIB Unlimited, Inc.)

in Borneo for hunting and as weapons in tribal wars. Using hollowed out bamboo tubes, which reach lengths of over 20 feet and darts made out of reeds, the Dyak are very capable hunters. In the tropical areas of Africa, the Pygmies use blowguns to hunt their prey of small game. Around 1500 in Japan, Ninja assassins killed in complete silence using poisoned darts from the blowgun. The Ninja also used the blowgun for diversions by shooting darts in different directions to make the enemy believe they were surrounded.

In North and South America, blowguns have been used for several thousand years by native Americans as survival weapons. Amazonian Indians today still rely on the extreme accuracy of the blowgun to hunt for wild game. Although rarely used as a weapon, blowguns do play an important role in tribal wars. North American Indians relied on the extreme accuracy of the blowgun for hunting and for skill games.

Many uses of the gun exist today. Hunters use blowguns to hunt small game and in pest control. Blowguns are used all over the world to help maintain wildlife by delivering tranquilizer darts in complete silence. The animals are then studied and released back into the wild.

Blowguns are increasingly being used in sport. With many different darts from which to choose, blowguns are finding their way into everyday society. With the introduction of soft-tip darts that can be used with electronic targets, the blowgun offers a wide variety of sporting activities.

EQUIPMENT

A number of gun and hunting manufacturers also carry a wide variety of blowguns and darts, including an increasing number of on-line dealers. Electronic and soft-tip targets are available at most sports retailers.

Accessible Dart Board

The Perkins Company of California has developed The E-Z Darts Accessible Dartboard as a solution to the problem of retrieving darts from regulation height dart boards by wheelchair users. The E-Z Darts allow players to lower the board to an accessible height to retrieve the darts. The board is easily pulled down and then returned to regulation height with a simple push.

Assistive Devices

Since many individuals with quadriplegia may be unable to hold the blow gun with their hands, a solution might be *The Third Hand* by Wirthco Engineering. *The Third Hand* is a clamping device that holds the blow gun at mouth level for participants unable to hold it in their hands.

Blowguns

Blowguns come in a variety of sizes and caliber's. Guns used for blowdarts do not have to be of high caliber or length. Generally a blowgun of 18" and .40 caliber will be suitable for targets up to 35'. Blowguns can reach a length of 72" with a range of about 250'. The blowgun that is light-weight, with a manageable mouthpiece and high level of accuracy will be suitable for people with disabilities. Assistance may still be required for some participants. Participants should not share mouthpieces without first disinfecting. Devices exist that allow the participant to fire numerous darts without having to reload one dart at a time. Most blowguns come with anti-inhalent devices.

Darts

Velcro or soft-tip tournament darts are recommended in the interest of safety. One on-line company (Self Defense Products) offers velcro darts and targets (see equipment resources). Although the darts are soft-tipped, they can be dangerous if shot at another person. Caution should be exercised at all times, and children should be well-supervised while playing.

EQUIPMENT SUPPLIERS

Blowguns Northwest
P.O. Box 13951
Mill Creek, WA 98082
(425) 741-8389
Website: http://www.blowgunsnw.com

Cajun Archery Blow Gun
2408 Darnell Rd.
New Iberiz, LA 70560
(800) 551-3076

Palco Marketing
13860 Industrial Blvd.
Plymouth, MN 55441
(763) 559-5539
(800) 882-4656
Email: info@palcomarketing.com
Website: http://www.palcomarketing.com

Self Defense Products
Email: email@selfdefenseproducts.com
Website: http://www.selfdefenseproducts.net

Target Zone Sports
PO Box 1244
Allyn, WA 98524
(360) 275-3312
Email: SALES@BLOWGUNS.NET
Website: http://www.blowguns.net

The Third Hand
Wirthco Engineering Inc.
6519 Cecelia
Minneapolis, MN 55439
(952) 941-9073

BIBLIOGRAPHY

Batavia, A.I. (1987). Blowdarts, Paraplegia News 41(10):43.

Blowdarts: A new sport for severely disabled persons (1987). Accent on Living 32(3):80.

Blowdarts-A new therapeutic recreation for high-level quads (1988). Occupational Therapy Forum 3(38):7.

Needed: Active therapeutic recreation for high-level quadriplegics (1988). Therapeutic Recreation Journal 22(2):8-11.

Rourke, L. (1994). Darts for everyone. *Sports 'n Spokes* 19(6):11.

Chapter 6

Boating

SPORT GOVERNING BODIES:
National: United States Sailing (USS)
                     USA Canoe/Kayak (USACK)
International: International Sailing Federation (ISAF)
                     Federation Internationale de Canoe (FIC)

Official Sport Of: _____DAAA   _____USABA   _____USCPAA
                       _____DS/USA   _____USADSF   _____WS/USA
                       _x__SOI

DISABLED SPORTS ORGANIZATION:
National: United States Sailing-Sailors with Special Needs (SWSN)
International: International Foundation for Disabled Sailing (IFDS)
                     Blind Sailors International (BSI)

PRIMARY DISABILITY: All

SPORT OVERVIEW

The topic of boating for people with disabilities is broad enough to fill hundreds of pages of this book. Boating can include everything form rowboats to sailboats, canoes to kayaks, and tall ships to motorboats. The overwhelming array of styles and types of boats in each class illustrates people's love for the water and the numerous inventions and adaptations used to pursue that love. Boating, whether by sail, motor, or manual power, is a recreational activity and competitive sport that people with disabilities can participate in side-by-side with their nondisabled peers.

Yachting has been a part of the Olympic Games since 1896, but it is one of the more recent competitions for individuals with disabilities with disability sailing organizations being formed in the 1990's. U.S. Sailing (the national governing body) was founded as the North American Yacht Racing Union, in October 1897, to promote yacht racing and unify the racing and rating rules in the United States and Canada and throughout the yachting world (see the following).

This chapter will discuss boating opportunities in kayaking, canoeing, and sailing. Program considerations for people with disabilities, competitive sailing opportunities, community-based programs, equipment suppliers, reference materials and additional resources will be covered.

KAYAKING

Kayaking is generally considered an easily accessible and wonderful boating activity for individuals with disabilities (Figure 6.1). There are two types of boats: the cruising kayak and the whitewater kayak. The cruising kayak is designed to navigate quiet waters as you become one with nature, while the whitewater boater is tugged by gravity and water in an explosion of spray along a river or down a mountainside. Both are enjoyable experiences. In some cases, boat modifications may be necessary to ensure proper positioning.

There are single boats (for the solo paddler) and the double kayak (for two paddlers). Each has its own advantages. One should have an idea of expectations and types

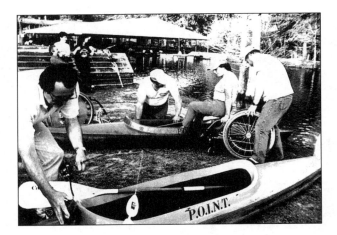

Figure 6.1. Certain Kayak models provide easy access for people with lower extremity impairments. (Courtesy of P.O.I.N.T.)

of water adventures before deciding to which to buy. Many sporting goods stores hold demonstration days where boats are on display and may be tried to determine preference.

Kayakers don't sit in their boats, they wear them. In order to paddle efficiently and with pleasure, the boat has to fit snugly and give support at the feet, knees, hips, rear, and back. Proper fit and positioning of the foot pegs, seat, and back support is a must. Balancing problems may prompt some kayakers to use seat belts for additional support. This is not recommended without extensive escape practice in a swimming pool before open water kayaking.

For the kayaker with lower extremity impairments, the following safety suggestions should be adopted:

- Use of a custom-made seat to counter the probable loss of knee and hip control.
- Use of ensolite to protect the buttocks.
- Use of a wetsuit to prevent hypothermia.
- Use of floats or foam inserts in pant legs to provide buoyancy to dangling legs and to prevent snagging on submerged objects.
- Use of a personal flotation devices (PFD) and helmet.
- Use of certified Red Cross boating instructors for training.

Individuals with lower extremity amputations will usually not wear prostheses while kayaking to avoid entrapment if capsized. Sponsons have been developed to aid with kayak and canoe stability. Sponsons are inflatable, rocket shaped floats that can be attached to the sides of kayaks and canoes. These floats can ensure both kayak and canoe safety.

A kayaker with an upper extremity amputation faces the difficulty of effectively holding the paddle. Conventional terminal devices that lock should never be used in aquatic activities. However, new technology in terminal devices (Figure 6.2 a-c) and simple modifications to the paddle, such as using tape to stabilize the grip and/or a rubber ring to prevent excess water from collecting on the paddle shaft, will enable an upper extremity amputee, with practice, to use the paddle (Figure 6.3).

CANOEING

Many of the suggestions for kayaking are applicable to canoeing (Figure 6.4a). The main differences involve the type of boat. The American Canoe Association manual *Canoeing and Kayaking for Persons with Physical*

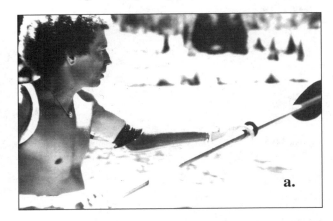

Figure 6.2 a-c. Paddle modifications make rowing easier for people with upper extremity prosthesis. (Courtesy of TRS)

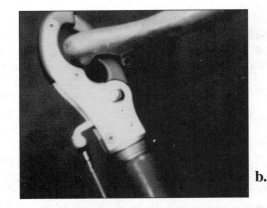

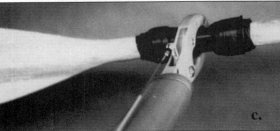

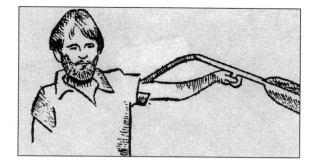

Figure 6.3. A one-armed paddle designed by Wilderness Inquiry and Gillette Children's Hospital.

Disabilities illustrates the similarities between the two sports. This 162-page manual covers all aspects of equipment, adapted equipment, specific disabilities, and implications for paddling. Canoes may appeal more to wheelchair users since canoers can take their wheelchairs along. It is also the preferred boat for multi-day trips, since equipment can be easily carried. The Rochester Rehabilitation Center's SportNet Program features canoe championships using outriggers (Figure 6.4 b)

The Canadian Recreational Canoeing Association has also produced a resource manual on canoeing for people with disabilities, as well as, a videotape titled *Canoeing is for Everyone*. Both focus on how people with disabilities can get involved in canoeing as a lifetime recreation (see additional resources for address).

The Special Olympics Rowing Sports Skills Program Guide is an excellent source for teaching rowing using a developmental progression.

USA Canoe/Kayak (USACK) is the national governing body for competitive kayaking and canoeing in the United States and was established to recruit, train and support athletes to compete in the Olympic Games in flatwater sprint and whitewater slalom canoe/kayak racing.

The United States Canoe Association (USCA) is a nonprofit educational and amateur athletic paddlesports organization. The USCA promotes marathon and sprint canoe/kayak racing and cruising, conservation, camping and camaraderie for youth, adults, clubs and other outdoor organizations (Figure 6.5 a and b).

SAILING

Sailing is one of the few sports where people with many different disabilities can compete against each other on an equal basis. In this sport, able bodied sailors compete alongside people with amputations, spinal cord injuries, and many other disabilities (Figure 6.6 and 6.7). The wind provides most of the necessary power in sailing which makes the sport very appealing to persons with disabilities. In addition, many of the physical motor skills of sailing have been eliminated or modified by recent technology designed for people with disabilities.

Sailing is an official competitive event in Special Olympics competition and offered as a Paralympic sport for people from all disability groups.

Accessible Sailboats

Currently there are six popular classes of accessible sailboats for recreation or competitive purposes. All are easily maneuverable with the Sonar and 2.4 metre being the most popular in sanctioned competitions in the Paralympic Games and Special Olympics competition. Manufacturers for each class can be found at the end of this chapter.

Sunbird : The Sunbird is a 15 ft. dingy designed to be

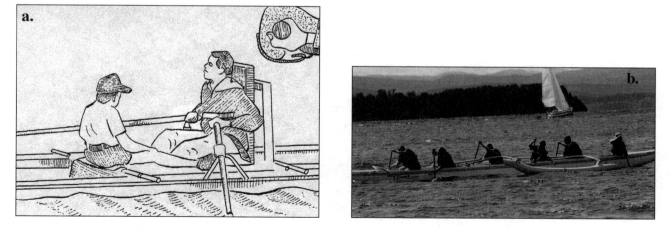

Figure 6.4 a and b. The Row-Cat catamaran can have its seating system designed to meet the individual needs of the rower. The Row-Cat Mitts assist in stabilizing weak wrists and in securing an insufficient grasp. Figure 6.4 b shows the Rochester Rehabilitation Center's Women's Outrigger Canoe team. The women's team includes three paddlers with disabilities of multiple sclerosis and spinal cord injury (level C-7) and three paddlers without disabilities (Photo by Marietta Tenny).

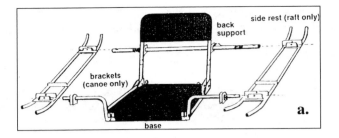

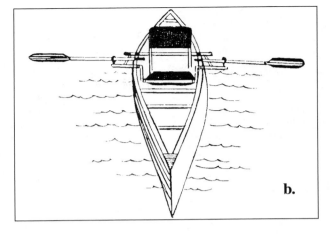

Figure 6.5 a and b. The Venture Rowing Seat fits most canoes and rafts.

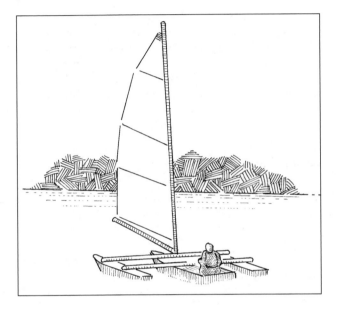

Figure 6.6. The Challenger is one of several boats designed for individuals with disabilities.

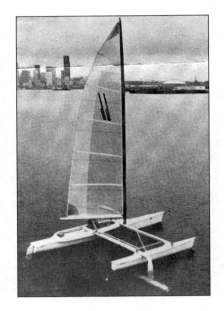

Figure 6.7. The Slatts-22 is a fast and very stable sailboat. (Courtesy of Hydro-Flight of Seattle and NOAP)

sailed solo from a single, seated position using a joystick rudder control.

Martin 16: The Martin 16 is built for both racing and recreation, and it can be sailed solo, or with a passenger with all controls (joystick steering device) accessible from a seated position. The "rider" seat, immediately behind the sailor, allows the sailing companion access to the sailing controls should the need arise. The stability of the keel makes it a very safe boat for people with severe disabilities. The high lift keel makes trailer launching simple from any ramp and can be easily rigged and sailed by one person. From its inception the Martin 16 was designed to be accessible to all sailors. Stability and adjustable seating as well as specialized control systems make the Martin 16 ideal for sailors with mobility im-

pairments. The Martin 16 offers optional automated systems for steering, sail sheeting and bilge pumping.

2.4mR (Norlin Mark III): The 2.4 metre class is a descendant of the America's Cup 12 Meter design, and is designed with racing in mind. It is stable, unsinkable, and comes equipped with all the sophistication and responsiveness of larger racing yachts. All the control lines are led under the deck to a console directly in front of the skipper. They are literally at the skipper's finger tips. Owing to it's design, where the sailor sits facing forward and all controls are led back to the cockpit, it was soon realized that the boat was particularly suitable for use by sailors with disabilities. At the same time it attracts top class able-bodied helmsmen. The Norlin Mark III was chosen by Sailing World Magazine as its 1994 Boat of the Year. The Disabled Sailing Committee of the International Sailing Federation (ISAF) selected the yacht for the Single Handed Class at the 2000 Paralympics in Sydney, Australia.

Freedom Independence: A popular recreational model for many years, and a favorite of many disabled sailing programs, this 20-foot daysailer makes sailing accessible by keeping it simple. The Freedom Independence (Figure 6.8 a-d)has been designed for extraordinary accessibility: freeboard is low and sidedecks are uncluttered to facilitate getting aboard. The Independence cockpit is equipped with two pivoting seats for helmsmen and one crew person. The specially-designed seats are counterweighted beneath the cockpit sole. Two wheelchairs may be accommodated in the cabin and there is adequate room for sails and gear. The Freedom Independence has added stability due to the ballast ratio and vertical center of gravity. The mainsail is fully battened for quiet, aerodynamic efficiency and the jib is self-tending. The unstayed Freedom spar eliminates troublesome standing rigging and the danger usually associated with an uncontrolled jibe. Freedom Independence is being built by Catalina Yachts in California

Sonar: The Sonar keel boat has a large cockpit designed for a crew of three. Since its introduction in 1980, yachts clubs and sailors across the country have come to appreciate the concept, and today, more than 500 boats are in circulation, with an active and enthusiastic owner-controlled class association.

Access Dinghies: Born out of the need to re-think entry level sailing, to simplify everything, to return to the basics, Access Dinghies are available in three deck configurations all based on the same hull. They are 2.3 m long, 1.2 m wide and around 36-48kg in weight depending on the model and accessories.

Tall Ship Sailing

Nothing is more exhilarating then sailing on a Tall Ship. Until recently, most tall ships were inaccessible to people with disabilities. Now two tall ships from England offer working cruises for individuals with and without disabilities. The Lord Nelson and Tenacious are owned and operated by the Jubilee Sailing Trust (JST), a UK national registered charity set up in 1978 with the aim of integrating able-bodied and physically disabled people through Tall Ship sailing (Figure 6.9 a-d). See Additional Resources at the end of the chapter.

The Lord Nelson is one of the best loved of all tall ships and has become world famous for being the first tall ship which crews of all abilities can sail. Due to her success a second ship, the Tenacious was built. The Lord Nelson is a 490 ton three-masted barque while the Tenacious is also a three-masted barque weighing in at 690 tons. Both ships offer comfortable facilities that are designed to accommodate people with physical disabilities.

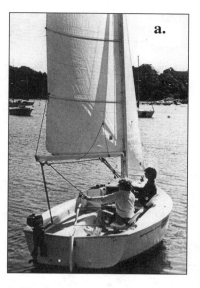

Figure 6.8 a-d. The Freedom Independence allows helmsmen and crew to be positioned within reach of all controls. (Courtesy of National Ocean Access Project)

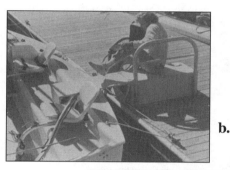

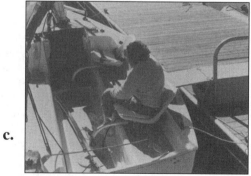

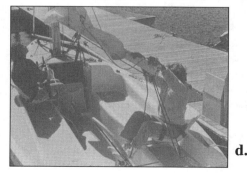

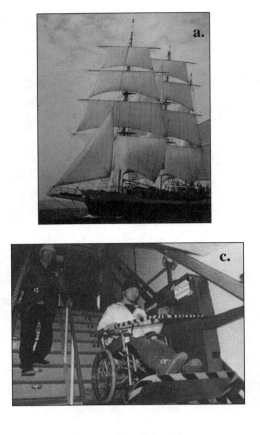

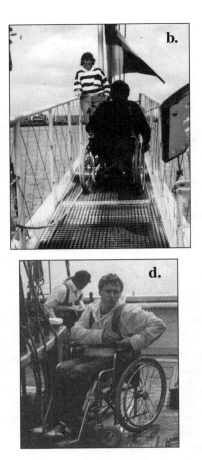

Figure 6.9 a-d. The Lord Nelson, a completely accessible $5 million vessel, offers a tall ship sailing experience for people with and without disabilities. (Courtesy of Operation NOAH)

Paralympic Sailing

Sailing competition is one of the newer Paralympic sports, being first offered at the 1996 Paralympic Games in Atlanta as a demonstration event. Due to its success the sport became a full medal event at the 2000 Sydney Paralympics. Athletes from all disability classifications are eligible to compete in Paralympic sailing competition. The classification system used is based on five factors—stability, hand function, maneuverability, visibility, and hearing.

The Yachts used in Paralympic competition have keels and are typically Sonar class and 2.4 metre boats, mainly because these designs provide greater stability and access to controls. The Sonar's have open cockpits to allow more room for the sailors. Sailors race under the fleet racing format, meaning all yachts race the course at the same time. Points are scored based on the yacht's finishing position with the yacht that possesses the least amount of points over the competition declared the winner.

Blind Sailing

Sailing is a very popular activity for individuals who are blind or who have visual impairments. Although blind sailors compete in Paralympic sailing competitions, they are also governed by their own association, Blind Sailors International (BSI) (see the following).

BSI uses the International Blind Sport Association (IBSA) classification of vision. B1, B2 and B3 sailors currently race in three separate divisions, according to the classification of the helmsman.

Blind sailors do not require special boats or special adaptive equipment to sail competitively. Twenty-three foot Sonar's is the boat of choice for blind sailing regattas. Competing blind sailing teams consist of four sailors on a boat, two of whom are blind. The two sighted sailors serve as guides. The helmsman must be a blind sailor, who must steer the boat independently unassisted by any sailor. The other blind sailor serves as crew, primarily trimming the sails. The sighted guide for the helm is not allowed to physically touch any of the controls on the boat, but is responsible for verbally guiding the blind helmsman. The four work together as a team with verbal communication skills and accurate execution of maneuvers being the key to success.

Special Olympics Sailing

Special Olympics Sailing was first included at the 1995 World Games in Connecticut. International Sailing Federation (ISAF) and National Governing Body (NGB) rules for sailing apply unless superceded by Official Special Olympics Sports Rules.

Special Olympics Sailing has training and competition opportunities for individual and teams of Special Olympics athletes; as well as, Unified Sports teams. Unified Sports allows athletes with and without mental retardation compete as part of a crew. There are four levels of competition within Special Olympics Sailing:

Level 1

Level 1 or development/introductory, is a Unified Sports™ event, where the Special Olympics athlete performs the crew duty of head sail trimming.

Level 2

Level 2 is also a Unified Sports™ event, where a Special Olympics athlete, in addition to the duties outlined in Level 1, will have control of the helm for fifty percent of the race. The teams may also use a spinnaker.

Level 3

At level 3 the entire crew consists of Special Olympics athletes.

Level 4

Level 4 is the highest skill class where Special Olympics athletes compete single-handed.

Special Olympics teams use dinghy boats, up to seven meters in length. At all national and international regattas both a monohull and a catamaran class boat are used.

SAILING RESOURCE ORGANIZATIONS

Sailing is fully integrated into the able bodied sporting community. A structure is in place within the various governing bodies to ensure that the needs of sailors with disabilities are met. A number of sailing organizations and programs ensure that many opportunities are available for sailors with disabilities. Some of the key organizations and sample programs are described on the following pages.

INTERNATIONAL AND NATIONAL GOVERNING BODIES

International Sailing Federation (ISAF)

The World Governing Body for Sailing is the International Sailing Federation (formerly the International Yacht Racing Union). They work with member organizations and disabled sailing organizations to promote sailing for people with disabilities.

The International Foundation Disabled Sailing (IFDS)

The International Foundation Disabled Sailing (IFDS) was established to promote sailing opportunities for disabled people all over the world and is the international governing body for sailing for people with disabilities. They are charged with organizing Paralympic sailing competition. Sailors with different levels of disability including mental, physical or sensory are included in IFDS programs. The IFDS works in conjunction with the International Sailing Federation (ISAF), the various national member organizations, and national disability sports organizations to promote the sport. The IFDS sponsors the World Disabled Sailing Championships using Sonar and 2.4 metre class boats. The IFDS has developed a Functional Classification System, to measure how a sailor's disability affects his/her functionality and to equalize competition among crews.

Additionally, the IFDS has two publications of interest to sailors with disabilities. The *World Disabled Sailor* is an informative newsletter, while the *Sailing Manual* provides a collection of ideas and strategies for facilitating sailing for people with disabilities.

United States Sailing (USS) Sailors with Special Needs (SWSN)

United States Sailing (USS) is the official governing body for sailing in the United States and is recognized by the United States Olympic Committee. USS is a member of the International Sailing Federation (ISAF) the world governing body for sailing. USS promotes sailing for individuals with disabilities through its subcommittee Sailors with Special Needs (SWSN). SWSN works closely with the International Foundation of Disabled Sailing in developing programs and competitions. US Sailing offers extensive information for sailors with disabilities on its website.

Blind Sailing International (BSI)

New Zealand is credited with the beginning of organized blind sailing in 1992 with the formation of the New Zealand Council for Sailing for Vision Impaired Persons. This led to the formation in 1994 of Blind Sailing International (BSI) that serves as the governing body for competitive international sailing for persons who are blind or visually impaired. World sailing regattas have been held every two or three years since 1992 with the number of countries and teams participating continuing to increase.

Local Adaptive Sailing Programs

Communities throughout the United States have developed sailing programs for individuals with disabilities. Space limitations precludes the inclusion of all of these programs. Below is a sampling of some of the specialized programs that are available. Contact Sailors with

Special Needs for information on programming within a specific geographic area.

Shake-A-Leg Programs

Shake-A-Leg, Inc. of Newport RI, is a non-profit 501(c)(3) charitable organization founded in 1982 to serve victims of physical trauma, with an emphasis placed on spinal cord and related nervous system impairments. The Adaptive Sailing Program was pioneered in 1986 and has been used as a model program throughout the United States. From the fully-accessible facility at Fort Adams State Park in Newport, Rhode Island, 5 custom designed Freedom 20's are available to people with physical and developmental disabilities for recreational, instructional and competitive sailing.

The Shake-A-Leg programs from Miami, FL and Newport RI are 2 programs that have received national recognition for their programming. Shake-A-Leg Miami, Inc. was created in 1990 to offer a universally accessible watersports facility for education and recreation. Operated in conjunction with the City of Miami Parks and Recreation, the facility is open to the public seven days a week with emphasis on people with disabilities, youth and families. Programs are offered in sailing, blind sailing and kayaking. See additional resources for addresses.

Other programs such as Sailing Alternatives, Inc. of Sarasota, FL, the Judd Goldman Adaptive Sailing Foundation of Chicago, the Buffalo NY Community Boating Center disabled sailing program, and the Y Knot sailing program in Lake George, NY typically offer supervised instructional clinics on accessible boats for individuals with and without disabilities. Some programs provide sip and puff rudder control and special seating.

EQUIPMENT

Specialized Seating and Cushions

The SS 2000 Strahle Seat has been specially designed for safety in the Sonar sailing boat. There is no chance of the seat or skipper falling out of the boat in heavy or light wind. Chest, leg and seat buckles are used and supplied. The seat is centered in the rear of the cockpit and is secured without drilling. Steering is done with left and right vertical levers on each side of the centered skipper. The seat has completed being tested using a C-5 quad skipper.

Cushions are vital pieces of equipment for sailors with disabilities. They are essential for skin protection for those with no sensation due to paralysis. They are important for the comfort of someone with limited movement, sitting for long periods and useful for someone with lack of trunk stability, or in need of support to maintain a particular position e.g. to reach winches or sheets.

A Jay Protector (JP) is fast becoming essential for the committed paraplegic sailor with no sensation in the

back-side. The JP is a small pad filled with a patented gel. The pad fits inside a sling which is strapped to the body to protect the sailor's buttock. The JP provides protection

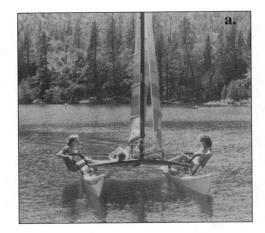

Figure 6.10 a and b. The trapseat quickly makes most catamarans accessible and safe for people with disabilities.

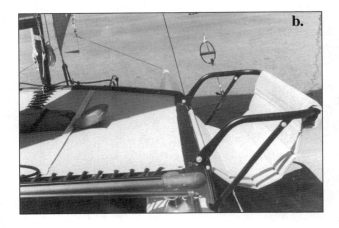

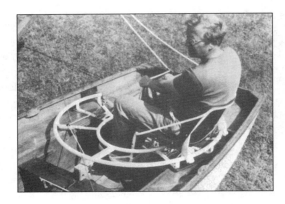

Figure 6.11. The Able-Sailor was designed to allow the mobility-impaired sailor to change sides within a boat without assistance. (Courtesy of Sailing Accessible, Inc., and Systems and Hardware LTD)

in the wheelchair, during transfer on the jetty and in the boat. It is designed to be worn outside protective clothing and will protect waterproof clothing. Some sailors wear a JP underneath their waterproofs to make sure it is not displaced during maneuvers.

A Roho is an inflatable rubber cushion (therefore unaffected by water) which has the appearance of an egg box. It provides excellent protection and comfort in the boat. Care must be taken to avoid punctures.

The Hobie Trapseat is a simple aluminum and canvas sling which clamps to the trampoline of a Hobie 16 thereby allowing severely disabled sailors to helm it in Comfort (Figure 6.10 a and b).

The Able-Sailor is a special seat was designed to allow the mobility-impaired sailor to change sides within a boat without assistance (Figure 6.11).

Personal Floatation Device (PFD)

The use of a personal floatation device (PFD) is essential for the safety of the boater and others who may be forced to rescue a boater who has failed to wear one. Wear a properly fitted personal flotation device at all times when on the water.

Audio Compass

The use of an audio compass such as the one available from Raytheon Marine is a useful device for individuals who are blind or visually impaired (see address at end of chapter).

EQUIPMENT SUPPLIERS

Many individuals with disabilities need few equipment modifications to participate in sailing programs. The use of accessible boats is the primary need of many individuals with disabilities.

Audio Compasses:

Raytheon Marine Europe LTD
Anchorage Park
Portsmouth PO3 5TD UK
Tel. 01705 694642

Accessible Boat Builders

Access Dinghy
Email: accessdinghy@msn.com.au
Website: http://www.accessdinghy.org

Catalina Yachts (Freedom Independence)
21200 Victory Boulevard
Woodland Hills, CA 91367
(818) 884-7700
(818) 884-3810 (fax)
Email: catalina@catalinayachts.com
Website: http://www.catalina.net

Martin 16
Martin Yachts Ltd.
302-2350 West 1st Avenue
Vancouver, B.C. V6K 1G2
(604) 731-7338
Website: http://www.canyacht.com

2.4 Metre
John W. Kruger
Gavia Yachts East Sales:
Glenbrook Road # 21
Stamford, CT 06906
(203) 327-7414
(203) 327-3193 (fax
Email: gavia@aol.com
Website: www.gaviayachts.com

Sonar International
100 Pattonwood Drive
Rochester, NY 14617
(716) 342-1040

Accessible Docks

VW Docks
P.O. Box 343
3050 16th Street
Spirit Lake, IA 51360
(800) 893-6257
(712) 336-1074 (fax)
Email: info@vwdocks.com
Website: http://www.vwdocks.com

Seats and Cushions

Roho Inc.
Website: http://www.rohoinc.com

The Strahle Seat
Email: trapseat@c-zone.net

ADDITIONAL RESOURCES AND WEBSITES

Individuals interested in boating and sailing activities will find many websites related to their sport. Because people with disabilities are easily included in most sailing clubs, few organizations have been developed specifically for people with disabilities. Because this sport is accessible for those with and without disabilities, most participants will find the following sites satisfactory for gathering information.

Kayaking And Canoeing

America Canoe Association
7432 Alban Station Blvd, Suite B-232
Springfield, Virginia 22150
(703) 451-0141

(703) 451-2245 (fax)
Website: http://www.acanet.org
   The United States governing body of paddlesport.

Canadian Recreational Canoeing Association
P.O. Box 398
446 Main St.
West Merrickville, ON KDG 1NO
(888) 252-6292
Website: http://www.crca.ca
   Official website of paddling in Canada.

Federation Internationale de Canoe (FIC)
Dozsa Gyorgy ut 1-3
1143 Budapest, Hungary
Email: icf_hq_budapest@mail.datanet.hu
Website: http://www.datanet.hu/icf_hq/

USA Canoe/Kayak (USACK)
P.O. Box 789 (421 Old Military Rd.)
Lake Placid, NY 12946
Email: USCKT@aol.com
Website: http://www.usacanoekayak.org

United States Canoe Association (USCA)
606 Ross Street
Middletown, OH 45044-5062
(513) 422-3739 (phone/fax)
Email: uscamack@aol.com

Sailing

Community Programs
Able Sail Ontario
65 Guise St. E.,
Hamilton, Ontario,
L8L 8B4 Canada
(416) 425 SAIL
(416) 425 5645 (fax)
Website: http://www.sailon.org/ablesail/

Access to Sailing
6475 E. Pacific Coast Highway
Long Beach, CA 90803
(562) 499-6925
(562) 437-7655 (fax)

Bay Area Association of Disabled Sailors
P.O. Box 77212
San Francisco, CA 94107
(415) 281-0212
Website: http://www.baads.org/

Buffalo Community Boating Center (BCBC)(disabled sailing program)
901 Fuhrmann Boulevard (Office Address)

Buffalo NY 14203
(716) 849-1174

Small Boat Harbor (Boating Center Location)
1111 Fuhrmann Blvd
Buffalo NY 14203
(716) 842-1276 (boating office)

Judd Goldman Adaptive Sailing Program
676 St. Clair, Suite 2150
Chicago, IL 60611
(312) 644-3200

Sailability
Website: http://www.sailability.org.au/
   Provides links to many sites for sailors with disabilities.

Sailing Alternatives, Inc.
7262 South Leewynn Drive
Sarasota, Florida 34240
(941)377-4986
Email: info@sailingalternatives.org
Website: http://wwww. sailingalternatives. org

Shake-A-Leg Miami, Inc.
2600 South Bayshore Drive
Coconut Grove, Florida 33133
(305)858-5550
(305)858-6262 (fax)
Email: SAL1Miami@aol.com
Website: http://www.shakealegmiami.org

Shake-A-Leg, Inc.
76 Dorrance Street, Suite 300
Providence, RI 02903
(401) 421-1111
(401) 454-0351 (fax)
Email: shake@shakealeg.org
Website: http://www.shakealeg.org/

Y Knot: Sailing Association for People with Disabilities
Lake George, NY
(518) 656-9462
Email: yknotsail@hotmail.comt
Website:
   http://www.timesunion.com/communities/yknot.htm

Governing Bodies

Blind Sailing International (BSI)
c/o The Carroll Center for the Blind
770 Centre Street
Newton, MA
(617) 969-6200
Website: http://www.blindsailing.org/

Blind Sailing International is the governing body for competitive international sailing for persons who are blind or visually impaired.

International Foundation for Disabled Sailors (IFDS)
Website: http://ifds.org/
International governing body for sailors with disabilities.

International Sailing Federation (ISAF)
Ariadne House, Town Quay
Southhampton
SO14 2AQ, United Kingdom
Email: sail@isaf.co.uk
Website: http://www.sailing.org

ISAF Disabled Sailing information.
Website: http://sailing.org/disabled/

Disabled Sailing Manual
Website:
    http://sailing.org/disabled/sailingmanual/default.asp
Ideas for potential sailors and includes the ISAF/IFDS Disabled Sailing Manual.

Special Olympics
1325 G Street, NW, Suite 500
Washington, DC 20005-3104
(202) 628-3630
(202) 824-0200 (FAX)
Email: SOImail@aol.com
Website: http://www.specialolympics.org

United States Sailing (USS)
Website: http://www.ussailing.org/

United States Sailing Association Sailors with Special Needs (USSA-SWSN)
Website: http://www.ussailing.org/swsn
National subcommittee of disabled sailors.

Sailing Class Organizations

The International Sonar Class Association (ISCA)
Website: http://www.sonar.org/
Organization for people who race in the Sonar class. This site provides information on all aspects of Sonar Class racing including builders, sailmakers, specialized equipment, and the latest information on Sonar races.

2.4 Metre Class
Email: 2.4m@fresk.pp.se
Website: http://www.sailingsource.com/24metre/
Organization for people who race in the 2.4 metre class. This site provides information on all aspects of 2.4

metre racing including builders, sailmakers, specialized equipment, and the latest information on 2.4 metre races.

Other Resources

John's Nautical & Boatbuilding Page
Website: http://www.boat-links.com/
Billed as the "Mother of All Maritime Links", this website has it all for the boating enthusiast.

Jubilee Sailing Trust (Lord Nelson and Tenacious)
Jubilee Yard
Hazel Road
Woolston
Southampton SO19 7GB
United Kingdom
Email: jst@jst.org.uk
Website: http://www.jst.org.uk/

Sailing Web: Options for Sailors with Disabilities
Website: http://www.footeprint.com/sailingweb/
Competitions, clubs, accessible sailboats.

States Organization for Boating Access (SOBA)
Guidelines for the Design of Barrier-Free Recreational Boating and Fishing Facilities.
P.O. Box 25655
Washington, DC 20007

BIBLIOGRAPHY

Armstead, L. (1997). *Whitewater Rafting in North America*. Connecticut: Pequot Press.

Bennett, J. (1996). *The Complete Whitewater Rafter*. Maine:Ragged Mountain Press, 1996.

Ray, S. (1992). *The Canoe Handbook*. Pennsylvania: Stackpole Books.

Rafter, D. (2000). Sharp as a TACK. *Sports 'n Spokes 26*(5)36-41.

Stuhaug, D. (1998). *Kayaking Made Easy*. Connecticut: Pequot Press.

Webre, A.W. & Zeller, J. (1990). Canoeing and Kayaking for Persons with Disabilities-Instructional Manual. The American Canoe Association.

Wilson, K. (1992). *Guidelines for the Design of Barrier-Free Recreational Boating and Fishing Facilities*. States Organization for Boating Access: Washington, DC.

Chapter 7

Boccia

SPORT GOVERNING BODIES:
National:
International: International Bocce Association (IBA)

Official Sport Of: __x__ **DAAA**   _____ **USABA**   __x__ **USCPAA**
                       _____ **DS/USA**   _____ **USADSF**   _____ **WS/USA**
                       __x__ **SOI**

DISABLED SPORTS ORGANIZATION:
National: United States Cerebal Palsy Athletic Association
International: Cerebral Palsy International Sports and Recreation Association

PRIMARY DISABILITY: All

SPORT OVERVIEW

Boccia (or Bocce) is a throwing game played either indoors or outside and is very similar to the Italian game of lawn bowling and the French game of petanque. The object of the game is similar to that of lawn bowling. A white target ball, (pallina, jack, or cue) is thrown on the court by one of the players, and opponents take turns attempting to get their red or green colored game balls as close to the target ball as possible (the indoor game uses blue and red balls). Once all the game balls have been thrown, points are awarded by the referee according to the placement of the ball nearest the target (Figure 7.1). Individual boccia is played with six balls per player for four rounds, while team boccia (3 players per team) is played using two balls per player for six rounds. The court dimensions vary depending on whether the game is played indoors or outside, but the strategy and object of the game remain the same.

Boccia is easily modified for individuals with disabilities, especially those with mobility impairments and is played at the Paralympic level by athletes with cerebral palsy as an indoor sport and within Special Olympics as an outdoor sport. Individuals with severe physical impairments or senior citizens can excel at the game. It is also an appropriate game for physical education classes since it fosters inclusion of individuals with disabilities. The International Bocce Association is the official governing body for boccia.

SPORT ORIGIN

Boccia has its origins as a throwing game in ancient Egypt and Greece who used to play at throwing a ball into a circle. Some of the earlier forms may have included throwing stones as close as possible to another stone. The Italians are credited with developing the game in its present form. The game saw it's international debut at the 1896 Olympic Games in Athens, Greece. The involvement of athletes with disabilities in boccia is attributed to organizations involved with sport for individuals with cerebral palsy. It was found that this sport could be an excellent competitive and recreational sport for athletes with severe disabilities. Later, the sport was adopted by Special Olympics as an event that would suitable for older athletes with mental retardation. It is also played as an official sport of the Dwarf Athletic Association of America.

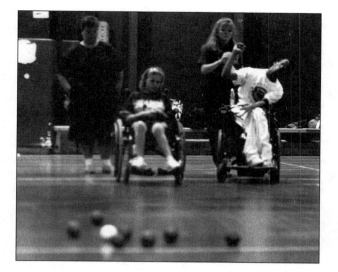

Figure 7.1. Success in boccia is often a matter of inches. Accuracy is the name of the game; the white target ball is always the point of concentration. (Courtesy of Rehabilitation Institute of Chicago's Wirtz Sports Program)

Paralympic Boccia

Paralympic boccia is limited to those athletes with cerebral palsy. International Boccia Association rules are followed (modified) within six divisions of play based on functional ability. This includes four individual divisions with division 3 being reserved for players who use assistive devices, pairs for players who use assistive devices and team competition. Each division is played by competitors of either sex. Official Paralympic Boccia Rules can be found on the International Paralympic Committee website <http://www.paralympic.org>.

USCPAA Boccia

Boccia has been modified specifically to include the more physically involved cerebral palsy athlete in a competitive sport. It is one of the few activities requiring a high degree of skill that can be mastered by individuals with disabilities (Jones, 1988). Boccia tests each competitor's degree of muscle control and accuracy (Figure 7.2 a and b). At the national and international levels, the game of boccia is currently open to only Class I and Class II athletes (wheelchair users) with cerebral palsy. The game is played one on one (individual boccia), three on three (team boccia), or in pairs for players who use assistive devices such as ramps, and is one of the few sports that are played on a coed basis. The athletes either throw, kick (Figure 7.3), or use an assistive device to propel the leather balls towards the jack.

The Court

The court used by athletes with cerebral palsy is quite different from the traditional boccia court. The surface should be flat and smooth such as a tiled or wood gymna-

sium floor. A boccia court for athletes with cerebral palsy consists of two areas, the players' boxes and the playing area (Figure 7.4 a,b). The playing area also includes two parts, the non-valid target area and the valid target area. The players' boxes consist of six equal-sized boxes. Each player must stay completely within his or her box during play.

Special Olympics Boccia

With the aging of the traditional Special Olympian and due to the needs of Special Olympics to reach a wider segment of the population, additional competitive

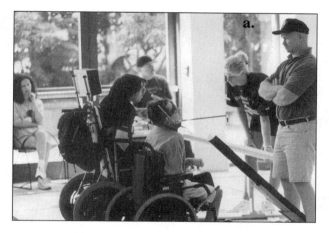

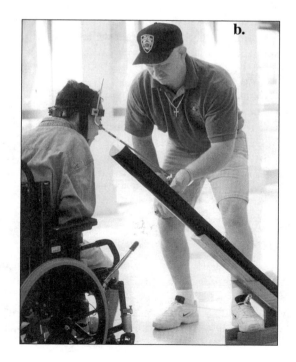

Figure 7.2 a and b. (a) USCPAA rules prohibit assistants from viewing the boccia court and communicating with players during a match. (b) Players must self-initiate the release of the ball. (Courtesy of USCPAA National Sports Festival and Ron Pacchiana)

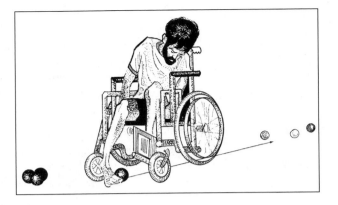

Figure 7.3. A number of athletes with cerebral palsy will choose to use their feet to compete in boccia. (Courtesy of Human Kinetics)

thrown across a wood floor are hard enough to still roll. Balls are available from Handi Life, the only authorized dealer for Paralympic boccia balls (see Additional Resources). For individuals without grasp difficulties, standard boccia balls are available from a variety of sports and recreational stores and manufacturers.

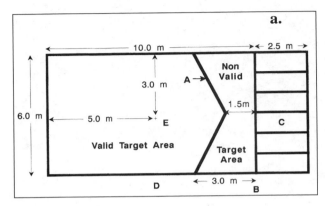

Figure 7.4 a and b. The boccia court (**a**) and precision boccia court (**b**) dimensions: (a) target ball throwing area, (b) throwing line, (c) sidelines of throwing box, (d) court boundary lines, (e) back line of throwing area, (f) non-valid area for target ball.

opportunities needed to be developed. Boccia was a perfect solution to these needs. Boccia was first played within Special Olympics as a demonstration sport at the 1991 International Summer Special Olympic Games in Minneapolis (Paciorek, 1992). Competition involved athletes in the seniors masters division (at least 30 years of age).

Although the objective of the game is similar to boccia played by athletes with cerebral palsy, the court and the balls are different. The game is played outside as competitors stand at opposite ends of long lanes and take turns throwing toward the jack. The balls are made of wood as opposed to the leather balls used by athletes with cerebral palsy. Special Olympics rules are used based on International Boccia Association rules. Special Olympics offers competition in singles, doubles, team (4 people) and Unified doubles and team competition. Unified competition combines athletes with and without mental retardation on the same team.

Precision Boccia

A Canadian version of the game called Precision Boccia, changes the objective from getting balls close to the jack to getting balls within designated areas of the court. Three separate areas within the standard boccia court are given different point values. Players are required to make two attempts at each area, with the player scoring the most points being declared the winner.

EQUIPMENT

Boccia Balls

Boccia balls for athletes with cerebral palsy and in Paralympic competition are different from traditional hard boccia balls. The indoor balls are comprised of handmade leather filled with plastic granulate and are about the size of a baseball. Since they are softer than the traditional boccia ball they are easily grasped and when

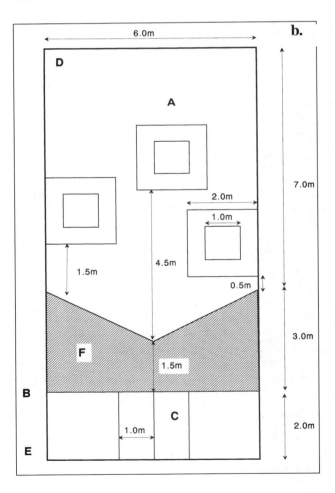

Chutes and Ramps

As in many sports, adapted equipment allows many individuals to participate who might otherwise be unable to compete. In USCPAA boccia, the use of chutes and ramps is restricted to a single division in which Class I and II athletes compete jointly (Figure 7.5 a and b). The assistive device is the equalizing factor. An individual's ability to effectively use a chute or a ramp depends on several factors, the type of ramp release mechanism or technique used by the athlete and the need for additional assistance. The most popular chute is made of plastic or aluminum pipe and be left whole or cut down the middle. A more complicated device includes a swivel base, height adjustments that control speed and distance and a release lever. In Paralympic competition, assistive devices should be contained within a size that when laid on its side fits into an area measuring 2.5m x 1m. Mechanical propulsion devices are not allowed, and the player must make direct physical contact with the ball immediately prior to its release into court. This includes using an aid attached directly to the player's head or hand.

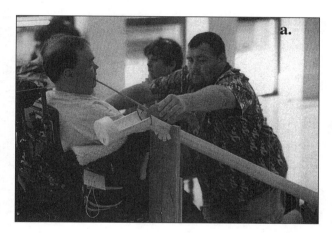

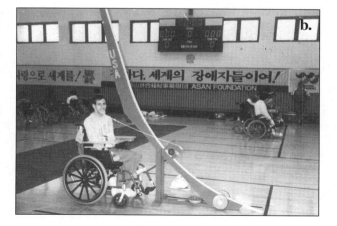

Figure 7.5 a and b. Boccia ramps can be easily made from materials found in most local hardware stores. (Courtesy of USCPAA National Sports Festival and Ron Pacchiana)

The type and variety of chutes is limited only by the imagination of the builder. Athletes should practice with and without chutes before deciding in which division to compete. Several factors should be evaluated when considering whether to use a chute, including the ability to grasp a ball, ability to release during the throw, and ability to place the ball accurately on all areas of the playing court. When determining the most efficient technique or playing style, one should not overlook the use of the lower extremities. Many players who have little or no functional use of their hands possess remarkable foot co-ordination.

ADDITIONAL RESOURCES AND WEBSITES

Boccia players will find many websites related to their sport. Because this sport is accessible for those with and without disabilities, most participants will find the following sites satisfactory for gathering information.

U.S. Bocce Federation
44 Park Lane
Park Ridge, IL 60068
(897) 692-6223
Website: http://www.bocce.com

Wonderful World of Bocce Association
C/O Rico Daniele
899 Main Street
Springfield, MA 01453
(800) 262-2354
Email: bocce54@aol.com
Website: http://www.sites2c.com/bocce

World Bocce Association
1098 West Irving Park Road
Bensenville, IL 60106
(630) 860-2623
(630) 595-2541 (fax)
Email: Mr. Bocce@worldbocce.org
Website: http://www.worldbocce.org

Collegium Cosmicum Ad Buxeas,
The preeminent international organization for the sport of bocce. This site include information on all aspects of bocce including history, rules, and links.
Website: http://www.bocce.org

Equipment Websites:

Boccia equipment can be purchased through many athletic vendors. Boccia balls for indoor or Paralympic competition is very different than the balls used in the traditional game. The following websites offer boccia equipment online.

Official Paralympic Boccia Balls (for indoor or Paralympic competition)
Handi Life
Blakke Moellevej
18B 4050
Skibby, Denmark
47 52 60 22
47 52 60 97 (fax)
Email: hls@handilifesport.com
Website: http://www.handilifesport.com

United States Cerebral Palsy Athletic Association
25 West Independence Way
Kingston, RI 02881
(401) 848-2460
(401) 848-5280 (fax)

Email: uscpaa@mail.bbsnet.com
Website: http://www.uscpaa.org
    USCPAA is also a distributor of official game balls.

BIBLIOGRAPHY

From Bowling to Boccia: The right equipment can make all the difference (2000). *Active Living* 9(1):14, 16.

Jones, J.A. (1988). Wheelchair boccia. In J.A. Jones (ed.), *Training Guide to Cerebral Palsy Sports* (173-181). Champaign, IL: Human Kinetics.

Paciorek, M.J. (1992). 1991 ISSOG: Bocce. *Palaestra* 8(2):28-29.

Chapter 8

Bowling

SPORT GOVERNING BODIES:
National: USA Bowling (USAB)
American Bowling Congress (ABC)
International: Federation Internationale des Quilleurs (FIQ)

Official Sport Of:

_____ DAAA	_____ USABA	__x__ USCPAA
_____ DS/USA	__x__ USADSF	_____ WS/USA
__x__ SOI		

DISABLED SPORTS ORGANIZATION:
National: American Wheelchair Bowling Association (AWBA)
American Blind Bowling Association (ABBA)
International:

PRIMARY DISABILITY: All

SPORT OVERVIEW

It has been estimated that over 100 million people in the world have bowled, with 60 million of those being in the United States. The tens of thousands of bowlers with disabilities involved in competitive bowling across the country, combined with the countless recreational bowlers involved in community-based programs, make bowling one of this country's most popular recreational activities. Modifications are minimal and specific to each individual. The American Bowling Congress (ABC) can provide a list of local leagues that offer competition for people with disabilities.

As with many sports, one of the greatest challenges facing a bowler with a disability is access to the bowling center. Bowling centers across the country are making access easier by ensuring ramps are available for access to lanes.

SPORT HISTORY

References to games similar to bowling have been traced to ancient Egypt and Polynesia where stones were rolled in an attempt to knock down objects. The modern day sport has its origins in Germany where it spread throughout Europe and finally to the United States in the early 1800's. The game became very popular throughout US cities with high concentrations of German immigrants in the mid 19th century, as many bowling alleys were constructed. The American Bowling Congress (ABC) was founded in 1895 to develop standard rules and equipment for the growing sport. Today the ABC and the Women's International Bowling Congress sanction many leagues around the country.

Although bowling was a demonstration sport at the 1988 Olympic Games and is one of the most widely played sports in the world by individuals with disabilities, it has yet to become an official Paralympic sport.

Federation Internationale des Quilleurs

The International Governing Body for bowling is the Federation Internationale des Quilleurs (FIQ). The FIQ was founded in 1952 succeeded the International Bowling Congress which had been formed in 1947 to foster worldwide interest in amateur tenpin and ninepin bowling. The FIQ has been recognized by the International Olympic Committee since 1979 as the world governing body for the sport of Bowling.

American Wheelchair Bowling Association

For athletes with physical disabilities, the American Wheelchair Bowling Association is a nonprofit organization composed of wheelchair bowlers dedicated to the encouragement, development and regulation of wheelchair bowling under uniform rules and regulations. They encourage all people who use wheelchairs to bowl for rehabilitation and recreational exercise in league and tournament competition. Although the actual founding of the AWBA did not occur until 1962, wheelchair bowling traces its roots to the end of World War II as bowling was found to be an excellent activity in rehabilitation programs for injured war veterans. Although many wheelchair bowling leagues exist across the country, athletes who use wheelchairs often bowl in ambulatory ABC sanctioned leagues.

American Blind Bowling Association

Many leagues for blind bowlers exist through the efforts of the American Blind Bowling Association (ABBA). Although most sighted bowlers are more effective if they throw a curve, an effective technique for blind bowlers is to throw a consistently straight ball. The use of a guide rail allows a bowler who is blind to make a straight approach when delivering the ball.

Deaf Bowling

The United States Deaf Bowling Federation (USDBF) is the National Sports Organization representing the sport of bowling for the USA Deaf Sports Federation. Individuals wishing to join this organization or to qualify for the US Deaf Bowling Team should access the website listed in the resource section of this chapter.

Special Olympics Bowling

Bowling has been a part of Special Olympics local programming for many years but was only first offered at international competitions since 1987. Bowling is the second largest participation sport in Special Olympics, with more than 100,000 athletes involved (Cloutier,1992). Events include singles, doubles (male, female, mixed), 4-person team (male, female, mixed), and unified doubles and team (mentally impaired and non-mentally impaired bowlers compete together). In Unified bowling, the scores of both athletes are averaged, and the best averaged score wins. Special Olympics conducts an annual National Unified Sports Bowling Championship in conjunction with the opening of the American Bowling Congress Tournament.

Two additional modified events, target bowl and frame bowl, are also offered for athletes with lower functional ability. These modified events are excellent activities for physical education classes. *Target bowl* uses regulation pins with a two pound ball and a lane half the length of a regulation lane. Carpet or Astroturf on the lane serves as a drag surface. Despite the modified length of the lane, all ABC rules apply. *Frame bowl* utilizes plastic pins and ball and a shortened lane of 16 feet 5 inches. Athletes roll two frames and have two rolls per frame to knock down the most number of pins.

United States Cerebral Palsy Athletic Association Bowling

The official sanctioned bowling competition offered by USCPAA is organized within four divisions, A through D. Divisions A and B are for athletes who use chutes or ramps. Division A allows for limited assistance from a coach, but division B permits none. Division C involves wheelchair and ambulatory athletes from CP classes 3 through 6. Division D includes classes 7 and 8. All competitions are coed.

EQUIPMENT

Generally, very little modified or adaptive equipment is needed to bowl beyond the standard equipment. The use of adapted equipment can make it possible for almost anyone to enjoy bowling and to experience its challenges, successes, and frustrations. Some of the more widely used modifications are described below. Individualization and experimentation by coaches are very important.

Bowling Balls

Many bowlers with physical disabilities bowl free arm and use standard bowling balls. For bowlers who want to bowl free arm but lack the finger dexterity to grip a standard ball, an alternative is available. A handle ball containing a spring-loaded retractable handle provides an easier and more comfortable way to grasp the ball (Figure 8.1). Upon release, the handle retracts flush to the ball, allowing a smooth, true roll. This ball can be ordered in various weights and is sanctioned by the American Bowling Congress.

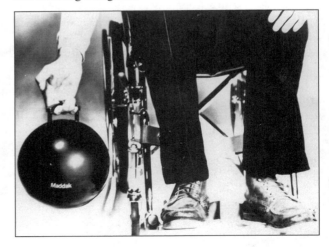

Figure 8.1. Spring-loaded handle bowling balls allow individuals with grasp difficulties to bowl. (Courtesy of Maddak, Inc.)

A bowling ball holder ring allows bowlers to keep their hands free to push their wheelchairs back and forth on the lane (Figure 8.2).

Bowling Sticks

Bowling sticks help bowlers who do not possess the strength or balance to bowl free-arm but do not wish to depend on the use of a ramp to bowl (McCole, McCole, & Patterson, 1988) (Figure 8.3). The use of bowling sticks is allowed by the AWBA in tournament play.

Bowling sticks come in different models. The adjustable two-pronged ball pusher is used in a similar manner as a shuffleboard stick. The triangular model is another type of design. Both models are fitted with a plastic coating to prevent scratching of the floor.

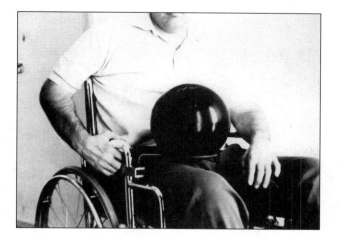

Figure 8.2. Snyder's bowling ball holder ring allows the use of hands for wheelchair mobility. (Courtesy of George Snyder)

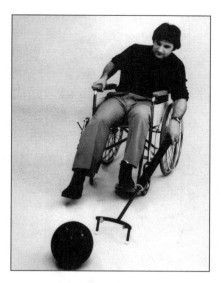

Figure 8.3. An adjustable bowling stick is an alternative to using a chute for those unable to bowl free-arm. (Courtesy of Maddak, Inc.)

Bowling Ramps

A variety of bowling ramps are available for individuals unable to bowl free arm or with bowling sticks (Figure 8.4 a-c). Ramps may be bought commercially or built from wood (Figure 8.5 a-c). Although special ramp divisions have been a part of Special Olympics and USCPAA bowling competition for many years, ramp bowling has only been recently added to official AWBA competitions. Ramp bowlers are placed in separate divisions and compete only against other ramp bowlers. Bowlers should consider cost, portability and individual bowling style when selecting a ramp.

Bowling style involves mostly delivery technique or the method in which the ball is pushed off the ramp. Most bowlers requiring a ramp are able to use their hands to push the ball. Individuals with more severe disabilities adopt alternatives such as using their feet. Other options can be as simple as using a head-stick or as complicated as employing a remote controlled release arm (Figure 8.6). Innovative Products of Grand Forks, ND has developed a battery powered bowling ball release that attaches to a metal bowling ramp. This device allows the bowler to release the bowling ball using an activation switch

Bowling Prosthesis

Nesbitt (1986) describes the bowling attachment as a device that attaches to any standard prosthetic wrist (120,thread) and fits into one of a bowling ball's finger holes. The release mechanism of the bowling attachment is activated as the expansion sleeve is stretched, which allows a conventional throwing motion and natural roll of the ball (Figure 8.7).

Bowling Rails

Most bowlers with visual impairments prefer not to use any assistive devices and will find their spot by using the ball return as a point of reference. Guide rails are the primary means of bowling for the blind or visually impaired who choose to use assistive devices. Made in 12 or 15 foot versions, guide rails provide a tactile reference for the bowlers and are aligned just to the side of the bowler's approach path.

Stanley and Kindig (1986) describe a makeshift improvised rail made by tying a rope between a chair and a high stool. The use of carpet strips can also be used as a guide for blind bowlers as well (Figure 8.8). A disadvantage of carpet strips is that they must be removed after each frame if visually impaired bowlers are playing with sighted bowlers.

EQUIPMENT SUPPLIERS

Adapted equipment is available from the following equipment companies.
a: Bowling sticks or pusher

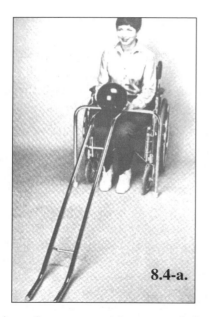

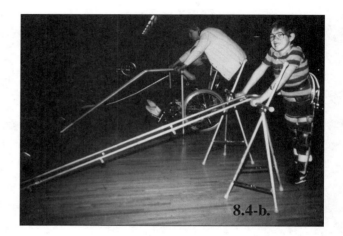

8.4-a.

8.4-b.

Figure 8.4 a-c. Some commercial ramps attach directly to the wheelchair for additional stability, while others attach to the bowler's walker. (Courtesy of Maddak and Specialized Sports Unlimited)

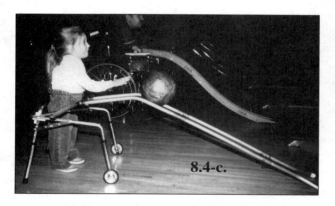

8.4-c.

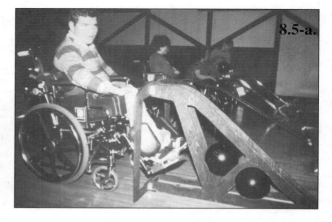

8.5-a.

Figure 8.5 a-c. Various wooden ramps can be easily made at home. (Courtesy of Specialized Sports Unlimited)

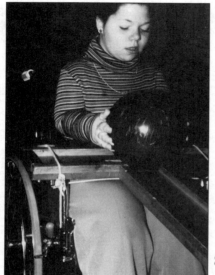

8.5-b.

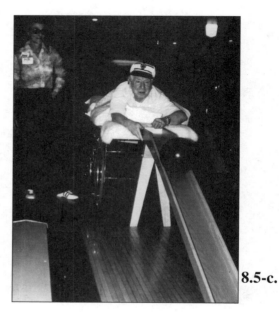

8.5-c.

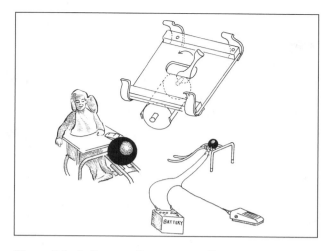

Figure 8.6. A diagram of a more complicated bowling device which allows individuals with severe disabilities to bowl.

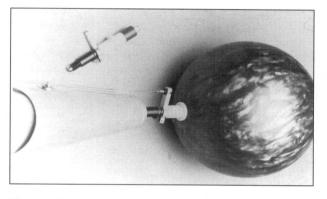

Figure 8.7. The interchangeable terminal device was designed especially for bowling. (Courtesy of TRS)

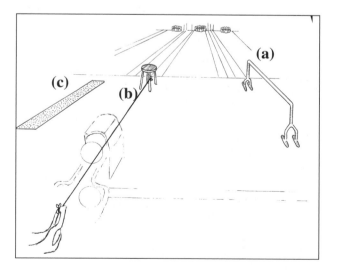

Figure 8.8. Blind or visually impaired bowlers may select from three methods of maintaining a straight approach: (a) commercial bowling rail, (b) makeshift guide rope, or (c) a carpet strip.

b: Prosthetic bowling attachment
c: Rails
d: Ramps
e: Ring ball holders
f: Snap handle balls

Access to Recreation, Inc. (a,d,e,f)
8 Sandra Court
Newbury Park, CA 91320
(800) 634-4351
(805) 498-8186 (fax)
Email: dkrebs@gte.net
Website: http://www.accesstr.com

Achievable Concepts (d,f)
P.O. Box 361
Moonee Ponds
Victoria 3039, Australia
03 9752 5958
03 9754 4798 (fax)
Email: sales@achievableconcepts.com.au
Website: http://www.achievableconcepts.com.au

American Foundation for the Blind (c)
11 Penn Plaza, Suite 300
New York, NY 10001
(212) 502-7600
Email: afbinfo@afb.org
Website: http://www.afb.org/

The Dragonfly Toy Co. (a,d)
291 Yale Ave.
Winnipeg, MB, Canada R3M 0L4
(800) 308-2208
(204) 453-2320 (fax)
Email: service@dragonflytoys.com
Website: http://www.dftoys.com

Erickson Creative Enterprise (d)
P.O. Box 8813
Rockford, IL 61126
(815) 962-6224
(815) 962-6253 (fax)

Flaghouse Inc. (a,d,f)
601 Flaghouse Drive
Hasbrouck Heights, NJ 07604-3116
(800) 793-7900
(800) 793-7922 (fax)
Email: sales@flaghouse.com
Website: http://www.flaghouse.com

Gould Athletic Supply Co. (a, c,d,f)
8101 Douglas Rd.

Glenside, PA 19038
(215) 836-9229

Hosmer Dorrance Corp. (b)
561 Division St.
Campbell, CA 95008-6905
(800) 827-0070
Email: filladv@usit.net
Website: http://www.hosmer.com

Handy bowl (d)
Jens Bangs Gade 13
DK 9000 Aalborg
45 98 77 08 44
45 98 77 08 34 (fax)
Email: flemminglyngo@handybowl.dk
Website: http://www.handybowl.dk

Innovative Products, Inc. (d)
830 South 48th Street
Grand Forks, ND 58201
(800) 950-5185
Email: jsteinke@iphope.com
Website: http://www.iphope.com

Maddak, Inc. (a,d)
(973) 628-7600
(973) 305-0841 (fax)
Email: custservice@maddak.com
Website: http://www.ableware.com

Sportime Supply Co. (d,f)
One Sportime Way
Atlanta GA, 30340
(800) 283-5700
(800) 845-1535 (fax)
Email: orders@sportime.com
Website: http://www2.sportime.com

ADDITIONAL RESOURCES AND WEBSITES

American Blind Bowling Association (ABBA)
315 N. Main
Houston, PA 15342
(724) 745-5986

American Bowling Congress (ABC)
5301 S. 76th St.
Greendale, WI 53129-1127
(414) 421-6400
(414) 421-1194 (fax)
Email: sjames@bowl.com
Website: http://www.bowl.com

American Wheelchair Bowling Association (AWBA)
6264 N. Andrews Ave.
Ft. Lauderdale, FL 33309
(954) 491-2886 (phone/fax)
Website: http://members.aol.com/bowlerweb/awba.htm

Federation Internationale des Quilleurs (FIQ)
1631 Mesa Ave., Suite A
Colorado Springs, CO 80906
Email: bowling@fiq.org
Website: www.fiq.org

The National Bowling Association Inc.
National Office Headquarters
377 Park Avenue, South, 7th Floor
New York, New York 10016
(212) 689-8308/8309
(212) 725-5063 (fax)
Website: http://www.tnbainc.org
    TNBA is one of the three major governing bodies for amateur bowling in the United States. Founded in 1939, operated by African Americans, and open to all, TNBA is committed to the principles of Sportsmanship, Fellowship and Friendship within its ranks and throughout the world of bowling.

United States Deaf Bowling Federation (USDBF)
Connie Marchione, Liaison and Coach
8071 Cherrystone Avenue
Panorama City, CA 91402-5414
(818) 785-1478 (TDD)
(818) 785-1478 (fax)
Website:
http://hometown.aol.com/kchodak/myhomepage/profile.html

Special Olympics Director of Bowling
Special Olympics Inc.
1325 G Street, NW, Suite 500
Washington, DC 20005-3104
(202) 628-3630
(202) 824-0200 (fax)
EMail: SOImail@aol.com
Website: http://www.specialolympics.org
    A copy of the Bowling Sports Skills Program Guide is available for purchase through SOI. This guide provides a developmental approach to teaching bowling.

United States Cerebral Palsy Athletic Association
Bowling Sports Technical Officer
Shelly LaBarre, CTRS
527 Frable St.
Nazareth, PA 18064

(610) 759-5655
Email: labarre1@enter.net

USA Bowling
5301 South 76th Street
Greendale, WI 53129-0500
E-mail: cpon@bowl.com
Website: www.bowl.com

Women's International Bowling Congress (WIBC)
5301 S. 76th St.
Greendale, WI 53129-1191
(414) 421-9000
(414) 421-4420 (fax)
Email: ssavet@bowl.com
Website: http://www.bowl.com

Young American Bowling Alliance (YABA)
5301 S. 76th St.
Greendale, WI 53129-1192
(414) 421-4700
(414) 421-1301 (fax)
Email: jjocha@bowl.com
Website: http://www.bowl.com

This organization attempts to work through every elementary school in the United States to increase the awareness of bowling as a desirable leisure time activity for children.

Publications

The Blind Bowler. Publication of the ABBA,
2211 Latham St. No. 120
Mountain View, CA 94040

The Eleventh Frame. AWBA National Newsletter
3620 Tamarack Drive
Redding, CA 96003
(916) 243-2695
(916) 244-6651 (fax)

Schaff, D. (1996). Wheelchair Bowling (available from The American Wheelchair Bowling Association (AWBA).

In addition to providing historical background, this 96 page book published by Jim Lane, includes principles of the game from keeping score through ball drilling for the wheelchair bowler. Through profiles of wheelchair bowlers, the text covers ball delivery, spare making techniques and special equipment that can be used.

BIBLIOGRAPHY

Cloutier, G (1992). ISSOG's: Bowling. Palaestra 8(2):21,22

Marsh, D. & Evans, E. (2000). Team Bowling, A great game for inclusion. *Palaestra 16*(2)32-33.

McCole, J,. McCole, J.B., & Patterson, J. (1988). Bowling. In J.A. Jones (ed),

Nesbitt, J. (1986). The International Directory of Recreation Oriented Assistive Device Sources. Marina Del Rey: Lifeboat Press.

Snyder, G.H. (1998). Strikes and Spares. *Active Living 7*(5)11-12.

Stanley, S.M., & Kindig, L.E. (1986). Improvisations for blind bowlers. Palaestra 2(2)38,39

Training Guide to Cerebral Palsy Sports (183,189). Champaign, IL: Human Kinetics.

Chapter 9

Cycling

SPORT GOVERNING BODIES:
National: USA Cycling (USAC) United States Cycling Federation (USCF)
International: Union Cycliste International (UCI)

Official Sport Of: _____DAAA   __x__USABA   __x__USCPAA
                           __x__DS/USA   __x__USADSF   _____WS/USA
                           __x__SOI

DISABLED SPORTS ORGANIZATION:
National: United States Handcycle Federation (USHF)
International:

PRIMARY DISABILITY: All

SPORT OVERVIEW

Cycling is one of this country's most popular recreational activities. Its popularity as a competitive sport has increased due to vast media coverage of the Olympic Games, the Tour de France, and other international events. Health-conscious citizens have also realized the great physical and psychological benefits cycling can provide. Extended bicycle tours are now available in almost every state documenting the increasing interest in this sport. Cycling encompasses many events such as off-road racing, track racing, time trials, mountain bike racing, and motorcross. Specific organizations exist to foster each of these pursuits. Bicycle riding whether for competitive or recreational purposes should never be done without a fully approved helmet (ANSI or Snell). Research has shown that head injuries can be reduced by 85% with the use of a helmet.

Internationally, the sport is governed by the International Cycling Union (UCI). The UCI is responsible for the promotion of the sport worldwide and for the development of rules and sanctioning of events. The counterpart to the UCI in the United States is USA Cycling.

Disability sport organizations generally follow the International Cycling Union UCI or USA Cycling rules with specific modifications related to each group. Cycling is offered as an official sport of the Paralympic Games for all athletes who have visual impairments, cerebral palsy, amputations and other physical disabilities, and through the World Games for the Deaf for individuals with hearing impairments. It was first offered as an event at the 1987 International Summer Special Olympic Games. Athletes with cerebral palsy compete using standard racing bikes and tricycles based on their classification. Athletes who are visually impaired compete on tandem cycles with a sighted teammate. Participation is in road and track races, and time trial events. Individuals with amputations and cyclists with permanent locomotor deficiencies compete in the individual road race events and time trials using cycles specifically constructed for their needs.

HISTORY

Cycling traces its roots back to 1816, when a German inventor created the swiftwalker (or draisine), a two wheeled contraption made of wood with a steerable front wheel. The absence of pedals meant that riders had to push themselves along using their feet. The activity quickly evolved into a competitive event throughout many larger cities of Europe.

An organizational structure was given to cycling in

the late 1800's beginning in England. The precursor to the International Cycling Union was The Bicycle Union, the oldest cycling federation in the world, founded in Great Britain in 1878. It changed its name in 1883 to the National Cyclists' Union (NCU) in order to encompass tricyclists. To serve an international community of cyclists, the NCU was reorganized in 1892 as the International Cyclists' Association prior to becoming the International Cycling Union.

Organized cycling began in the United States in 1920 with the formation of the Amateur Bicycle League of America. The name was changed in 1975 to the United States Cycling Federation. In 1995, a new organization, USA Cycling (USAC), was incorporated, and shortly thereafter, the two corporations merged, with USA Cycling being the umbrella corporation. Today, USA Cycling is the official national governing body of the sport and serves to promote and expand cycling opportunities for all. USA Cycling offers programs and training for cyclists with disabilities and works with the United States Handcycling Federation in competitive events. In 1995, USAC, in conjunction with its national championship program, held national championships for three of seven USOC-recognized disabled sports organizations: Disabled Sports USA, United States Association for Blind Athletes and U.S. Cerebral Palsy Athletic Association. USAC also serves as a resource for the disabled cycling community by identifying active organizations whose sole purpose is to serve athletes with disabilities.

The popularity of cycling has increased for individuals with disabilities as well. Continuing advances in bicycle and tricycle design have made cycling a realistic activity for many disability sports organizations (Figure 9.1). Cycling competitions are relatively new for athletes with disabilities and have evolved only within the last 20 years or so. In the early eighties, the visually impaired were the first group of athletes with disabilities to compete, and athletes with cerebral palsy and amputations began racing at the International Games for the Disabled

in 1984. Up until the 1992 Paralympics, the competitions for each of these groups were held separately. Then at the Barcelona Games, spectators witnessed intense competitions in both track and road races between athletes in all three disability groups.

Competitive cycling is offered by Disabled Sports USA, the United States Cerebral Palsy Athletic Association (USCPAA), the United States Association for Blind Athletes (USABA), Special Olympics, USA Deaf Sports Federation (USADSF), International Paralympic Committee (IPC), and by the United States Handcycle Federation (USHF). Distances range from 400-meter races for some junior cerebral palsy events to 40-to-135-kilometer races for blind tandems (Figure 9.2), amputees, and deaf athletes.

Special Olympics has offered cycling as an official sport since 1988. Competition takes place in three ability levels. Events include time trials, and road races at various distances. Both events also include Unified competition divisions. Unified tandem time trials have been offered since the 1991 International Games in Minneapolis (see the following).

Cyclists who are deaf or hearing impaired belong to the United States Deaf Cycling Association (USDCA), an association of the USA Deaf Sports Federation. With a strong affiliation with the USCF, the organization is responsible for developing, training, coaching and selecting cyclists to compete in various deaf sports championships. The group also promotes cycling for juniors and conducts clinics in such areas as training techniques, racing rules and bicycle maintenance.

CYCLING COMPETITIONS

Various forms of cycling competitions exist, although not all disability sport organizations offer each form. Cycling competitions generally involve time trials (team and individual), track racing, road racing, tandem cycling, and hand cycling. Athletes compete in various divisions

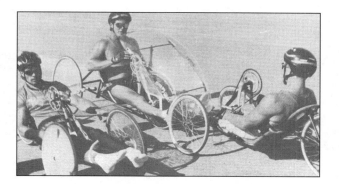

Figure 9.1. Handcycling is a fast growing sport, due to the advancements in bike technology. (Courtesy of *Sports 'n Spokes* 9/92:38)

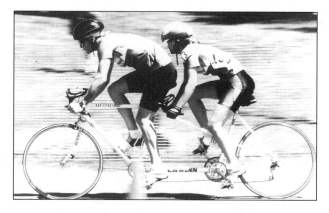

Figure 9.2. Tandem cycles have raised cycling to an international sport for the blind. (Courtesy of USABA)

based on their classification and type of cycle being used. Cyclists with amputations and other limb disabilities compete under the auspices of the USA Cycling and are affiliated with Disabled Sports USA, (DSUSA). Riders choose to compete in divisions for upper or lower limb disability, with or without prostheses (Figure 9.3 a-d). It is generally recommended that riders with lower limb amputations use a prosthesis if at all possible. The use of a prosthesis can also serve to exercise the residual limb. Use is based on the preference of the rider however. The classification system is based on the amount of lower limb disability. At the Paralympic level, locomotor disabled athletes compete in four different classes, LC1-LC4. Each rider must hold a valid license from their national federation to compete. Class LC1 is for riders having minor or no lower limb handicaps. LC2 is for riders with handicaps in one leg but who are able to pedal normally using 2 legs with or without prostheses. LC3 is for riders with handicaps on one lower limb (with or without upper limb handicaps) although most riders pedal with one leg. LC4 is for riders with handicaps affecting both legs.

Athletes with cerebral palsy compete in one of four divisions. Division 1 and 2 is for tricycles with distances of 1,500 meters to 5,000 meters; and divisions 3 and 4 are for bicycles with distances ranging from 5,000 meters to 20,000 meters. Athletes compete in both time trials and road races.

Time Trials

Time trials involve a rider or a team of riders racing a prescribed distance against the clock. At the end of the competition all riders times are compared, with the fastest rider(s) being declared the winner. Team time tri-

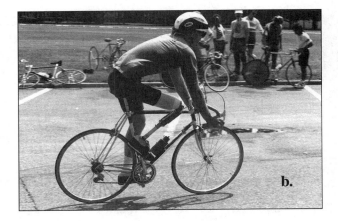

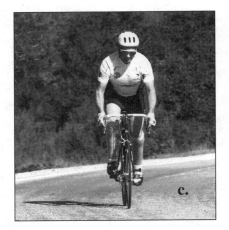

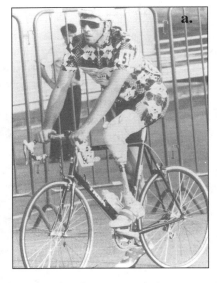

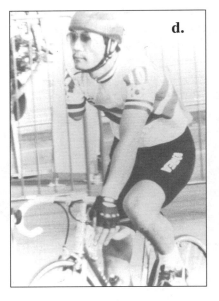

Figure 9.3 a-d. (a-c) Advancements in lower extremity prosthetics have made cycling a viable international sport for amputee athletes. (d) Many upper extremity amputees chose to ride without their prosthesis. (Photo by Oscar Izquierdo, Michael J. Paciorek, and Hosmer Dorrance Corp.)

als involve 3-4 racers working together over a long distance (Figure 9.4a and b). Cyclists remain in a straight line with most of the cyclists drafting behind the leader who is doing the bulk of the work. At various intervals the leader switches places with one of the trailing cyclists. This rotation continues until the end of the race. The efficient switching of leaders is a key to success. Athletes with hearing impairments may need to rely on visual signals to switch rather than auditory signals, thus potentially affecting efficiency. All of the disability sport organizations who compete in cycling offer time trials racing as an official event.

Tandem Racing

Tandem or double bike is bicycle riding by two people. The popularity of tandem cycling as a recreational family activity has increased dramatically in recent years, especially in the able-bodied community. Tandem riding fosters inclusion opportunities, with individuals with and without disabilities being able to ride together. Dozens of companies now manufacturer tandem bikes due to its increased popularity (Figure 9.5). Tandem racing is typically associated with athletes who have visual impairments and the sport is offered through the United States Association for Blind Athletes (USABA). The blind ath-

lete or "blind stoker" sits on the back of the bike while the sighted guide, pilot, or captain, sits on the front of the bike and steers. Both athletes pedal and must work in unison to be successful at high levels of competition.

In blind tandem racing, the men compete over distances ranging from 100 to 135 km, on circuits of 5 or 10 km, or races between two towns, while the women compete in similar events over shorter distances. A mixed category allows males and females to compete together.

Although tandem riding is generally associated with athletes who are blind, tandem racing is also an event in Special Olympics Unified Sports competition. Athletes without mental retardation compete as a partner with a Special Olympian. Tandem competition is offered in time trial format only.

Track Racing

Track racing is done on a velodrome; a wooden racing track in the shape of an eclipse with straight steep sides and semi-circular banked corners. Track racing is offered for different disability groups at the Paralympic level. Track racing for blind athletes using tandems was first offered at the 1996 Paralympic Gamers in Atlanta (Figure 9.6). Track racing consists of different events including Sprint, Pursuit, and Time Trials. Sprint is an event in which two cyclists compete over a distance of 1,000 meters. Individual pursuit is an event in which only two riders start at a point marked half way along the opposing straights of the track. From the start gun to the finish, the purpose of the race is to catch the other rider. If a rider catches his or her rival before the designated race distance, the race ends immediately. Otherwise the pursuit is decided by the rider who completes the distance in the shorter time.

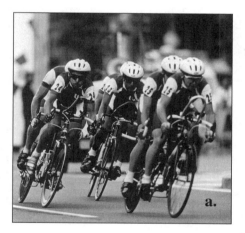

Figure 9.4 a and b. The first ever tandem team time trials for blind cyclists were at the 1992 Paralympic Games in Barcelona, Spain. (Courtesy of USABA and Michael Paciorek)

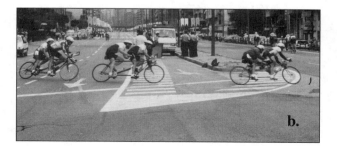

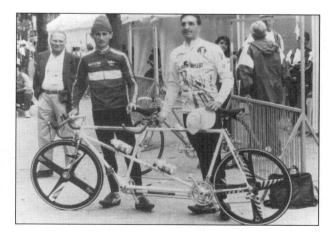

Figure 9.5. The use of carbon fiber spoked wheels is an example of how tandem cycle technology has kept pace with that of conventional racing cycles. (Courtesy of Michael J. Paciorek)

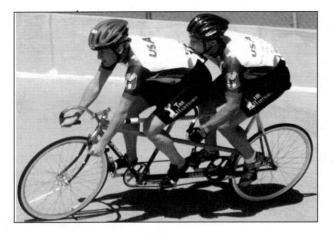

Figure 9.6. Tandem track racing on a velodrome. (Courtesy of USABA)

Road Racing

Road racing is an event of all the disability sport organizations in which a group of athletes compete over a long distance on a prescribed course on the open road closed to traffic. As with all competitions, athletes are grouped according to a classification system to equalize competition. Tandem road racing for athletes with visual impairments was first offered at the 1992 Paralympic Games in Barcelona.

HANDCYCLING

The number of websites devoted to a sport may be a good indication of its popularity. If this is the case, then handcycling appears to be very popular. Many exceptional websites exist related to all aspects of this sport. Handcycling has the potential to become more popular than wheelchair racing for individuals with physical disabilities. Individuals can realize a very strong cardiovascular and upper body workout, without having to worry about the techniques required for wheelchair racing. Although not yet an official Paralympic sport, it appears that it will not be long before it is added. Handcycling is a technique where individuals use arm power to propel a bicycle. Although the sport has been popular for quite a few years, it was not until 1998 that an organizing body was formed. Prior to this time, handcyclists were caught somewhere in-between wheelchair racing and bicycle racing. This is no longer the case. The United States Handcycling Federation (USHF) was formed to foster and promote the development of handcycling in both recreational and competitive natures. USHF is the official national governing body for handcycling in the United States and is recognized by Wheelchair Sports USA and the United States Olympic Committee. For competitions, the USHF shares the role of governance with USA Cy-

cling. The USHF is working hard to provide an outlet for handcyclists in this country who want to race, tour or just have fun in their handcycles.

EQUIPMENT

With a few exceptions, the needs of most cyclists with disabilities can be accommodated at any good cycle shop. The purchasing of handcycles and other adapted equipment has been made easier in the last few years due to the increased number of manufacturers carrying such equipment. This increase is due to the growth of the sport and increase in demand for equipment. Various models of handcycles are on the market. Two of the more popular suppliers are Freedom Ryder and Top End although other brands exist. Handcycles come in high-rider and low-rider designs. Since the high-rider is not as aerodynamic as the low-rider, it is not the cycle of choice for competitive cyclists. It does make for an excellent recreational cycle, however. Some representative equipment suppliers are listed at the end of this chapter.

Tandems

The popularity of tandem bicycles has increased dramatically in recent years for all individuals (Figure 9.7a and b). Conventional tandems are manufactured by dozens of U.S. companies and are used primarily to enable blind and visually impaired people to participate in

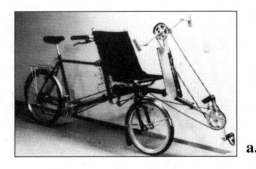

a.

Figure 9.7 a and b. Recent developments in tandems enable nondisabled and mobility impaired people to ride together. (Courtesy of Angle Lake Cyclery)

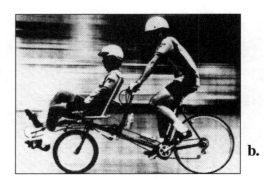

b.

competitive and recreational cycling. A national organization founded in 1976, the Tandem Club of America (TCA), keeps track of the growing number of tandem, cycling clubs throughout the United States (see additional resources).

Handcycles

Arm-driven mechanisms, or handcycling; have opened the cycling roads to individuals with lower extremity impairments (Figure 9.8). A variety of handcycle models, including 2, 3, and 4-wheeled are available. Most of the models have multiple gears similar to any bicycle. Selection should be based on ones preference and intended use of the cycle for recreation or competition. Individuals should test ride a variety of models before selection. The nature of the rider's disability will be a factor in choosing the best handcycle.

The three-wheel model usually has the single wheel in front with a drivetrain on the front wheel, however some models reverse this with the single wheel in back and drive train in the rear (Figures 9.9 a-d).

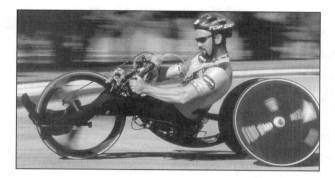

Figure 9.8. Handcycling has grown from a very popular recreational activity to a world-wide sport. (Courtesy of *Sports 'n Spokes* 1999 25/6: 50)

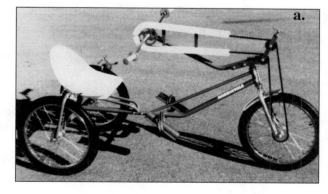

Figure 9.9 a-d. Arm-driven tricycles have opened cycling to individuals with lower extremity impairments. (Courtesy of For Fun Cycle Corp., Quantum Leap All-terrain Hand Cycle, and Magic in Motion)

The introduction of 2-wheeled handcycles is relatively new and still in development (Figure 9.10). The obvious benefit of a 2-wheeled handcycle is the added maneuverability over a 3- or 4-wheeled cycle.

Handcycles have already taken the next step with the introduction of an all-terrain handcycle by Titaniumarts.com. This is the first hand cycle to bridge the gap between today's road only hand cycles and the chair-lift dependent downhill racers. With bicycle cranks for propulsion and a steering similar to the downhill racers, this vehicle can climb slopes and descend at speed with safety. This cycle is also an effective road bike as well.

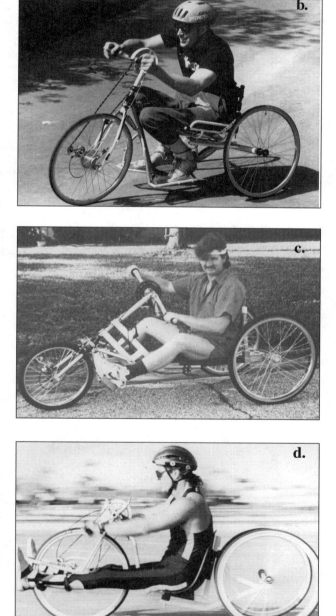

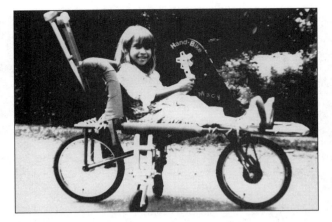

Figure 9.10. The Hand-Bike arm-driven bicycle independent cycling for children and adults. (Courtesy of Physically Challenged Co.)

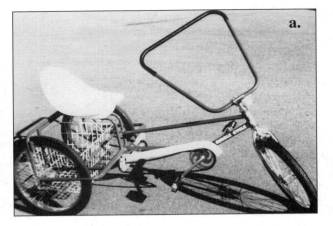

Figure 9.11 a. Single cycle foot-powered adult tricycle. (Courtesy of For Fun Cycles Corp.)

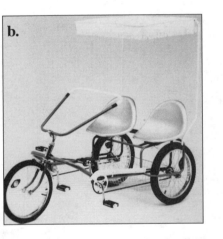

Figure 9.11 b. The Duo-cycle adult tricycle allows non-disabled and disabled individuals to ride together. (Courtesy of For Fun Cycles Corp.)

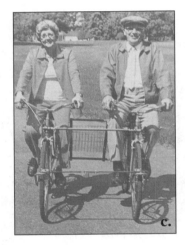

Figure 9.11 c. The Pedal Partner Kit easily attaches to any two bicycles with the same wheel size. (Courtesy of Gandy)

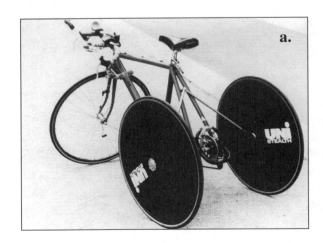

Figure 9.12 a and b. Much of the same technology used in two-wheel cycling is also used with competition tricycles. (Photo by Michael J. Paciorek)

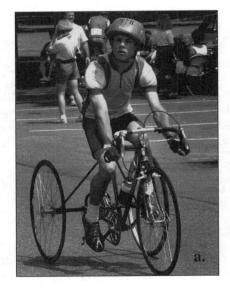

Adult Tricycles

Adult tricycles have long been used by senior citizens and other adults who cannot use a conventional two-wheel bike (Figure 9.11 a-c). Their popularity and effectiveness in providing quality and stable cycling has carried over to individuals with disabilities.

Technological advances have produced a new breed of lightweight; high-speed racing tricycles that are being seen more often at USCPAA competitions (Figure 9.12 a and b). Individuals who require additional stability may choose to use a recumbent tricycle that virtually eliminates balance difficulties with its low clearance. Recumbent bikes are generally for recreational use only and are not eligible for USCPAA competition.

Bikes for Short-Statured People

For many years, the only option for short-statured individuals was to modify an existing bike or to use a children's bike. Now there is another option. Atherton Bicycles (see Equipment Suppliers) is a builder of custom bicycles and racing frames. They build bicycles for people of short stature, as well as high quality custom racing frames for any individual.

Wheelchair Attachments

There are also 7-speed modular arm-driven units that attach directly to wheelchairs provided by Sunrise Medical (Quickie brand). Versatility, transition, and ease make this detachable unit very popular. In addition to allowing the individual to remain in the wheelchair, the detachable unit provides efficient transportation and easy transition to wheelchair mobility (Figure 9.13 a and b). These are designed strictly for the recreational athlete, but can be an inexpensive alternative for a beginning rider.

Adaptations for Amputees

Cycling for individuals with hand or arm amputations has provided a unique challenge (Figure 9.14). In the past, single-handed individuals had to compromise safety while riding due to inability to brake both front and rear wheels. However, a system called the dual bicycle brake hand lever is available for either mountain bikes or road bikes developed by Therapeutic Recreation Systems, Inc. (Figure 9.15 a and b). The dual bicycle brake level mounts easily to standard bicycle handle bars and operates both the front and rear brake calipers simultaneously, when operated with only one hand. The single lever is convenient, powerful, and efficient. The rider can use prosthesis (if applicable) for handle bar control and balance and activate the brake lever with the sound hand.

Training

Arm ergometers, commonly used by wheelchair athletes for upper body training, help cyclists stay in condition during the off season or in bad weather. Many have the versatility to he powered by the arms or by the legs. For more information on arm ergometers, see the Fitness Programs chapter in this book.

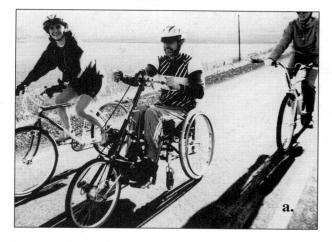

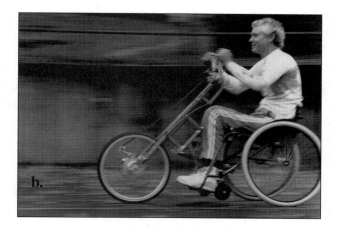

Figure 9.13 a and b. Cycle-One attaches directly to the wheelchair and makes cycling available to most wheelchair users. (Courtesy of Shadow Cycle-One Magic in Motion)

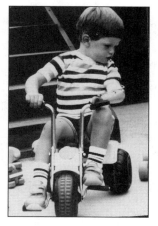

Figure 9.14. A specialized terminal device makes cycling easier for people with upper extremity amputations. (Courtesy of TRS)

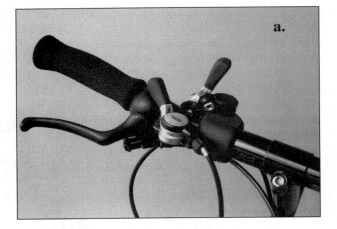

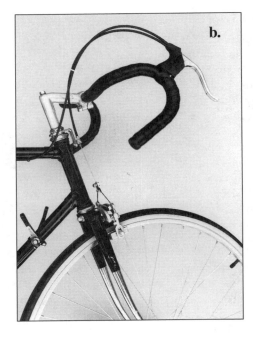

Figure 9.15 a and b. (a) The dual bicycle brake hand lever attaches to standard handle bars and operates both the front and back brakes. (b) Mountain bike dual brake lever with "clustered" gear shifters. (Courtesy of TRS)

EQUIPMENT SUPPLIERS

Readers will find the following selection of equipment suppliers to be a good start when researching the various handcycling, tandem and tricycle models available.

Advanced Mobility Products Ltd.
Unit # 111-2323 Boundary Rd.
Vancouver, B.C., V5M 4V8
(604) 293-0002
(800) 665-4442
(604) 293-0005 (fax)
Email: mobility@mobilityproducts.com
Website: http://www.mobilityproducts.com

Ann Arbor Cyclery (recumbent bikes)
224 Packard St.
Ann Arbor, Michigan 48104
(734) 761-2749
(734) 761-3146
Email: a2cyclery@provide.net
Website: http://www.a2bike.com/recumbents_set.htm

Atherton Bicycles (Bikes for short statured people)
6101 Big Springs
Arlington, Texas 76001
817-478-5509
Email: wheelthg@flash.net
Website: http://home.flash.net/~wheelthg

Bike Route.com
http://www.bikeroute.com/
This is an excellent site providing information on recumbents, handcycles, adult trikes and tandems.

Bike-On.com
22 Jennifer Lane
Coventry, RI., 02816
(888) 424-5366
(401) 821-7544
Email: Info@bike-on.com
Website: http://www.bike-on.com
An excellent on-line company to find new and used handcycles and equipment.

Co-Motion Cycles (Tandems)
222 Polk Street
Eugene, Oregon 97402
(541) 342-4583
(541) 342-2210 (fax)
Email: info@co-motion.com
Website: http://www.co-motion.com

Freedom Ryder
Website: http://www.freedomryder.com
(800) 800-5828

GT Bicycles
2001 East Dyer Rd.
Santa Ana, CA 92705-5709
888-GT-BIKES
Email: speedshop@gtbicycles.com
Website: http://www.gtbicycles.com

Haverich Adaptive Cycles
Haverich Ortho-Sport Inc.
165 Martell Court
Keene, NH 03431

(800) 529-9444
(603) 358-0438
(603) 358-0453
Email: info@haverich.com
Website: http://www.haverich.com

Invacare Top End
Sports & Recreation Products
4501 63rd Circle North
Pinellas Park, FL 33781
(800) 532-8677
(727) 522-8677
(727) 522-1007 (fax)
Email: ask.top.end@invacare.com
Website:
    http://www.invacare.com/sports_and_rec/handcycling

Just Two Bikes (JTB®, Inc.)
15449 Forest Blvd N. #C
Hugo, Minn. 55038
(651) 426-1548
(800) 499-1548
(651) 653-9444 (fax)
Website: http://www.justtwobikes.com

Lightning Handcycles
360 Sepulveda Blvd, Suite 1030
El Segundo, CA 90245
(888) 426-3292
(310) 335-1543 (fax)
Email: information@handcycle.com
Website: http://www.handcycle.com

Mobility Engineering
9104 W Pooler
Pasco, WA 99301
(509) 545-0659
Website: http://www.mobilityeng.com

New Halls Wheels
P.O. Box 380784
Cambridge, MA 02238
Email: newhalls@tiac.net
Website: http://www.newhalls.com

People Movers
980 N. Main St.
Orange, CA 92867
(714) 633-3663
Email: peplmvrs@primenet.com
Website: http://www.recumbent.com

Rhoades Car Division
125 Rhoades Lane
Hendersonville, TN 37075

(800) 531-2737 x2754
(615) 822-2737 x104
(615) 822-4129 (fax)
Website: http://www.rhoadescarshowroom.com

Rowbike
Sky Fitness Inc.
P.O. Box 114
Waconia, MN U.S.A. 55387
(800) 203-2541
(612) 442-7046
(612) 442-8637 (fax)
Email: sales@rowbike.com
Website: http://www.rowbike.com

Sammon Preston Pediatrics
4 Sammons Ct.
Bolingbrook, IL 60440
(800) 323-5547
(800) 547-4333 (fax)
Email: sp@sammonspreston.com
Website: http://www.sammonspreston.com

Spinlife.com
(800) 850-0335
Website: http://www.spinlife.com/
    A comprehensive online source for sport products.
Save on brands like Top End, Quickie, New Halls Wheels
and more.

Spokes 'n Motion
2225 South Platte Dr.
Denver, CO 80223
(303) 922-0605
(303) 922-7943 (fax)
Email: info@spokenmotion.com
Website: http://www.spokesnmotion.com

Sportaid
78 Bay Creek Rd.
Loganville, GA 30052
Email: Stuff@sportaid.com
Website: http://www.sportaid.com
(800) 743-7203
(770) 554-5944 (fax)

Step 'N Go Cycles
6 Linden terrace
Burlington, VT 05401
(800) 648-7335
(802) 862-2980
(802) 864-6156 (fax)
Email: info@stepngo.com
Website: http://www.stepngo.com

Sunrise Medical (Quickie Products)
Website: http://www.sunrisemedicalonline.com

TherAdapt Products Inc.
17W163 Oak Lane
Besenville, IL 60106
(800) 261-4919
(630) 834-2478 (fax)

Titaniumarts.com (All-Terrain Handcycle)
221 Pine Street
Florence, MA 01062
(413) 585-5913
Email: oneoffti@javanet.com
Website: http://www.titaniumarts.com

Trailmate
2359 Trailmate Dr.
Sarasota, FL 34243
(800) 777-1034
(800) 477-5141 (fax)
Email: Info@Trailmate.com
Website: http://www.trailmate.com

Prosthetic Devices

Therapeutic Recreation Systems Inc.
2450 Central Avenue, Unit D
Boulder, CO 80301-2844
(800) 279-1865
(303) 444-4720
(303) 444-5372 (fax)
Website: www.oandp.com/trs

ADDITIONAL RESOURCES AND WEBSITES

Cyclists will find many websites related to their sport. Quality websites related to handcycling are increasing rapidly. Selected sites providing links to others are listed below. Because this sport is accessible for those with and without disabilities, most participants will find the following sites satisfactory for gathering information.

Handcycle Racing.com
Email: superfrog@handcycleracing.com
Website:
    http://www.mindspring.com/~superfrog/index.html
This site is devoted to the racing enthusiast and provides information on all aspects of handcycle racing and competitions.

Handcycling.com
Website: http://www.handcycling.com/
This excellent website provides information on news, sale of equipment, personalized training, and many additional links.

International Cycling Union (UCI)
Casa Postale 84 (37 Route de Chavannes)
1000 Lausanne 23, Switzerland (1007)
Email: Admin@uci.ch
Website: http://www.uci.ch

National Association for Bikers with a Disability
Website: http://www.nabd.org.uk
This United Kingdom based organization provides advice on adaptations to bikes and trikes to suit a variety of disabilities.

The Tandem Club of America (TCA)
Website: http://www.tandemclub.org

United States Handcycling Federation
(831) 457-7747 (for general information)
C/0 Wheelchair Sport USA
3395 E. Fountain Blvd., L-1
Colorado Springs, CO 80910
(719) 574-1150 (for membership information)
(719) 574-9840 (FAX)
Email: info@ushf.org
Website: http://www.ushf.org
This should be the first stop for any handcycling enthusiast. From this site, an interested person will be able to link to any other site related to the sport.

USA Cycling
One Olympic Plaza
Colorado Springs, Co 80909-5775
Tel: (719) 578-4581
Fax: (719) 578-4596
Email: usac@usacycling.org
Website: http:// www.usacycling.org

United States Deaf Cycling Association (USDCA)
C/0 USA Deaf Sports Federation
3607 Washington Blvd., Suite 4
Ogden, UT 84403-1737
(801) 393-7916 Office (tty: use your state relay service)
(801) 393-2263 (FAX)
Email: usadsf@aol.com
Website: http://www.usadsf.org
Website: http://home.earthlink.net/~skedsmo/usdca.htm
(for USDCA)

BIBLIOGRAPHY

Gabriel, R.A. (1999). Purchasing tips for today's handcycles. *Active Living* 8(2)14-18.
Hoek, M.V. (1999). Bike riding, does limb difference make a difference? *In-Motion* 9(4)12-14.
Lawless, I.L. & Vogel, B. (1999). handcycling gains momentum. *Sports 'n Spokes* 25(2)44-46.

Chapter 10

Equestrian

SPORT ORIGIN

The association between man and horse dates back to prehistoric times. Historically, the therapeutic benefits of the horse were recognized as early as 460 BC although equestrian sports as we know them today did not develop until the 20th century. The Greeks used the horse as treatment for their injured soldiers in the belief that it would improve their health and well-being. Later, the British would do the same thing by putting their injured WWI veterans on horseback. Therapeutic riding centers opened in North America in the 1960's and therapists have continued to use the gentle rhythmic movement of the horse to relax the rider's muscles and stimulate the development of muscle tone, coordination, mobility and flexibility. The use of the horse for therapy quickly branched off into competitive opportunities after Liz Hartel, a Danish rider with polio, won the Olympic silver medal in dressage at the 1952 Helsinki games. Equestrian became part of the Paralympic competition program for the first time at Atlanta in 1996. Modern competitive dressage for riders with physical disabilities began in the 1970's in Scandinavia and Europe.

This is the only sport that brings together two athletes, the horse and the rider, each relying on the success of the other. Similar to sailing, it also allows men and women to compete equally and to share the same podium.

Paralympic equestrian athletes compete in dressage and are judged on their display of superior horsemanship skills as they maneuver their horse through a series of commands during the walk, trot and canter gaits. Riders develop creative ways to communicate with their horses if they are unable to give signals with their legs, such as utilizing a dressage whip or other aids. Competitors are divided into grades that range from high levels of paralysis to those who are blind or visually impaired.

A challenge for the athletes at Paralympic and Special Olympic International competition is having to perform on borrowed horses. Riders and horses have only days to familiarize themselves with each other, with the team developing the strongest working bond often winning.

Equestrian rules and procedures for competition are overseen internationally by the Federation Equestre International (FEI) and in the United States by the American Horse Shows Association (AHSA).

Federation Equestre Internationale (FEI)

Founded in 1921 the Federation Equestre Internationale (FEI) is the international governing body for equestrian. It establishes rules and regulations for the conduct of international equestrian events in the Jumping, Dressage, Three-Day Event, Driving, Vaulting and Endurance Riding.

American Horse Shows Association (AHSA)

Founded in 1918, the American Horse Shows Association (AHSA) is the national governing body for equestrian sports in the U.S. It is the regulatory body for the Olympic and World Championship equestrian sports - Combined Driving, Dressage, Endurance, Show Jumping, Eventing, and Vaulting - as well as 18 other breeds and disciplines of competition.

The AHSA Rule Book has become the definitive guide to equestrian competition, and is so universal its specifications are enforced even at unrecognized competitions. Disability sport organizations follow AHSA rules in their competitions

SPORT OVERVIEW

Horseback riding has long been recognized as a great therapeutic tool for individuals with physical or mental impairments (Figure 10.1), but it is also recognized as an excellent activity for competition. This chapter will provide information on both forms of equestrian activity. It will describe the benefits of riding as means of therapy, and will identify resources who provide these services. Competitive programs offered by three disabled sports organizations will be reviewed in addition to adaptations and modified equestrian equipment.

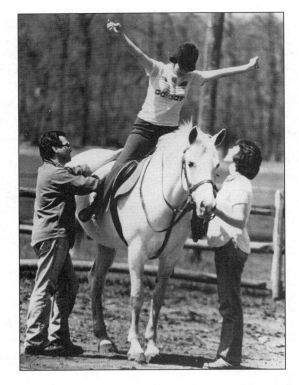

Figure 10.1. Therapeutic exercise are often a part of equestrian programs. (Courtesy of Specialized Sports Unlimited)

North American Riding for the Handicapped Association (NARHA)

The North American Riding for the Handicapped Association (NARHA) is an organization which fosters safe, professional, ethical and therapeutic equine activities through education, communication, standards and research for people with and without disabilities.

NARHA was founded in 1969 to promote and support therapeutic riding. Divided into 11 regions throughout the United States and Canada, there are approximately 600 NARHA riding centers, where more than 30,000 individuals with disabilities find a sense of independence through horseback riding. NARHA is the accrediting organization for Easter Seals' camps with equine activities. Other organizations participating in NARHA riding programs include the Muscular Dystrophy Association, Multiple Sclerosis Society, Special Olympics, Spina Bifida Association and United Cerebral Palsy.

A state by state list of the centers by regions can be found on the NARHA website or by contacting their office. NARHA conducts the following services:

- Establishes standards and techniques for teaching riding to people with disabilities.
- Provides a wide range of resource materials including videos, manuals, and other literature for individuals interested in starting riding programs.
- Advises and accredits existing NARHA-member operating centers to ensure the highest safety standards at riding centers, and instructor certification. About 28% of NARHA affiliated programs have earned accreditation through this voluntary process that recognizes operating centers that have met established industry standards:
  a) Maintains contacts with members of the medical profession to ensure the safety and well-being of riders with disabilities, and to gain approval and to promote riding as a valuable therapeutic activity.
  b) Publishes a newsletter to keep members abreast of trends in riding for people with disabilities.
  c) Provides a wide range of educational services while promoting responsible research and making resulting data available to members, special interest groups, and the general public.
- Assists riders in being included into open competitions.

NARHA has developed three special interest sections that focus on different aspects of therapeutic riding.

American Hippotherapy Association (AHA)

Hippotherapy, from the Greek word "hippos" meaning horse, is a treatment that uses the movement of the horse to assist individuals with motor dysfunction. Formed in 1993, the American Hippotherapy Association's mission is to promote research, education and communication among physical and occupational therapists and others using the horse in a treatment approach based on principles of classic hippotherapy. Hippotherapy should not be confused with therapeutic riding programs, since the purpose is not to teach specific riding skills but rather to facilitate sensory processing through the rhythmical movement of the horse in a casual and enjoyable environment.

Individuals with almost any type of disability can enjoy the benefits associated with hippotherapy. Hippotherapy has shown positive results in improving balance, posture, mobility and may also affect psychological, cognitive, behavioral and communication functions.

Competition Association of NARHA (CAN)

The Competition Association of NARHA (CAN) is the competitive riding branch of NARHA. CAN works with disability sport organizations to promote standards related to the education and training of coaches, judges and riders, to advocate access to competitions for CAN members, and to establish NARHA as a leading authority in competition for those with disabilities, to name a few. CAN has a strong educational component and works with horse show organizers, judges and breed associations to aid in the incorporation of riders with disabilities to their shows. The CAN web page can be accessed through the NARHA website.

Equine-Facilitated Mental Health Association

The Equine-Facilitated Mental Health Association involves therapeutic riding instructors working with, or as mental health professionals to deal with emotional, mental, physical, social or spiritual needs.

Therapeutic Programs

Children and adults riding at the hundreds of NARHA riding centers experience a wide range of benefits including improved flexibility, balance, confidence, self-esteem and other benefits related to mental, emotional and physical needs. Individuals report an increase in general well-being, and increased interest in the outside world and in one's own life. Being able to work with and control a large animal gives the rider confidence in risk-taking activities and becoming empowered to control events in their own lives. These benefits are often reported in conjunction with friendships formed during the therapeutic riding experience with people ranging from the van driver, to the volunteer side walker, to the horse itself.

COMPETITIVE PROGRAMS

Competitive riding programs for individuals with disabilities is facilitated by several groups including the Competition Association of NARHA (CAN), the American Competition Opportunities for Riders with Disabilities (ACORD), the United States Cerebral Palsy Athletic Association, Special Olympics, the Dwarf Athletic Association of America, and the International Paralympic Committee.

Competition Association of NARHA (CAN)

See description above.

American Competition Opportunities for Riders with Disabilities (ACORD)

ACORD is the umbrella non-profit organization for competition for riders with any disability in the United States. ACORD strives to provide safe, quality horse shows for riders with disabilities similar in scope to competitions for able-bodied riders.

USCPAA

The United States Cerebral Palsy Athletic Association (USCPAA) Equestrian program has a working relationships with ACORD and CAN in coordinating competitive riding opportunities for their members. USCPAA offers competitive equestrian events under two categories, cerebral palsy (CP) and les autres (LA) (including spinal cord-injured, multiple sclerosis, muscular dystrophy, arthrogryposis, amputee, etc.) Events are offered in two main sections, A for assisted and B for unassisted. "Assisted" refers to the use of a leader or sidewalker. Only riders in section B are considered for international competitions. Events are offered in dressage, handy rider (obstacle course), equitation for the following five functional classes/profiles for CP or LA riders.

Functional Classes/Profiles for Riding

CP	LA
CP1 and 2	LA1
CP3	LA2
CP4 and 5	LA3
CP6	LA4
CP7 and 8	LA5

The combination of 10 riding classes and different events for each main category (dressage, handy rider, equitation) results in 46 different riding events being conducted in a USCPAA-sanctioned riding competition.

Special Olympics

Equestrian sports events have been a part of Special Olympics since 1983, when the first competition was held in Baton Rouge. Equestrian became an official Special Olympics sport in 1988. Today more than 200 athletes from over 30 countries participate in Special Olympics International Equestrian competition. Special

Olympics Equestrian rules are based upon Federation Equestre Internationale (FEI), American Horse Shows Association (AHSA), and American Quarter Horse Association (AQHA) rule for Equestrian Sports competition.

Special Olympics offers the following 11 official events:

1. Dressage
2. Prix Caprilli (jumping)
3. English Equitation
4. Stock seat Equitation
5. Western Riding
6. Working Trails
7. Showmanship at Halter/Bridle Classes
8. Gymkhana Events
    a) Pole Bending
    b) Barrel Racing
    c) Figure 8 Stake race
    d) Team relays
9. Drill Teams of Twos and Fours
10. Unified Sports Team Relays
11. Unified Sports Drill Teams

Divisioning

According to the Official Special Olympics Summer Sports Rules, male and female riders compete together based on age and ability (assistance needed and skill level). Riders are grouped on the amount of assistance that is required and placed into divisions based on skill level.

Assistance Needed

Support (S): Rider needs the physical support of one or two sidewalkers and or the presence of a leader. Any help in the arena is considered supported.

Independent (I): Rider receives no assistance while competing.

Physical Limitations: Rider is unable to post the trot or sit the jog.

Divisions

A Level: Walk, Trot/Jog, Canter/Lope-Independent only. Rider is expected to compete with no modifications to NGB rules.
1) A = can perform any class requirements
2) AP = riders that have a physical disability prohibiting them from posting the trot or sitting the jog

B Level: Walk and Trot/Jog
1) B-I = Independent , can perform any class requirements
2) B-IP = Independent riders that have a physical disability prohibiting them from posting the trot or sitting the jog
3) B-S = Supported, can physically perform any class requirements
4) B-SP = Supported riders that have a physical disability prohibiting them from posting the trot or sitting the jog

C Level: Riders will ride at the walk only
1) C-I = Independent
2) C-S = Supported

Rider's Division Level

	C-S	C-I	B-S/B-P	B-I/BIP	A/AP
Dressage		x		x	x
Prix Caprilli					x
English Equitation	x	x	x	x	x
Western Equitation	x	x	x	x	x
Western Riding				x	x
Working Trails	x	x	x	x	x
Showmanship		x		x	x
Team Relays	x	x	x	x	x
Pole Bending				x	x
Barrel Racing				x	x
Figure 8 Stake Race				x	x
Drill Team 2 or 4	x	x	x	x	x

INTERNATIONAL PARALYMPIC COMMITTEE

Equestrian competition is an official Paralympic sport and is open to athletes with cerebral palsy, physical disabilities, visual impairments, blindness or mental disabilities. All riders are grouped according to their functional profiles and are judged on their ability to control and maneuver the horses. The complete classification and rules can be found on the International Paralympic Committee webpage.

Riding for Individuals Who are Blind

Riders who are blind are eligible to compete in Paralympic Competition and face even more significant challenges due to their lack of sight. The use of "living letters" has been documented in dressage. A team of nine callers stand at each of the eight dressage letters in a regulation ring and call out the letters as the rider approaches. One stands in the middle of the ring for the "X" (an invisible mark). The riders complete the event entirely by hearing, without sight.

EQUIPMENT

Equipment is designed specifically to ensure the safety and enjoyment of the rider as well as the horse. Many riders who have disabilities are capable of riding without the use of modified or adapted equipment. Many riders develop their own adaptations as the need requires. Some riders with arm dysfunction may strap their arm for support. Riders with Reflex Sympathetic Dystrophy may ride without stirrups because of the pain in their legs caused by the pressure. Riders who are not able to sit astride a horse may select to ride sidesaddle. The use of specialized equipment should only supplement a well-organized and well-staffed program. The equipment listed below is not standard for every rider and does not represent the only equipment available. Only the proper combination of horse, rider, instructor, and tack (equipment) will ensure a successful riding experience.

Helmets

Riding is a sport with potential risk for serious injury or death. To lessen the risk of acquiring severe head injury, the simplest and most important piece of equipment used by each and every rider will be the safety helmet. Regardless of the style preferred, only helmets that meet or exceed standards approved by the Safety Equipment Institute should be used, and the strap should be securely fashioned at all times. Specially designed helmets other than equestrian, may provide more protection than equestrian helmets. Riding should not be permitted unless a helmet is worn.

Walker Belts

A waist belt can be used to assist the rider in maintaining balance (Figure 10.2). Approximately four inches wide, the belt has a leather handhold on each side that enable sidewalkers to hold on to riders without grabbing clothes. Various models are available. The use of a safety vest is a possible alternative to a safety belt (Figure 10.3).

Saddles

Numerous modifications and alternatives to standard saddles have been developed for the safety and comfort of riders with disabilities. For riders with extremely tight adductors, the use of a bareback saddle instead of a standard saddle is initially recommended (Figure 10.4). A vaulting surcingle (Figure 10.5), designed for therapeutic riding programs, should always be used when with a bareback saddle in order to ensure the rider has something other than the reins to use for stability .

Riders with spinal cord-related disabilities, reduced seat and lower extremity sensation will often use saddle fleece pads in addition to the saddle for extra protection (Figure 10.6). An alternative to the fleece pad is the saddle cushion by ROHO, Inc. the makers of wheelchair seat cushions. ROHO's unique air flotation design involves small flexible air cells and produces cushions for Western and English style saddles (Figure 10.7).

Figure 10.8 a and b illustrate the differences between the English and Western saddles.

For riders with extreme balance difficulties, the use of a Western saddle or the incorporation of various modifica-

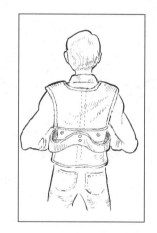

Figure 10.3. A safety vest can be a homemade option to a waist belt body harness.

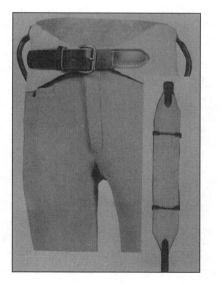

Figure 10.2. A waist belt with handles providing side walkers with a secure method of Spotting a rider. (Courtesy of Courbette Saddery Co., Inc.)

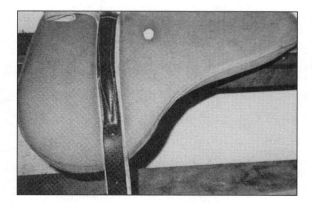

Figure 10.4. A bareback saddle may initially be more appropriate for a rider with tight adductors. (Courtesy of Cheff Center for the Handicapped)

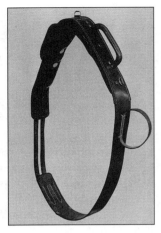

Figure 10.5. A vaulting surcingle is usually used in conjunction with a bareback saddle. (Courtesy of Courbette Saddlery Co., Inc.)

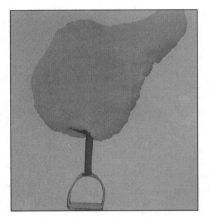

Figure 10.6. Saddle fleece pads are used by many spinal cord-injured riders to prevent body sores. (Courtesy of Courbette Saddlery Co., Inc.)

tions that can be attached across and in front of the pommel of the saddle is recommended (Figure 10.9). Saddles with deeper seats also offer greater stability for the rider.

Therapeutic saddles are available in custom and semi-custom models. The seat can be raised in specific areas to accommodate a rider's disability. Double foam seats, thigh blocks, longer or shorter flaps and panels are all available. Some riders find it more comfortable to ride aside than astride. Entry level English style leather side saddle has a leaping horn and balance strap. The flat padded seat, comes with stirrup leather and iron, and cotton girth . The Suede Western Sport Saddle saddle made by Circle Y has pommel and cantle on treeless body. It is very comfortable with the suede acting as a gripper to hold the rider securely. This saddle gives a rider a great feel of the horse. A saddle that is very popular in therapeutic riding programs is the Tots-in-Tandem saddle specifically designed for two. The saddle has a pommel safety, and uses standard English fittings. It allows instructors ro ride along with the participant. Freedom

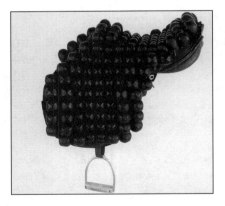

Figure 10.7. ROHO's air flotation design provides flexible air cells in the shape of an English saddle. (Courtesy of ROHO, Inc.)

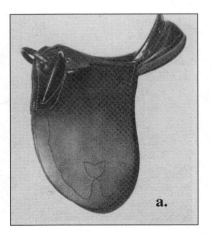

a.

b.

Figure 10.8 a and b. English saddle (left) and Western saddle (right). (Courtesy of Cheff Center for the Handicapped)

Rider and the 1824 Therapeutic Riding Catalog offers many of these products (see Equipment Suppliers).

Reins

Modified reins are available for riders with upper extremity difficulties. Selection will depend on the individual needs of the rider. Ladder reins (Figure 10.10) provide a rider with grasp problems or use of only one hand the ability to control the horse. An adapted rein bar functions similarly to ladder reins but only provides one alternative length compared with the several variations in the ladder reins.

Humes reins provide another alternative for riders with grasp difficulties (Figure 10.11 a and b). Adjustable, with looped hand holds, they allow the rider's hands to slip easily into position. At times, additional neck straps for the horse may be appropriate when riders require more stability. Use of these straps will eliminate a rider's need to use the reins for balance and thus prevent injury to the horse's mouth. Overhead checks (anti-grazing devices) are also suggested, especially for horses with riders who have balance difficulties. They keep horses from reaching down to eat, which could cause riders with poor stability to be pulled off balance.

Stirrups

A number of safety stirrups are available for therapeutic riding programs including the popular Peacock Stirrup (Figure 10.12), STI Western Breakaway Stirrups and SideStep Safety Stirrup are all designed to release the foot of a rider when falling.

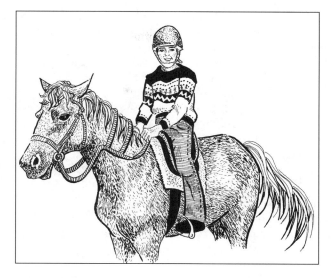

Figure 10.10. Ladder reins are used for riders with grasp difficulties. (Courtesy of Human Kinetics Publishers)

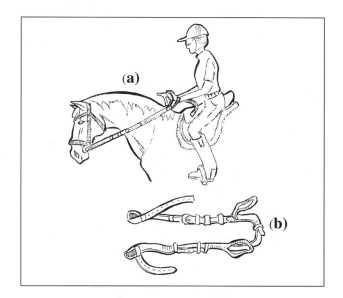

Figure 10.11. The adapted rein bar (a) and the Humes Reins (b) are alternative for riders with grasp difficulties.

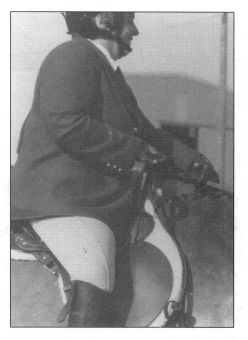

Figure 10.9. A spinal cord injured rider uses an adapted support attached to the front of the saddle for additional support.

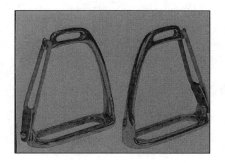

Figure 10.12. Peacock stirrups incorporate a breakaway rubber support for safety. (Courtesy of Courbette Saddlery Co., Inc.)

Some riders will be faced with the problem of keeping the feet properly positioned in the stirrups. This will usually occur with riders who have either tight heel cords or weak ankle muscles. The use of rubber soled boots and a rubber insert on a pair of Peacock Stirrups may provide a solution. If the problem persists, the rider should use a pair of Hooded Stirrups or Devonshire Boots (Figure 10.13). These modified stirrups, with a front cover and solid base, keep the foot from slipping through, prevent rubbing sores to the ankle, and maintain the foot in proper.

Finally, for the above the knee amputee, Kegel (1985, pp.24-25) suggests the use of a residual limb stirrup to assist riders in maintaining balance. Use of other tack such as breastplates, stirrup leathers, hand hold mounting straps and German side reins will depend on the individual needs of the rider.

Mounting Blocks

Mounting blocks vary from small two-step blocks to major full-size mounting ramps (Figure 10.14). Program managers should consider the needs of each rider when determining which mounting device is more appropriate. Plans for building a mounting ramp are available from Freedom Rider.

EQUIPMENT SUPPLIERS

1824 Therapeutic Riding Catalog
1824 Arnott Mason Corporation
12644 Chapel Road
Clifton, VA 20124
(703) 818-1517
(703) 818-1518 (fax)
Email: Info@1824catalog.com (to request catalog)
Website: http://www.1824catalog.com
   Provides an extensive line of adapted and therapeutic riding equipment for individuals with disabilities.

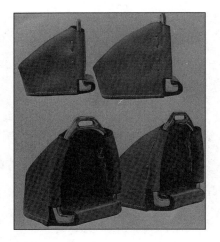

Figure 10.13. Devonshire Boots help maintain feet position. (Courtesy of Courbette Saddlery Co., Inc.)

Freedom Rider
PO Box 4188
Dedham, MA 02027-4188
(888) 253-8811
Email: info@freedomrider.com
Website: http://www.freedomrider.com
   Provides an extensive line of adapted and therapeutic riding equipment for individuals with disabilities.

ROHO, Inc.100 Florida Avenue
Belleville, IL
62221-5430
(800) 851)-3449
(618) 277-6518 (fax))
Website: http://www.rohoinc.com
   Custom saddle.

ADDITIONAL RESOURCES AND WEBSITES

Hundreds of equine websites are available. The sites listed below are primary sites from which other sites of interest may be accessed.

Associations

American Competition Opportunities for Riders With Disabilities (ACORD) Inc.
5303 Felter Road
San Jose, CA 95132
(408) 261-2015
(408) 261-9438 (fax)

American Horse Shows Association Inc.
4047 Iron Works Parkway
Lexington, Kentucky 40511
(606) 258-2472
(606) 231-6662 (fax)
Website: http://www.ahsa.org

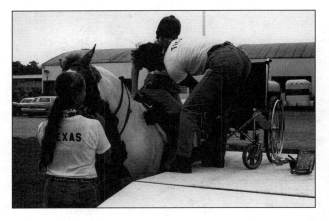

Figure 10.14. Full-size loading ramps take a lot of lifting out of mounting riders on horses. (Courtesy of Cheff Center for the Handicapped)

American Quarter Horse Association (AQHA)
P.O. Box 200.
Amarillo, TX 79168
Website: http://www.aqha.org
(806) 376-4811

Canadian Therapeutic Riding Association (CanTRA)
P.O. Box 24009
Guelph, Ontario
Canada N1E 6Z8
(519) 767-0700

Equiworld.net
Email: info@equiworld.com
Website: www.equiworld.net
    Equiworld is a comprehensive provider of global on-line equine information and resources located in Aberdeen, Scotland.

Federation Equestre Internationale (FEI)
Avenue Mon-Repos 24
P.O. Box 157
1000 Lausanne 5
Switzerland
(41) 21 310 47 47
(41) 21 310 47 60 (fax)
Website: http://www.horsesport.org

International Paralympic Committee
Adenauerallee 212
D- 53113 Bonn
Germany
Email: info@paralympic.org
49-228-2097 200
49-228-2097 209 (fax)

International Paralympic Committee
Equestrian Chairperson
Mrs. Jonquil Solt
Blackdown Farm
Leamington Spa
Warwickshire, CV32 6QS
United Kingdom
44-1926-422-522
44-1926-450-996 (fax)

North American Riding for the Handicapped Association
P.O. Box 33150
Denver, CO 80233
(800) 369-RIDE (7433)
(303) 452-1212

(303) 252-4610 (fax)
(303) 457-8496 (Fax-on-Demand)
Email: Narha@narha.org
Website: http://www.narha.org

Video Resources

Kerry
    The story of Kerry Knaus-Hardy, born with a serious neurological disability and not expected to live past her sixth birthday. Beating the odds, she now operates a 10 acre horse ranch which offers trail rides and camping trips for people with differing abilities. Offers a candid insight into what it is like to have one's abilities and intelligence questioned because of a physical challenge. (available from Freedom Rider)

Ability, Not Disability
    Award winning documentary of the Cheff Center for the Handicapped in Michigan. Demonstrates how therapeutic riding provides exercise, improves coordination, and builds self-esteem. Covers the Center's certification program for therapeutic riding instructors. (available from Freedom Rider)

Driving For The Disabled—Getting Underway Video
    This video is a basic driving how-to for individuals with disabilities. Some of the techniques shown apply only to wheelchair users, however there are also sections on harnesses, training, horse selection and safety. (available from NARHA)

A New Freedom: Therapeutic Horseback Riding.
    Features President and Mrs. Ronald Reagan and focuses on the rider. (available from NARHA)

A Parent's Story: Therapeutic Horseback Riding.
    Features actor William Christopher and focuses on the parents of riders. (available from NARHA)

BIBLIOGRAPHY

Heine, B. (1997). Introduction to Hippotherapy. *NARHA Strides Magazine*, 3(2).

Kegel, B. (1985). Sport and recreation for those with lower limb amputations or impairments. *Journal of Research and Development*, Clinical supplement No. 1. Washington D.C.: Veterans Administration.

Official Special Olympics Summer Sports Rules (1996-1999). Special Olympics International: Washington, D.C.

Chapter 11

Fencing

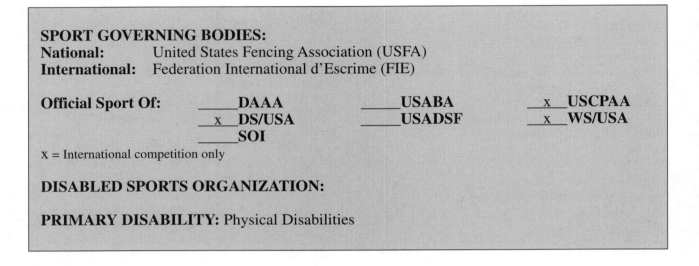

SPORT GOVERNING BODIES:
National: United States Fencing Association (USFA)
International: Federation International d'Escrime (FIE)

Official Sport Of: ____DAAA   ____USABA   _x_USCPAA
                         _x_DS/USA   ____USADSF   _x_WS/USA
                         ____SOI
X = International competition only

DISABLED SPORTS ORGANIZATION:

PRIMARY DISABILITY: Physical Disabilities

SPORT OVERVIEW

Traditionally a European sport, fencing is not as popular in the United States as the more conventional sports of track, field, or even shooting (Figure 11.1). It is however, an international sport for three disabled sports organizations, the United States Cerebral Palsy Athletic Association, Wheelchair Sports USA, and Disabled Sports USA. Participants from these organizations participate through the Cerebral Palsy-International Sports and Recreation Association (CP-ISRA), International Stoke Mandeville Wheelchair Sports Federation (ISMWSF), or the International Sports Organization for the Disabled (ISOD) respectively. Founded in 1981, the United States Fencing Association is the recognized national governing body for fencing and selects the wheelchair fencing team that participates in international competition.

SPORT ORIGIN

Fencing was one of the original sports of the modern Olympic games, and enjoys a rich history dating back to ancient Egypt. In later times, dueling with swords was a popular means of settling disputes. By the 1800's the emphasis on mortally wounding an opponent declined due to the threat of jail terms. Emphasis was now on wound-

ing the opponent in the arms or legs. This formed the basis for modern fencing.

For individuals with disabilities, wheelchair fencing originated at Stoke Mandeville Hospital in England in 1953 by Sir Ludwig Gutmann. A Paralympic sport since 1960, The Wheelchair Fencing Committee of the International Stoke Mandeville Wheelchair Sports Federation (ISMWSF) sets forth the rules for the sport. The ISMWSF Official Rules for Fencing are designed to accommodate the special needs of the wheelchair fencer and are to be used in conjunction with the Federation Internationale d'Escrime (FIE) Rules for Fencing.

WHEELCHAIR FENCING
ISMWSF/ISOD Competition

Events:

The Olympic and Paralympic sport of fencing is comprised of three weapons: foil, epee, and sabre. A competitive fencer may compete in all events but will generally specialize in one of the three events. The rules governing these three weapons are determined by the FIE . The object of a fencing bout is to score 15 points (in direct elimination play) or five points (in preliminary pool play) on your opponent before he scores that number on you. Each time a fencer scores a touch, a point is received. Direct elimination matches consist of three three-minute periods.

Briefly, the FIE weapons are described as follows:

Foil: The foil comes from the 18th century small sword can be one of the more physically demanding events. The foil has a flexible rectangular blade, approximately 35 inches in length, weighing less than one pound. Fencing foil, the competitors may only touche with the point and the right to score is at the fencer who first starts an attack. The opponent must defend himself before he can score. Foil technique emphasizes strong defense and the killing attack to the body.

Epee: Similar to the dueling swords of the mid-19th century, epees are similar in length to the foil, but weigh more (27 ounces), and have stiff blades with a triangular cross section, and large bell guards to protect the hand from a hit. Fencing epee, the competitors may only touche with the point, with the fencer who touches first scoring. Epee technique emphasizes timing, point control, and a good counter-attack and is considered a game of tactics and precision.

Sabre: Sabres came from the late 19th century, and is the modern version of the slashing cavalry sword. Sabres are similar in length and weight to the foil but have a light, flat blade and a knuckle guard. The sabre is both a thrusting weapon (use of the tip) and a cutting weapon (use of the blade). Fencing sabre, competitors touch with the whole blade and the right to score is at the fencer who first starts an attack. The opponent must defend himself before he can score. Sabre technique emphasizes speed, feints, and strong offense.

Modifications to FIE Rules

Since all competitors entered in ISMWSF competition are classified in and compete in wheelchairs (spinal cord-injured, amputees, etc.), it is understandable that ISMWSF

rules for wheelchair fencing apply to any sport involving competitors who use wheelchairs. ISMWSF modifications to nondisabled rules include safety requirements, equipment modifications, and terminology changes that provide specific instruction for wheelchair fencing. Scoring with an electronic apparatus is identical to the process used in sabre competitions in traditional fencing.

Since the wheelchair is fixed in position, certain modifications are made for wheelchair fencing involving the positioning and distance of fencers.

The wheelchair is secured to a frame on the floor that gives the fencer's body freedom of movement allowing for exciting and fast action (Figure 11.2). Wheelchairs are set on angles of @110 degrees to the central bar.

The distance of the fencers depends on the length of their arms. The fencer with the shortest arm decides whether the fight will be at his distance or that of his opponent. Technical information can be found in the wheel-

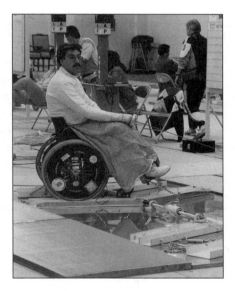

Figure 11.2 a and b. Elaborate wheelchair tie-down systems are used in wheelchair fencing. (Courtesy of Specialized Sports Unlimited)

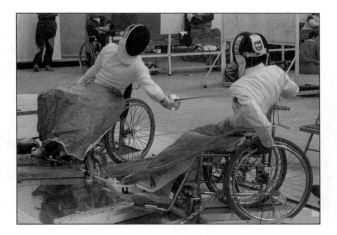

Figure 11.1. Primarily a European sport, wheelchair fencing is beginning to gain popularity in the United States. (Courtesy of Specialized Sports Unlimited)

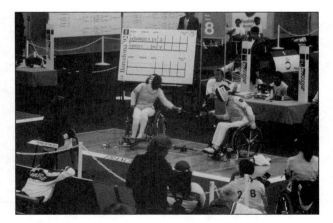

chair fencing rule book available from the USFA or on their website.

Wheelchair Fencing Classification

Individuals eligible for wheelchair fencing must have a permanent disability that does not allow for participation in able-bodied fencing. Women compete in foil and epee while men compete in foil, epee, and sabre. Three categories of classification are used for spinal cord injuries, A, B, and C for spinal cord injuries:

Class A: Fencers have full sitting balance, and many are still ambulatory.

Class B: Fencers lack full sitting balance but have full use of their arms and hands.

Class C: Fencers lack full use of their arms and hands.

Technical information on classification can be found in the Official Rules for Wheelchair Fencing.

Cerebral Palsy

In international fencing competition for athletes with cerebral palsy there are four divisions for both men and women. Placement in divisions is based on the competitor's sport classification. Men compete in three events: foil, epee and sabre. Women compete only in foil. Divisions one, two, and three follow International Stoke Mandeville Wheelchair Sports Federation (ISMWSF) rules that reflect wheelchair fencing modifications for the disabled. Division four competitors follow Federation International d'Escrime rules without modifications.

Class and Division Breakdown for Cerebral Palsy Athletes

Division	CP-Class	Event	
		Women	Men
One	3	Foil	Foil
Two	4,5,7	Foil	Foil
Three	6	Foil	Foil, Epee, Sabre
Four	8	Foil	Foil, Epee, Sabre

Other Disabilities

Amputees

Individuals with arm amputations have generally fenced from a standing position according to FIE rules with no modifications, while those with leg amputations have been more successful using a wheelchair following ISMWF rules. With the advancements in prostheses it is conceivable that ambulatory fencing for leg amputees will soon be common.

Blind and Visually Impaired

Fencing for individuals who are blind or visually impaired is not very common, however, documentation ex-

ists of blind fencers in Britain and France, with epee the weapon of choice. In Britain the fencers align themselves with one another using a line or spool wire, whereas in France the fencers have sighted guides or "seconds" to keep them aligned. The rules are exactly the same as able-bodied epee rules.

EQUIPMENT SUPPLIERS

The following suppliers are listed in this section because they are USFA Corporate Members.

American Fencers Supply
1180 Folsom St.
San Francisco, CA 94103
(415) 863-7911
(415) 431-4931 (fax)
Website: http://amfence.com

Blade Fencing Equipment Inc
245 West 29th Street
New York, NY 10001
(800) 828-5661
(212) 244-3090
(212) 244-3034 (fax)
Website: http://www.blade-fencing.com

Blue Gauntlet Fencing Gear Inc.
479 North Midland Ave.
Saddle Brook, NJ 07663
(201) 797-3332
(201) 797-9190 (fax)
Website: http://www.Blue-Gauntlet.com

George Santelli Inc.
465 S. Dean St.
Englewood, NJ 07631
(201) 871-3105
(201) 871-8718 (fax)
Website: http://www.santelli.com

Get the Point
1007 Cherry Lane
Cinnaminson, NJ 08077-2307
(609) 786-9255
(609) 786-7755 (fax)

Physical Chess, Inc.
336 West 37th Street
New York, NY 10018
(800) 336-2464 ((800) FENCING)
(212) 216-9684
(212) 216-9540 (fax)
Website: http://www.physicalchess.com

The Fencing Post
1004 Bird Ave.
San Jose, CA 95125
(408) 297-4448
(408) 275-8060 (Fax)
Website: http://www.thefencingpost.com

Triplette Competition Arms
101 East Main St.
Elkin, NC 28621
(336) 835-7774
(336) 835-4099 (fax)
Website: http://www.triplette.com

Zivkovic Modern Equipment Inc.
77 Arnold Rd.
Wellesley Hills, MA 02481-2820
(781) 235-3324
(781) 239-1224 (fax)
Website: http://www.zivkovic.com

ADDITIONAL RESOURCES AND WEBSITES

Canadian Fencing Federation
1600 Prom. James Naismith Drive
Gloucester, ON K1B 5N4
(613) 748-5633
(613) 748-5742 (fax)
Website: http://www.fencing.ca

Federation International d'Escrime (FIE)
Avenue Mon Repos 24
Case Postale 2743
1002 Lausanne, Switzerland
(41-21) 320-3115
(41-21) 320-3116 (fax)
Website: http://www.fie.ch

International Wheelchair Fencing Committee:
Alberto Martinez Vassallo, President
Somatenes 3
08950 Esplugas (Barcelona)
Spain
34-3-4736083 (phone/fax)

Northeast Passage (Wheelchair Fencing)
P.O. Box 127
Durham, NH 03824-0127
(603) 862-0070

Shepherd Fencing Club (Wheelchair Fencing)
Sheperd Center
Promotions Fitness Center

2020 Peachtree Rd., NW
Atlanta, GA 30309
(404) 352-2020

United States Fencing Association (USFA)
One Olympic Plaza
Colorado Springs, CO 80909-5774
(719) 578-4511
(719) 632-5737 (fax)
Email: usfencing@aol.com
Website: http://www.usfa.org

USFA National Wheelchair Fencing Coach
Leszek Stawicki
1609 Ellwood Avenue, #C4
Louisville, KY 40204
(502) 568-6781

Chairman, USFA Wheelchair Fencing Committee
Marcella Denton
4009 Woodgate Lane
Louisville, KY 40220
(502) 582-5734 (Day)
(502) 491-6883 (Evening)
Email: Marcella.M.Denton@lrl02.usace.army.mil

University of New Hampshire Fencing Club (Wheelchair Fencing)
C/o John Moss, Coach
Hamel Recreation Center
128 Main Street
Durham, NH 03824-2534
(603) 862-2038

Wheelchair Sports-USA
US Fencing - Disabled Committee
Mario Rodriguez
2023 Steber
Houston, TX
(713) 946-1780
Email: usfencer@hotmail.com

BIBLIOGRAPHY

Belson, M. (2000). Duelign Eagles. *We Magazine* 4(3):66-71

Chapter 12

Fishing

SPORT OVERVIEW

A bad day of fishing is better than a good day at work. Whether it is a lazy summer afternoon at the local fishing hole or an exciting day on a charter boat, fishing is one of today's most popular recreational activities throughout North America. In the stressful world, fishing allows one to escape from the daily routine for a few hours.

Fishing also represents one of the easiest activities to adapt to the individual needs of the participant with a disability. This section will discuss a variety of resources, specialized equipment including rods, reels, line, rod holders, specialized tackle, and some ways to enjoy fishing without buying expensive equipment for the novice adaptive fisherman.

SPORTS ORGANIZATIONS AND RESOURCES

Most fishing related organizations welcome and encourage people with disabilities. A variety of disability sport organizations and resources are available to assist people in accessing fishing opportunities and in promoting the sport.

Accessing Fishing Areas

Outfitting a person with a disability with proper fishing equipment is the easy part of a fishing trip. Unfortunately for individuals who use wheelchairs, one of the biggest barriers to participation is accessibility . Fish cannot be caught in living rooms! Solutions to this problem are both immediate and long-term. Immediate solutions include locating an accessible fishing area or pier (Figure 12.1) (such information is usually available through your state's Fisheries Division of Department of Natural Resources or Fish and Game Department), or using a wheelchair accessible boat. Pontoon boats are easily accessible and make loading and unloading wheelchairs easy. A va-

riety of accessible boats are available through most retailers. See the boating chapter in this book for additional information on accessible boats.

Long-term solutions include working to increase the number of accessible fishing sites available as *Project Access* is doing (see the following). Many of the Department of Natural Resources (DNR) in each state have lists of accessible fishing areas. Some accessible fishing sites in each State are listed on the *Project Access* website. One in four people in the United States could benefit from accessible recreation areas due to various physical limitations. With the aging of the American population, we cannot continue to ignore the great number of potential users when designing our recreational areas.

Project Access

Project Access is an example of what is possible in accessibility. Started in the Catskill Mountains of New York, *Project Access* is a volunteer organization that provides accessible paths to trout fishing streams. *Project Access* has no formal national organization. The website (see Additional Resources) is meant to serve as a database and starting point for other independent projects developed across the country. This information is available to anyone who needs it, not just project planners, but also those fishers who need special access. The group hopes that by describing the very simple methods and success in creating several access sites on three Catskill rivers, others will be encouraged to create additional sites on good rivers nationwide. This website provides "how to" information to those interested in initiating a project. A 12-minute "how to" video is available for purchase. The *Project Access* website also provides a section on accessible fishing. The information supplied by various states identifies those fishing opportunities nationwide that are accessible for the individual with a disability. The site is being continually updated.

Fishing Has No Boundaries

The goal of Fishing Has No Boundaries is to open the great outdoors for people with disabilities through the world of fishing. Founded in Wisconsin in 1986, this organization sponsors many fishing trips specifically for individuals with disabilities (see additional resources).

Paralyzed Veterans of America (PVA) National Bass Trail

The Paralyzed Veterans of America sponsors a variety of bass fishing tournaments for fishers with disabilities (Figure 12.2). The concept began in 1987 with the sponsoring of the Annual U.S. Open Bass Tournament by the Central Florida Chapter of PVA. Due to the success enjoyed by this tournament, interest was sparked throughout the country. In 1994, the PVA Sports and Recreation Program, expanded bass fishing into the National Bass Trail of five tournaments. Locations of these tournaments and other information about the National Bass Trail can be found on the National Bass Trail website (see Additional Resources).

Each tournament consists of an Open/Team Competition for those who wish to fish from a boat and a Bank Competition for those who prefer to fish from the shore.

Anglers with disabilities in the Open/Team Competition are paired with able-bodied boat captains and fish as a team on Saturday. On Sunday, only the anglers with disabilities compete. The boat captains serve as guides and help in finding fishing locations and choosing baits. Although only the anglers with disabilities are fishing on Sunday, the boat captains whose anglers place in the top ten also win. Awards and prizes are given to both anglers and boat captains.

Anglers in the Bank Competition are paired with volunteers who assist them in whatever needs they have while fishing. Prizes are awarded based on the total weight for both days of fishing.

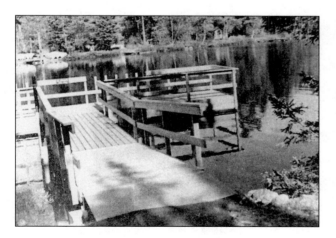

Figure 12.1. Fishing and boating piers provide access to many great fishing spots. (Courtesy of *Disabled Outdoors*)

Accessible Fishing Lodges

A number of fishing lodges and wilderness outfitters are making their services available to people with disabilities. Although primarily a resource for hunters, the Buckmasters website provides excellent resources for the sports-person with a disability including accessible lodges.

EQUIPMENT

Many individuals with disabilities will find little need in modifying typical fishing equipment. However, those individuals with upper limb amputations, high level spinal cord injury and/or various hand disorders affecting grasp will find adaptive equipment readily available from most retailers to meet their needs.

Rods

The selection of an appropriate rod is based on the type of fish desired. There is generally no difference in the rods utilized by fishers with and without disabilities, although adaptations such as rod holders, may need to be made to hold and maneuver the rod. Those fishing for pike, muskie, channel cats will require a good long stiff fishing rod. Those going after pan fish, bass, and trout and a lot of action will find a light or ultra light rod suitable. These rods will give you that fight and still allow you to land the fish. Adaptive reels generally fit on any type of standard rod.

Harness Rod Holders

Another alternative for the hemiplegic or single-arm amputee who requires some assistance in rod stability is the Freehand Recreation Belt (Figure 12.3). Various makes and models fulfill the same basic function of se-

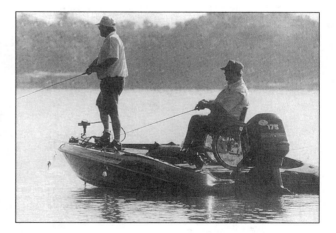

Figure 12.2. The Paralyzed Veterans of America sponsor the PVA National Bass Trail, which involves a series of competitive fishing bass tournaments across the country. (Courtesy of Sports 'n Spokes 1998, 24/6, p. 49)

curing the rod and freeing the hand or hands to reel fish in, finesse, or jig.

Attachable Rod Holders

Devices are available that attach directly to an individual's wheelchair or to the side of a boat. They vary in size, function, and price, so comparison shopping is essential. These can be found at Wal-Mart and other large tackle distributors. Access to Recreation also distributes one that attaches directly to the wheelchair.

Line

The line chosen should be sensitive to feel the fish. Many fishers find it a good idea to go 2lbs lighter on the test that is normally used. When fishing for toothy critters, the use of a leader to cut down on the number of knots that need to be tied is appropriate.

Fishing Reels

Individuals with upper extremity disabilities face obvious challenges when attempting to operate most standard fishing reels. Some simple solutions are readily available. Those who have difficulty turning the handle may add an extension to the reel handle for easier turning. Individuals with amputations may select the Ampo Fish 1 (Figure (12.4) There are also options to use electric reel in devices.

Electric and/or electronic fishing reels provide an excellent solution for the one-handed fisher or the person with a grasp problem (Figures 12.5 a-d). These reels provide one-hand fingertip control with all the functions of standard reels through battery-operated controls. The reels can be used with fresh-water or salt-water fish and most come with a coiled cord with plug for a battery pack, a cord with solid copper alligator clips that can be attached directly to a 12 volt battery on a boat, car, or power wheelchair. Reels vary in sophistication and price and are available from a variety of fishing distributors. Most electric reels are more than just "fishing winches". They still allow the fisher to play the fish, and to experience the feel of the fight. Electronic fishing reels can also be mastered with home-made or adapted devices. Cecotti (1982) documents his efforts in developing a pneumatic (sip and puff) system that controls an elaborate fishing device for a person with high level quadriplegia (Figure 12.6).

Grasping Devices

Several simple, inexpensive devices may assist individuals with holding the fishing rod more securely. The *Batick Bracket* is designed with pieces of foam to allow an individual to hold a rod without gripping or bending the hand (Figure 12.7). Although not available commercially, a similar device can be easily made at home. Access to Recreation distributes various types of rod holding devices. The *Strong-Arm* (Figure 12.8) and *Reel-Eze* both attach to the wrist. The *Strong-Arm* is for the fisher with very limited or no grasp ability allows for unassisted casting. The *Reel-Eze* is made from leather with a metal brace to support the wrist. A piece of 3/4" tubing fits over the reel handle to aid in cranking.

Those who require an even greater amount of stability can try grasping splints. Similar in concept to an archer cuff, these splints come in various sizes and can be used on either hand.

Casting Devices

Individuals with severe upper extremity disabilities may be faced with more than just reeling difficulties. The

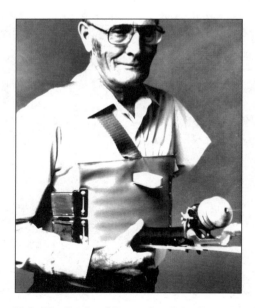

Figure 12.3. The Freehand Recreation Belt allows the user to bait a hook, cast, troll, and reel entirely with one hand. (Courtesy of Free Handerson Co.)

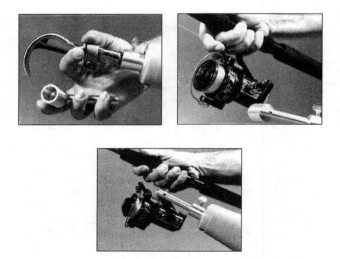

Figure 12.4. The Ampo Fish 1. (Courtesy of Bassmatic)

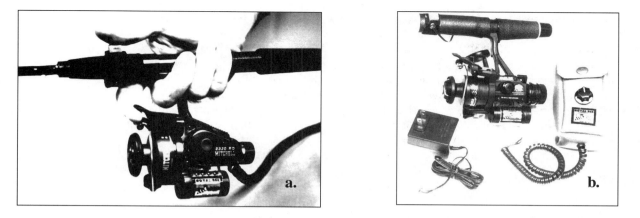

Figure 12.5 a-d. Three pictures (a,b,c) show different types of electric fishing reels featuring push-button control, rapid retrieve, and one-hand operation. Picture (d) shows the incorporation of a microcomputer system that increases the number and sophistication of features. (Courtesy of Royal Bee Corp., and Miya Epoch)

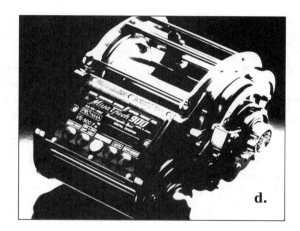

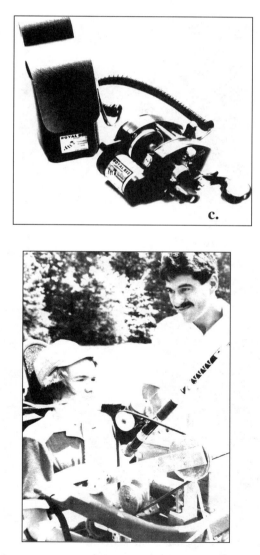

Figure 12.6. A sip and puff fishing reel for high-level quadriplegics. (Courtesy of *Sports 'n Spokes* 7/82:18)

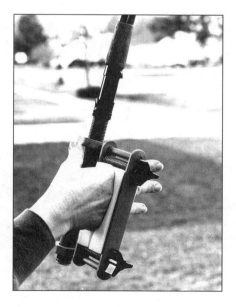

Figure 12.7. The Batick Bracket is padded with foam rubber to help provide a secure and comfortable method of holding a lightweight fishing rod.

mobility and coordination required for casting may also be absent. Fortunately, there are easy solutions to this problem as well. Of the mechanical casting devices available, *Van's E-Z Cast* (Figure 12.9) is the most popular. Designed by a person with quadriplegia, the device requires only a small amount of upper body movement to activate. It is distributed through Access to Recreation and other retailers. The "medical glove" provides quadriplegics with an altwernative to other rod holders (Figure 12.10).

Automatic Tying Device

The tying of knots can provide a significant challenge for the one-handed or grasp impaired fisherman. An appropriate solution is the Ty-All, from Access to Recreation. This device aids the one-handed fisherman in threading hooks, tying knots, and cutting line.

Fishing Tackle

It is beyond the scope of this chapter to describe all of the different innovations and adapted devices available in the broad category of fishing tackle. Some are designed specifically for the disabled fisherman, while others were developed to help anyone with some of the more troublesome tasks of fishing. Special tackle include heated rod handles, "no knots" fishing hooks, line threaders, fish grapplers, cuffed cutting tools, and even a motorized battery operated bobber that allows the fisher to direct the bait to any location without casting.

EQUIPMENT SUPPLIERS

For the individual with a disability who wishes to fish, most equipment suppliers and retailers will be suitable. Many new online companies offer an extensive line of equipment. Some representative companies follow.

Access to Recreation, Inc.
8 Sandra Court
Newbury Park CA 91320
(800) 634-4351
(805) 498-7535
(805) 498-8186 (fax)
Email: dkrebs@gte.net
Website: http://www.accesstr.com

Dolphin Electreel, Inc.
2819 62nd Avenue East
Bradenton, FL 34203
(941) 758-9369
(800) 717-3716
Email: electrel@gte.net
Website: http://www.dolphinelectreel.com

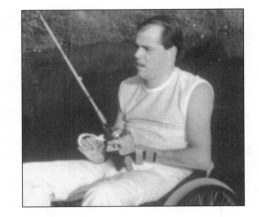

Figure 12.9. Van's E-Z Cast is a mechanical casting device that is easily operated by fishing enthusiasts with upper extremity impairments. (Courtesy of the Creative Shop)

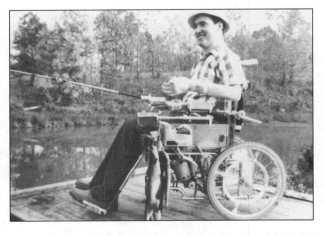

Figure 12.10. The "medical glove" provides quadriplegics with an alternative to other rod holders. (Courtesy of Patton Enterprises)

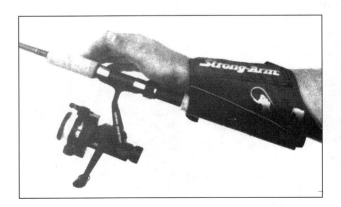

Figure 12.8. The Strong-Arm rod holder. (Courtesy of Strong-Arm Fishing Products)

Electric Fishing Reel Systems, Inc.
P.O. Box 2041
1700 Sullivan Street
Greensboro, NC 27420
(336) 273-9101
Email: info@elec-tra-mate.com
Website: http://www.elec-tra-mate.com

Hunting Fishing, Inc.
12010 Fruitwood Dr.
Riverview, Florida, 33569
813-672-9472
877-275-9955
Website: http://www.huntingfishinginc.com
    Complete online equipment outfitter.

BigFishTackle.Com
(877) 982-2553
(562) 430 – 9177 (fax)
Email: bigfish@bigfishtackle.com
Website: http://www.bigfishtackle.com
    Complete online equipment outfitter with disability section.

ADDITIONAL RESOURCES AND WEBSITES

Fishermen will find many websites related to their sport. Because this sport is accessible for those with and without disabilities, most participants will find the following sites satisfactory for gathering information.

Buckmasters Online
Website: http://buckmasters.rivals.com/
    Although primarily a site for hunting, Buckmasters Online offers information on various outdoor activities, including fishing. A special section for the sports-person with a disability is included.

Fishing Has No Boundaries, Inc.
P.O. Box 175
Hayward, WI 54843
Email: info@fhnbinc.org
Website: http://www.fhnbinc.org/
(800) 243-3462
(715) 634-3185
    This organization, with chapters in 13 states and England, sponsors many fishing events for individuals with disabilities who wish to fish.

Fishing Schools.com
Website: http://www.fishingschools.com/
    This website provides an incredible amount of fishing

resources from fresh water to salt water. Also listed are resources for boats, equipment and supplies and related organizations.

Outdoor Guides.com
Email: guide@crosstel.net
Website: http://www.outdoorguides.com/
    This is one stop shopping for the online outdoor enthusiast. This site provides a complete list of equipment manufacturers and over 4,000 outdoor guides listed Worldwide. The site also provides a guide to state regulations on fishing and hunting, and public and private outdoor usage areas.

Paralyzed Veterans of America (PVA)
Sports and Recreation Program
900 Seventeenth Street, NW
Suite 400
Washington, DC 20006
(800) 424-8200 ext. 752
(202) 955-8358 (fax)
Email: info@pva.org
Website: http://www.pva.org

PVA National Bass Trail
Website: http://www.pva.org/basstrail/index.htm

Project Access
Website: http://www.projectaccess.com/

Project Access Video
Catskill Fly Fishing Center and Museum
Old Rte 17, PO Box 1295
Livingston Manor, NY 12758
    The Project Access video is a 12-minute "how-to", which describes the methods employed by volunteer work crews, using hand tools, to create natural-looking pathways down otherwise non-negotiable banks. The cost is $10 (includes s&h).

Turning Point
C/o Shorty Powers
4144 N. Central Exprssway
Suite 515
Dallas, TX 75204
(214) 827-7404
    Every Mother's Day for over 16 years, Turning Point has hosted the National Bass Championships for the Physically Challenged at Crips Camp in Uncertain, Texas.

The U.S. Fish and Wildlife Service
Department of the Interior

1849 C Street NW
Washington DC 20240
Email: Contact@fws.gov
           (see FAQ before using email)
Website: http://www.fws.gov/

This United States agency website provides excellent information the on best fishing holes, conserving wildlife, and a variety of links to related organizations.

BIBLIOGRAPHY

Cecotti, F. (1982) Electronic fishing reels: A fishing reel for the severely disabled. *Sports 'n Spokes* 8(2):18-19.

Chapter 13

Fitness Programming

ACTIVITY OVERVIEW

Within the last few years greater attention has been placed on physical fitness and physical activity levels of United States citizens by the federal government. The Surgeon General's Report of 1996 was one of the most important policy statements regarding physical fitness and physical activity released by the United States Government. The statement definitively linked physical activity to numerous health improvements. It also identified physical inactivity as one of the four major causes of cardiovascular disease and linked it to many other health disorders. Physical activity and acceptable levels of physical fitness greatly reduces the risk of dying from coronary heart disease and reduces the risk of developing diabetes, hypertension, and colon cancer: enhances mental health; fosters healthy muscles, bones and joints; and helps maintain function and preserve independence in older adults. Health related physical fitness refers to having appropriate levels of aerobic capacity, muscular strength, muscular endurance, joint flexibility, and body composition.

Healthy People 2000 and Healthy People 2010 are also ambitious governmental policy statements that set specific goals for physical activity and reduction of obesity in the American population.

Physical inactivity is pervasive in our society as over 60 percent of American adults are not regularly active. This percentage is no doubt increased for people with disabilities due to lack of access to programs and opportunities for physical activity. People with disabilities have increased health concerns and susceptibility to secondary conditions. Having a long-term condition increases the need for health promotion that can be medical, physical, social, emotional, or societal. It is important that we promote the health of people with disabilities, prevent secondary conditions, and eliminate disparities between people with and without disabilities in the U.S. population. People who have activity limitations report having had more days of pain, depression, anxiety, and sleeplessness and fewer days of vitality during the previous month than people not reporting activity limitations. Many health clubs throughout the United States are now opening their doors to people with disabilities and accommodating their specific needs (Figure 13.1 a and b).

Until recently the medical system in the United States has been one of the treatment of disease as opposed to a more proactive approach of prevention of diseases. Billions of dollars are being used on disease treatment while a far less amount is being used for disease prevention. If more emphasis were placed on disease prevention (as advocated by the Surgeon General's Report and Healthy People 2010) health care costs in this country would show a dramatic decline. Rehabilitation has traditionally been specific to treatment (prevention or correction of a problem), physical restoration, therapy, self-help skills, and vocational education (Saari, 1981). Recreation offered by rehabilitation programs to supplement treatment has involved such things as hobby and crafts. With the surge of interest in sports and recreation, professionals began including sports- and recreation-oriented fitness exercises in individual rehabilitation programs. This chapter is included in this book to reinforce the Surgeon General's Report and Health People 2010, and because a certain level of fitness is required for successful participation in many of the activities presented in this book.

Studies continue to report the decline of physical fitness of our nondisabled youth due to inactivity and poor diet. Although studies with youths who have disabilities are less frequent, data indicates that they run a greater risk at have lower levels of fitness due to sedentary living and a lack of access to activities that may improve fitness. Winnick and Short (1982) have long reported that sensory and orthopedically impaired youth are significantly behind the nondisabled in many fitness measurements. Although improved fitness is important to these individuals for health and physical performance, it may also boost social and emotional development. It can be assumed that those who do have attain appropriate levels of physical fitness will be less likely to participate in potentially beneficial physical activities.

For individuals who have acquired disabilities and whose rehabilitation periods are over, maintenance of physical fitness is critical. Curtis et al. (1986) reported fewer physician visits and trends toward fewer complications and fewer rehospitalizations by spinal-cord injured athletes compared to their non-athlete counterparts.

Disease Prevention

Since 1970 a greater percentage of Americans have assumed more responsibility for their own health care and for their families. This movement towards greater individual responsibility range from regular exercise and proper diets to personally monitoring temperature, pulse, and blood pressure. Many businesses have opened health fitness facilities on-sight for their employees or have included health club membership as part of their incentive packages. The emergence of Health Maintenance Organizations (HMO's) with the emphasis on prevention of disease has yet to see the impact that was anticipated. The government has finally taken a more active role with their policy statements including the Surgeon General's Report and Health People 2010. Litigation towards tobacco companies have attempted to put pressure on these groups to pay some of the cost for the lives they have destroyed through the use of their deadly products. In the final say however, it will be each individual's personal decision as to their own diet and exercise routine and whether they choose to smoke or not.

The role of physical education and health education programs in our schools is critical for helping people make wise decisions. Children with and without disabilities will likely to be more active as adults if they are more active as children. They are more likely to be physically fit as adults if they were physically fit as children. They will be more likely as adults to engage in regular physical activity as adults if they have developed the critical skills needed for participation during their physical education classes as children. Physical education and health classes

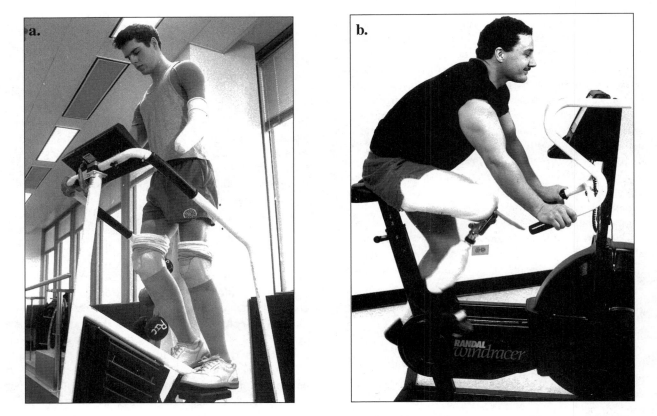

Figure 13.1 a and b. Stepping machines and stationery bikes are commonly found in most fitness programs. (Courtesy of Rehabilitation Institute of Chicago's Wirtz Sports Program and Oscar Izquierdo)

should not be viewed as "extra" classes or as a time for the teachers break. They should be viewed as disease prevention classes that will have a dramatic impact on the quality and productivity of lives. Physical education teachers and programs must be given the support they need to implement quality programs and they should be held to high standards once this support is established. Physical activity must be taught to be a normal part of every day life. Typical sedentary habits can be easily eliminated with awareness and education. Autoholics must leave the car in the driveway and have their children walk the one block to school. Parents may wish to walk with their children if concerned about safety. Individuals should park farther away from work to gain benefits from the walk. Stairs should be taken instead of elevators. These simple changes in habit can potentially serve to increase levels of fitness to a moderate level. Those who exercise to a greater degree will enjoy greater benefits. Sedentary habits are learned during childhood. Once learned, the ability to change is more difficult.

Individualized Exercise Programs

Individualized exercise programs for people with and without disabilities have enjoyed great popularity during the past three decades. Workouts reflect an individual's interests, disability, restrictions, time, equipment, and transportation options.

The choice of activity (jogging, swimming, aerobics, weight training, gardening) determines the type of exercise and routine. It is critical to choose an activity that is enjoyable to keep interest and motivation at high levels. Issues of specificity (intensity, duration, frequency, progression, and consistency), and the need for strength, power, endurance, and flexibility will depend on the activity and the participant. All exercise programs should be reviewed with a personal physician for modification and approval and should include regular stretching and flexibility procedures. This can reduce the risk of injury, enhance performance, and increase overall range of motion.

Nutrition

Without a doubt, American citizens are probably one of the most malnourished societies in the world. Our population is generally overweight due to lack of physical activity and reliance on over eating and fast foods high in fat content. Nutrition is the study of how consumed carbohydrates, fats, proteins, water, vitamins, and minerals provide the necessary energy to maintain body functions both at rest and during physical activity . Nutrition involves the proper balance of these six classes of nutrients. Attention to exercise without equal attention to nutrition will limit the benefits derived from a program. Consult a physician or nutrition specialist if necessary.

PROGRAM RESOURCES

Much information is available for starting and maintaining a fitness program. Organizations such as the National Strength and Conditioning Association (NSCA) and the American College of Sports Medicine (ACSM) are two such examples of excellent resources.

The National Strength and Conditioning Association

Founded in 1978, the National Strength and Conditioning Association (NSCA), is a non-profit, worldwide authority on strength and conditioning for improved physical and athletic performance. The National Strength and Conditioning Association (NSCA) facilitates a professional exchange of ideas in strength development as it relates to the improvement of athletic performance and fitness. The NSCA also provides its members with a wide variety of resources including professional journals, conferences, scholarship and grant opportunities, and educational texts and videos. A listing of specific articles related to strength and conditioning for a wide variety of disabilities can also be accessed from this organization.

American College of Sports Medicine (ACSM)

The American College of Sports Medicine is another excellent resource for information on maintaining and enhancing physical performance, fitness, health, and quality of life. Articles may be accessed on physical fitness for children and adults with cerebral palsy.

Disabled Fitness Programs

A number of programs across the country have begun to place more emphasis on fitness for specific disability groups. Lasko-McCarthey and Aufsesser (1990) outline very specific suggestions for the establishment of community-based fitness programs for adults with physical disabilities. Assessment forms and training routines used within the San Diego University based program are used as examples. Community-based fitness programs have also been established at Arizona State University, New Jersey's Kessler Institute for Rehabilitation, the YMCA of Eugene, Oregon, and the Center for Health and Fitness at the Rehabilitation Institute of Chicago (Figure 13.2 a and b), to name a few.

The interest in providing exercise options for people with disabilities has even extended to programs like the American Heart Association's *Jump Rope for Heart*. Lavay and Horvat (1991) suggest that with a few modifications, jumping rope can benefit children with disabilities as much as it does their nondisabled peers. With the wide variety of disabilities and health conditions, specific fitness and exercise programming is critical.

Many national associations have developed fitness material for their members. The Multiple Sclerosis Society offers printed material in addition to fitness videos. The United States Cerebral Palsy Research and Education Foundation has developed a set of exercise principles and guidelines. Most of the established disability sport organizations have also produced fitness information for their members including Disabled Sports-USA.

Since 1990, Disabled Sports USA has presented adapted fitness workshops for health care and fitness professionals. More than 800 professionals, including personal trainers, fitness instructors; occupational, physical and recreation therapists; and adapted physical education teachers have been trained in adaptations of aerobic, resistance and strength exercises for people with physical disabilities. The primary goal of the workshop is to increase the availability of exercise instruction for people with physical disabilities. Disabled Sports-USA has also produced a series of videotapes that present aerobics, strength and flexibility exercises for individuals with paraplegia, quadriplegia, cerebral palsy and amputations.

Disabled Sports-USA has also established regional workshops in which individuals can be certified to teach these specially designed exercise programs. Presently, one-day adapted fitness workshops are available on a contractual basis. Any workshops offering enrollment to the general public are posted on their website. Refer to the resource listing at the end of this chapter for more information.

Orthotic & Prosthetic Athletic Fund

The Orthotic & Prosthetic Athletic Fund supports year-round fitness and education programs that enable persons with disabilities to enjoy the rewards of physical fitness, social interaction, and personal achievement. The O&P Athletic Fund exists for the O&P profession and the individuals it serves. The Fit for Life initiative for older patients and others who may not want to participate in demanding aerobic exercise activities. This fitness pro-

gram focuses on golf, a lifetime sport that can be enjoyed by disabled persons of all ages and abilities. Programs for juniors have also been instituted to help young children with amputations to become physically active and fit.

Special Olympics Conditioning

Special Olympics has always been concerned about the fitness of its athletes. Some events, primarily distance events, can harm an athlete who has not completed a proper conditioning program. To reduce these risks, many Special Olympic programs require certificates of training from coaches before athletes are allowed to enter certain events. In conjunction with the National Strength and Conditioning Association (NSCA), SOI has published *Total Conditioning for the Special Olympian* for coaches.

Special Olympics is the only disability sports organization that offers fitness events as part of its official activities. Various fitness events including modified push-ups, sit-ups, and exercycle (riding a stationing bicycle one-kilometer for time). One-arm and two-arm curls and chin-ups are offered under powerlifting competition.

Exercise Videos

Many exercise videos are now available for individuals with disabilities. While we have listed names and addresses where these may be purchased at the end of the chapter, we caution our readers to be selective in their choice of videos. The qualifications of consultants or celebrities should be investigated.

SPECIALIZED EQUIPMENT

Typically, little specialized equipment will be necessary to begin and maintain a fitness program. Changes in lifestyle such as increased walking and dietary changes can have dramatic improvement on ones health. Some specific equipment is available for those with disabilities.

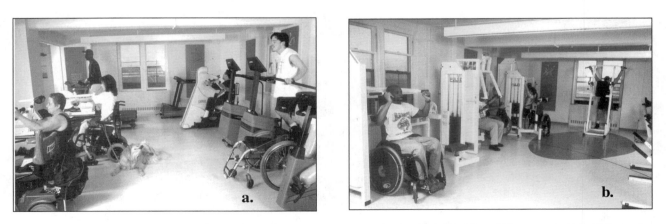

Figure 13.2 a and b. Community-based fitness programs such as the one at the Center for Health and Fitness at the Rehabilitation Institute of Chicago offer programming for individuals with and without disabilities. (Courtesy of Chicago's Wirtz Sports Program)

Ergometers

Designed for individuals requiring the use of wheelchairs, ergometers allow the person with a physical disability to improve upper body strength and aerobic capacity. Various models are available by the manufacturers listed in this chapter, including table and floor models, and models that are adapted for wheelchair users (Figure 13.3 a). The Saratoga Cycle offers a quick release interchangeable hand grip to suit individuals with varying degrees of hand function (Figure 13.3 b-d. The MotoMed Viva allows individuals to passively work their lower extremities. It is a motorized movement trainer that allows passive, active and active-assist exercise. Certain models combine upper and lower extremity exercise in one machine such as the SCIFIT Power trainer (Figure 13.4 a and b). While the upper extremities are at work, the lower extremities are stabilized by support boots and are moving passively at the same ratio.

Wheelchair Ergometers

Similar in concept to arm ergometers, the wheelchair ergometer accurately simulates normal wheelchair wheeling while stationary.

Wheelchair Rollers

Similar to a treadmill for individuals who are ambulatory, the wheelchair roller offers a popular way to train indoors (Figure 13.5). The wheelchair is placed securely on top of one or two steel rollers while the individual practices free wheeling or endurance training. This device also allows the coach to video tape the athlete and to make adjustments in stroke mechanics.

Upright Exercisers

The EasyStand 6000 Glider distributed by Altimate Medical provides dynamic leg motion for individuals who are unable to stand upright or walk on their own. The ergonomically designed glider handles are linked allowing one leg to move forward while the other moves

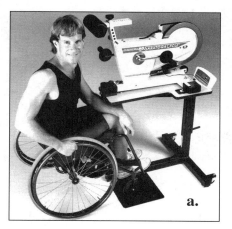

Figure 13.3 a. The Saratoga Cycle is one of the most popular pieces of fitness equipment used in disabled fitness programs. A specially designed table and stand provides easy access for wheelchair users. (Courtesy of Saratoga Access and Fitness, Inc.)

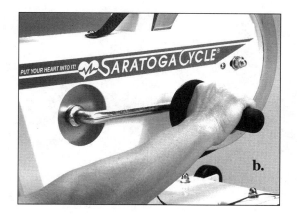

Figure 13.3 b-d. A quick release interchangeable hand grip system allows individuals with various degrees of hand function to use the Saratoga Cycle: (a) standard hand grips, (b) adjustable-loop hand grips, (c) limited-grasp hand grips, (d) grip cuffs. (Courtesy of Saratoga Access and Fitness, Inc.)

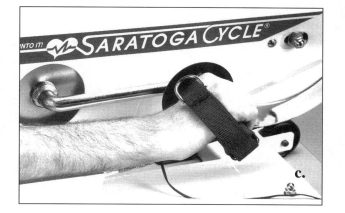

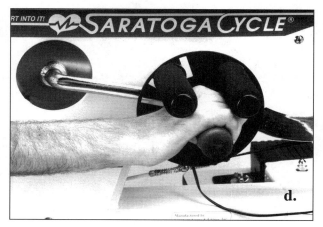

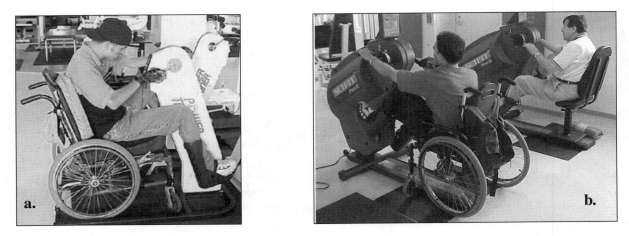

Figure 13.4 a and b. The SCIFIT Power Trainer (a) and the SCIFIT Pro II (b) combine arm and leg action in one machine. (Rehabilitation Institute of Chicago's Center for Health and Fitness)

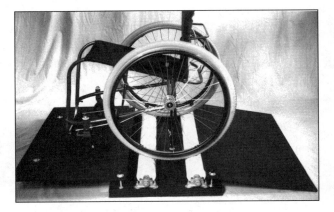

Figure 13.5. Wheelchair rollers are today's wheelchair treadmill. (Courtesy of Magic in Motion)

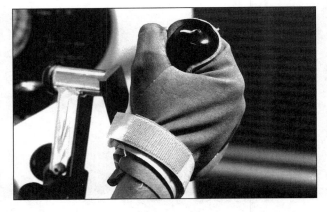

Figure 13.6 a. Commercially made activity mitts assist many individuals in using hand-activated fitness equipment. (Courtesy of Rehabilitation Institute of Chicago's Wirtz Sports Program, Oscar Izquierdo and Patton Enterprises)

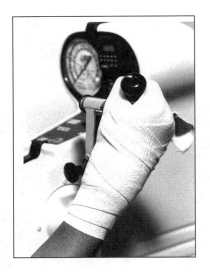

Figure 13.6 b. Ace bandages are effective when activity mitts are not available. (Courtesy of Rehabilitation Institute of Chicago's Wirtz Sports Program and Oscar Izquierdo)

back. The geometric design of the leg support system prevents vertical shearing while legs are in motion. With its adjustable resistance, users can enjoy a mild or vigorous workout while enhancing the therapeutic benefits of standing.

Activity Mitts

Individuals with limited hand function use a variety of means to participate. Activity mitts or medical gloves are used with free weight or exercise machines (Figure 13.6 a). Another effective technique is to wrap an ace bandage to secure the hand to the apparatus (Figure 13.6 b).

Wheelchair Fitness Trail

Fitness trails have been popular for people without disabilities for some time, but many are not accessible to those with physical disabilities. A fitness trail for wheelchair users can be set up in a space as small as 100 feet by 100 feet. The trail can consist of 10 or more exercise stations with instructions at each station.

EQUIPMENT SUPPLIERS

The number of reputable weight training equipment suppliers is tremendous. The following is a sample of some of these companies and is not meant to be inclusive. See additional equipment in the Weight Training chapter.

Ergometers

Access To Recreation
8 Sandra Court
Newbury Park CA 91320
(800) 634-4351
(805) 498-7535
(805) 498-8186 (fax)
Email: dkrebs@gte.net
Website: http://www.accesstr.com

CYBEX International, Inc.
10 Trotter Drive
Medway, MA 02053
(508) 533-4300
(508) 533-5500 (fax)
Email: info@cybexintl.com
Website: http://www.cybexintl.com

Endorphin Corporation
6901 90th Avenue North
Pinellas Park, Florida 33782
(800) 940-9844
(727) 545-9848
(727) 546-0613 (fax)
Email: endorph@gte.net
Website: http://www.endorphin.net

Flaghouse Rehab
601 Flaghouse Drive
Hasbrouck Heights, NJ 07604-3116
(800) 793-7900
(800) 793-7922 (fax)
Email: sales@flaghouse.com
Website: http://www.flaghouse.com/

Great Lakes Medical
Website: http://www.motomed.com/
(888) 843-8480

Invacare Corporation
One Invacare Way
P.O. Box 4028
Elyria, OH 44036-2125

(800) 333-6900
Website: http://www.invacare.com/

No Boundaries
12882 Valley View Street #5
Garden Grove CA 92845
(800) 926-8637
(714-) 91-5899
(714) 891-0658 (fax)
Website: http://www.powertrainer.com/

Saratoga Access and Fitness, Inc.
PO Box 1427
Fort Collins, Colorado 80522-1427
(800) 474-4010
(970) 484-4010
(970) 484-4092 (fax)
Email: adegraff@saratoga-intl.com
Website: http://www.saratoga-intl.com/

SCIFIT, Inc.
5616A. S.122nd E. Ave.
Tulsa, OK 74143
(800) 278-3933
(918) 254-4189 (fax)
Email: scifit@busprod.com
Website: http://www.scifit.com/

Therapeutic Alliances Inc.
333 North Broad Street
Fairborn, Ohio 45324
(937) 879-0734
(937) 879-5211 (fax)
Email: TAIinfo@aol.com
Website: http://www.musclepower.com/

Easy Stand Glider

Altimate Medical Inc.
P.O. 180, 262 W. 1st St.
Morton, MN 56270
(800) 342-8968
(507) 697-6393
(507) 697-6900 (fax)
Email: info@easystand.com
Website: http://www.altimatemedical.com/

Activity Mitts

Abilitations/Sportime
One Sportime Way
Atlanta, GA 30340-1402
(800) 850-8603

Access To Recreation
(see above)

Exercise Tubing

M-F Athletic Company
11 Amflex Drive
P.O. Box 8090
Cranston, RI 02920-0090
(800) 556-7464
(800) 682-6950 (fax)
Email: mfathletic@mfathletic.com
Website: http://www.mfathletic.com/

Other Cardio Equipment

Nu Step
Life Plus, Inc.
3770 Plaza Drive, S1
Ann Arbor, MI 48108-1654
(800) 322-2209
(313) 769-8180 (fax)

Thera-band

Micro Bio-Medics Inc.
(800) 713-8388
Website: http://www.microbiomedics.com
Check website or call for closest regional office.

Fitness Videos

Aerobics for Quadriplegia, Aerobics for Cerebral Palsy, Aerobics for Paraplegia, Aerobics for Amputees
Disabled Sports-USA (see address above)

Armchair Fitness
CC-M Productions
8512 Cedar Street
Silver Spring, MD 20910
(800) 453-6280
(301) 585-2321
Email: cc-m@cc-m.com,
Website: http://www.cc-m.com/fitness.html
Armchair Fitness is series of 4 videos for people who limit vigorous activity because of preference, lifestyle, age, or disability. Featuring a complete fitness program, each video is designed with advice from physical educators and therapists.

Chair Dancing International
2658 Del Mar Heights Rd.
Del Mar, CA 92014
800-551-4FUW
Website: http:// www.chairdancing.com
Chair Dancing International distributes a 3 part Chair Dancing series. Chair Dancing, Chair Dancing Around the World, Sit Down and Tune Up

Fitness For All
SJD Inc.

PMB 331
8895 Towne Centre Dr., Ste. 105
San Diego, CA 97122
(619) 558-1105
Email: bonnie@sjd.com
Website: http://www.sjd.com/bva.htm

Keep Fit While You Sit
Amputee Coalition of America
(888) AMP-KNOW

Lisa Erickson's Seated Aerobic Workout
Accent in Living
(800) 787-8444

ROM Institute
3601 Memorial Dr.
Madison, WI 53704
(800) 488-4940
ROM Dance: A range of motion exercise and relaxation program.

Seat-A-Robes
TherEd Resources
(800) 610-4278
Email: thered@rcanect.net
Website: http://www.advancedrehabtherapy.com

Sit and Be Fit
Karen and Mark Wilson
10201 North 58th Place
Scottsdale, AZ 85253
(602) 998-8455

Thera-Fit While You Sit
Sportime
(800) 850-8602

ADDITIONAL RESOURCES AND WEBSITES

The Aerobics and Fitness Association of America
15250 Ventura Blvd., Suite 200
Sherman Oaks, CA, 91403-3297
(877) 968-2639
(818) 788-6301 (fax)
Website: http://www.afaa.com
The Aerobics and Fitness Association of America, founded in 1983 is the world's largest fitness educator. AFAA produces a wide variety of educational materials including a journal, textbooks, reference manuals and videos.

American College of Sports Medicine (ACSM)
401 W. Michigan St., Indianapolis, IN 46202-3233
(317) 637-9200
(317) 634-7817 (fax)
Website: http://www.acsm.org/

American Council on Exercise
5820 Oberlin Drive, Suite 102
San Diego, CA 92121-3787
(858) 535-8227
(858) 535-1778 (fax)
Website: http://www.acefitness.org/

The American Council on Exercise (ACE) is a non-profit organization committed to promoting active, healthy lifestyles and their positive effects on the mind, body and spirit. ACE pledges to enable all segments of society to enjoy the benefits of physical activity and protect the public against unsafe and ineffective fitness products and trends. ACE accomplishes this mission by setting certification and education standards for fitness instructors and through ongoing public education about the importance of exercise.

The American Orthotic and Prosthetic Association
O & P Almanac
P.O. Box 18052
Merrifield, VA 22118-0052

Keeping Fit: Resources for Active Living is a 16-page, full color booklet with information about aerobics, weight training, swimming, jogging, and other activities to maintain healthy living.

American Running Association (ARA)
4405 East West Highway, Suite 405
Bethesda, MD 20814
(301) 913-9517
(800) 776-2732
(301) 913-9520 (fax)
Email: run@americanrunning.org
Website: http://www.americanrunning.org/

The American Running Association (formerly the American Running and Fitness Association) is a non-profit, educational organization dedicated to providing educational support to runners through programs and sound information on training, nutrition, and injury prevention, treatment, and rehabilitation.

Disabled Sports USA (Fitness Department)
451 Hungerford Drive Suite 100
Rockville, MD 20850
(301) 217-0968 (fax)
(301) 217-0963 (TDD)
(301) 217-9839

Email: programs@dsusa.org
Website: http://www.dsusa.org/

Healthy People 2010
Website: http://www.health.gov/healthypeople/

This website provided information on all the goals and objectives of Healthy People 2010.

National Center on Physical Activity and Disability (NCPAD)
University of Illinois-Chicago
1640 W. Roosevelt Rd.
Chicago, IL 60608-6904
(800) 900-8086 (voice and tty)
Email: ncpad@uic.edu
Website: http://www.ncpad.org

NCPAD is a national information center funded by the Centers for Disease Control (CDC) and prevention, and operated by the University of Illinois-Chicago, The Rehabilitation Institute of Chicago (RIC), and the National Center on Accessibility (NCA). NCPAD has a variety of print material available on a wide range of health-related and sport topics.

National Strength and Conditioning Association
1955 N. Union Blvd.
Colorado Springs, CO 80909
(719) 632-6722
(800) 815-6826
(719) 632-6367 (fax)
Email: nsca@nsca-lift.org
Website: http://www.nsca-lift.org/

O&P Athletic Fund Inc.
1650 King St., Suite 500
Alexandria, VA 22314
(703) 836-7116, ext. 3007
(703) 836-0838 (fax)
Email: opaaf@opoffice.org
Website: http://www.oandp.com/resources/sports/opaaf/

PE4U
The PE4U website offers dozens of links to exceptional websites relate to health and fitness issues
Website: http://www.pelinks4u.org

Other Resources

Disability Mall
Disability mall is an online resource that features many companies that provide exercise equipment as well as other products for individuals with disabilities
Website: http://www.medmarket.com

Professional American Academy of Health, Fitness & Rehabilitation
The Medical Exercise Specialist
Website: http://www.medicalexercisespecialist.com

The Medical exercise Specialist is an excellent publication with articles related to fitness and weight training for people with disabilities.

Turnstep.Com
Website: http://www.turnstep.com/

This website provides articles and advice for integrating all people into your aerobics classes, regardless of ability or disability.

BIBLIOGRAPHY

American College of Sports Medicine (1997). *Exercise Management for Persons with Chronic Disease and Disabilities*. Champaign, IL:Human Kinetics.

Healthy People 2010- Conference Edition Chapter 6, November 30, 1999.

Lockette, K.F. and Keyes, A.M. (1994). *Conditioning with Physical Disabilities*. Champaign, IL: Human Kinetics.

Miller, P. (ed) (1995). *Fitness programming and physical disability*. Champaign, IL: Human Kinetics.

Rimmer, J. (1994). *Fitness and rehabilitation programs for special populations*. Madison, WI: Brown & Benchmark.

United States Department of Health and Human Services (1996). *Physical Activity and Health: A Report of the Surgeon General*.

Saltin, B., Boushel, R., Secher, N., & Mitchell, J. (2000). *Exercise and Circulation in Health and Disease*. Champaign, IL: Human Kinetics.

Seaman, J. (1995) ed. *Physical Best and Individuals with Disabilities*. The American Alliance for Health, Physical Education, Recreation and Dance: Reston:VA.

Winnick, J.P. and Short, F.X. (1999). *The Brockport Physical Fitness Test Manual*. Champaign, IL: Human Kinetics.

Chapter 14

Flying

SPORT GOVERNING BODIES:
National: Federal Aviation Administration (FAA)
International:

DISABLED SPORTS ORGANIZATION:
National: Freedom's Wings International
International: The American Wheelchair Pilots Association

PRIMARY DISABILITY: Individuals with physical/sensory disabilities

SPORT OVERVIEW

Technological advancements have made it possible for thousands of individuals with disabilities to fly. The persistence of individuals with disabilities who want to fly and the impact of advocacy organizations that promote flying for the disabled have boosted the number of disabled flyers over the past 20 years.

This chapter will focus on gliders or sail planes, ultralights, and standard motor-powered aircraft to provide a variety of references for these air vehicles.

ORGANIZED EFFORT

As with most of the sports discussed in this book, flying has several interest groups that concentrate on "spreading the word," and assisting individuals with disabilities in their quest to fly. Providing access to FAA-certified instructors and finding adapted equipment and hand-controlled aircraft are key functions of Freedom's Wings International (Figure 14.1), a New Jersey-based group to which most hand-control glider pilots belong.

International Wheelchair Aviators (IWA), formerly The California Wheelchair Aviators (CWA), comprises a group of pilots from throughout California and the United States that sponsors monthly fly-ins at different airports around the country.

Other groups involved in providing flying opportunities for people with disabilities include The Canadian Paraplegic Association, The Soaring Society of America,

and The American Wheelchair Pilots Association. Addresses for these organizations, equipment suppliers, and flight schools with hand-controlled aircraft can be found in Additional Resources.

TYPES OF AIRCRAFT

Gliders

Hand-controlled gliders that do not need rudder pedals have not always been as prevalent as they are today. An extensive period of trial and error and equipment modifications were required before the FAA approved hand controls that could safely replace foot-operated pedals. Hand controls have made it possible for thousands of mobility-impaired individuals to operate gliders.

Ultralights

Ultralights are a special class of lightweight, primarily single-occupant, air sport vehicles recognized by the FAA (Figure 14.2 a and b). Operating the low-cost ultralights requires neither a license nor a medical examination, making them popular with individuals with and without disabilities. Design features include fixed seats, a single joy stick flight control (no need for rudder pedals), and an engine and pull starter well within reach of the seated pilot. These features are ideal for pilots with mobility impairments. Extra instrumentation, rear brakes, parachutes that will bring down both pilot and ultralight, and either pontoons or wheels can be added).

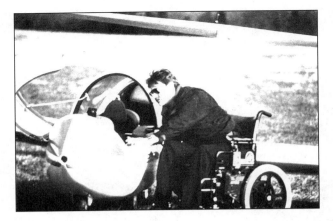

Figure 14.1. The New Jersey based group Freedom's Wings International specializes in opportunities with hand-controlled gliders. (Courtesy of *Sports 'n Spokes* 5/93:43)

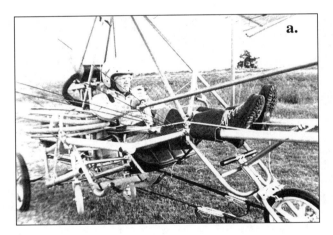

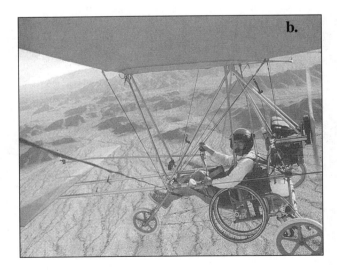

Figure 14.2 a and b. Ultralights are low-cost alternatives to flying for many, including people with disabilities. (Courtesy of *Sports 'n Spokes* 11/83:17 and 23/7: 62)

Motor-Powered Aircraft

For many years physical standards for licensing have prevented individuals with physical disabilities from becoming pilots. Numerous individuals with disabilities have fought for the opportunity to fly aircraft. Rulings in the late 1970s led to FAA approval and increased use of hand controls in motor-powered aircraft. Rings can be added to existing controls, or a complete set of hand controls can be installed for individuals with lower extremity disabilities (Figure 14.3).

EQUIPMENT SUPPLIERS

Hand Controls

Aero Haven, Inc
P.O. Box 2799
Big Bear City, CA 92314
(909) 585-9663

A.R. Allen
2252 Barbara Dr.
Clearwater, FL 33546
(813) 535-1153

Aircraft Inspection & Maintenance
2680 East Wardlow Rd.
Long Beach, CA 90807
(213) 595-5738

Charles City Aeromatic
Charles City, IA
(515) 228-3553

Union Aviation Hand Control
Union Aviation, Inc.

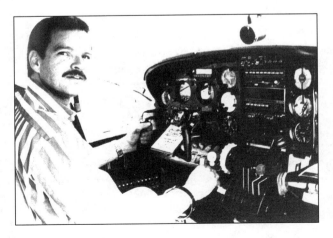

Figure 14.3. The FAA has approved various types of hand controls for motor-powered aircraft. (Courtesy of *Sports 'n Spokes* 7/90:65)

Sturgis Airport
P.O. Box 207
Sturgis, KY 42459
(270) 333-5633

Driving Ring
Hosmer-Dorrance Corp.
561 Division St.
P.O. Box 37
Campbell, CA 95008
(408) 379-5151

Ultralights

Dan Buchanan
333018 Anzara St.
Union City, CA 94587

Pterodactyl, Ltd.
P.O. Box 191
Watsonville, CA 95076

ADDITIONAL RESOURCES AND WEBSITES

At this time, the number of websites related to flying for individuals with disabilities is limited. By accessing the following sites, readers will have links to most other sites. Most participants will find the following sites satisfactory for gathering information.

Flight schools with hand-controlled aircraft

Aero Haven Aviation
Big Bear City, CA
(909) 585-9663

Charles City Aeronautics
Charles City, IA 50616
(515) 228-3553

Double Eagle Aviation
6961 South Apron Dr.
Tucson, AZ 85706
(520) 294-8214
Website: http://www.2-eagle.com

Flying Nunn's Aviation
Clinton County Airport
10 A Airport Rd.
Plattsburgh, NY 12901
(518) 561-3822

Lucky Mindy Aviation
Litchfield, MN
(612) 485-3454

Flying Organizations

Aircraft Owners & Pilots Association (AOPA)
421 Aviation Way
Frederick, MD 21701-4798
(800) USA-AOPA
(301) 695-2000
(301) 695-2375 (fax)
Website: http://www.aopa.org

American Wheelchair Pilots Association (AWPA)
c/o Dave Graham
1621 East Second Ave.
Mesa, AZ 85204
(602) 831-4262

Federal Aviation Administration (FAA)
National Headquarters
Flight Standards Service
800 Independence Ave., SW
Washington, DC 20591
(202) 267-8441
Website: http://www.faa.gov

Challenge Air
Love Field Airport - North Concourse
8008 Cedar Springs Rd., N106-LB24
Dallas, Texas 75235
(214) 351-3353
(214) 351-4565 (fax)
Website: http://www.challengeair.com
Challenge Air for Kids and Friends, a not-for-profit organization, joins with communities and families to host exciting special events nationwide, where we inspire physically challenged and seriously ill children and young adults by providing the opportunity to fly in small airplanes piloted by both wheelchair and non-wheelchair aviators.

Experimental Aircraft Association
EAA Aviation Center
3000 Poberezny Road
Oshkosh, WI 54903-3086
(920) 426-4800
Website: http://www.eaa.org

International Wheelchair Aviators (IWA)
Big Bear Airport
500 W. Meadow Lane
P.O. Box 2799
Big Bear City, CA 92314
(909) 585-9663
(909) 585-7156
Email: aero.haven@bigbear.com
Website: http://www.aerohaven.com

Gliders/Sail Planes

Canadian Paraplegic Assoc.
c/o David Byers
520 Sutherland Dr.
Toronto, Ontario M4K 2J8
Canada
(416) 422-5644
(416) 422-5943 (fax)

Freedom's Wings International
Ray Temchus
1832 Lake Ave.
Scotch Plains, NJ 07076
(908) 232-6354
Email: raydt@earthlink.net
Website: http://www.freedomswings.org

Sky Sailing
31930 Highway 79
Warner Springs, CA 92086
(760) 782-0404
(760) 782-9251 (fax)
Email: soar@skysailing.com
Website: http://www.skysailing.com

The Soaring Society of America, Inc.
P.O. Box 2100
Hobbs, NM 88241-2100
(505) 392-1177
(505) 392-8154 (fax)
Website: http://www.ssa.org

U.S. Hang Gliding Association
559 E. Pitco Peak Ave., Ste. 101
Colorado Springs, CO 80903
(719) 632-8300

Ultralights

Bob Busic
3215 University St.
Memphis, TN 38127
(901) 357-7384

Beneficial Design, Inc.
5858 Empire Grade Rd.
Santa Cruz, CA 95062
(408) 429-8447

Freedom Flyers, Inc.
c/o Gary Vicks
P.O. Box 479
2802 Singleton St.
Rowlett, TX 75088
(214) 475-8870

Lookout Mountain Flight Park
P.O. Box 273
Lookout Mountain, TN 37350
(800) 688-LMFP
Email: airwave@voy.net
Website: http://www.hanglide.com

Tennessee Air Cooperative, Inc.
c/o Bob Busic
3215 University St.
Memphis, TN 38127
(901) 357-7384
(901) 725-5349

DFE Ultralights, Inc.
Box 185
Vanderbilt, PA 15486
(412) 529-0450
(412) 529-0596 (fax)

Videos

How to Fly with a Hand Control
A Look Back at IWA
Both videos are available from:
International Wheelchair Aviators
Big Bear Airport
500 W. Meadow Lane
P.O. Box 2799
Big Bear City, CA 92314
(909) 585-9663
(909) 585-7156 (fax)
Email: aero.haven@bigbear.com
Website: http://www.aerohaven.com

Chapter 15

Football

SPORT NATIONAL GOVERNING BODIES:
National: NCAA or Your Local State High School Football Association

Official Sport Of: _____DAAA   _____USABA   _____USCPAA
                             _____DS/USA   __x__USADSF   _____WS/USA
                             __*__SOI
*prohibited

DISABLED SPORTS ORGANIZATION:
National:
International:

PRIMARY DISABILITY: Amputee, Blind, Cerebral Palsy, Deaf, Les Autres,
Spinal Cord-Injured

SPORT OVERVIEW

Football is a popular competitive and recreational sport that can be easily modified whenever enough interested players are available. Various versions of the game are played including tackle, touch, flag, and wheelchair football. The fact that the game can be played inside or outside by people using either manual or power chairs makes it a popular choice for adapted physical education or competitive sport experiences. The amount of aggressiveness allowed during a game is up to the competitors to determine before the game begins. Some players like to play very rough although in most cases it is technically a "touch" game.

SPORT ORIGIN

Football for individuals with disabilities can be considered a fledging sport in terms of organizational structure. Individual teams are located throughout the country but without a true national governing body, the sport has been slow to develop, although traditional tackle football has been played by the deaf for over 100 years. The development of the football huddle is credited to Paul Hubbard, a deaf quarterback at Gallaudet University from 1892-1895. Hubbard did not want his sign language signals intercepted by the defense, so he devised a strategy to shield the signals by having the players turn their backs to the one of scrimmage a few yards away. Players could then communicate freely without fear of giving away their plans. Football clubs around the nation then adopted the huddle.

Wheelchair Football

Although not nearly as popular as wheelchair basketball or wheelchair rugby, wheelchair football has been organized since 1948 when it began at the University of Illinois (Hamilton, 1990). Rule modifications vary from league to league and situation to situation. A rugged, highly maneuverable wheelchair is desirable for individuals wishing to play this sport.

The Recreation Department of Santa Barbara, California is well known for its leadership in the sport as they conduct an annual football tournament attracting teams from around the country (Figure 15.1 a and b). Known as *The Blister Bowl*, the competition allows some rule modifications although a regulation ball is used. Teams consist of 6 players (including at least one female and one quadriplegic athlete) using a 60x22-yard hard surface playing field divided into 15-yard segments. End zones are eight yards long (Figure 15.2).

Other events are beginning to be organized throughout the country. For instance, The Warm Springs Sports Program in San Antonio has sponsored a "Spoke Bender Bowl" for many years. The annual event brings teams together from all over Texas.

The game consists of four 15-minute quarters. Play is started from the 15-yard line with the "kicking" team throwing the ball downfield to simulate a kick. Players advance the ball by the quarterback handing off for running plays or passing the ball downfield (all players are eligible receivers). A first down is achieved after passing the 15-yard marker line and two-hand touch tackles are used.

Touchdowns count as 6 points with extra points being taken from the 3-yard line. Extra points are earned by running (2 points) or by passing (1 point).

Universal Wheelchair Football Association (UWFA)

Recently, individuals in the Cincinnati area have attempted to provide a greater organizational structure to the game and have developed greatly modified and flexible rules that allow participation for all abilities. Played since 1991 by Northern Kentucky Wheelchair Sports, in 1997 the Universal Wheelchair Football Association (UWFA) was formed to promote the sport on an international level. In 1998, the Cincinnati Recreation Commission formed Greater Cincinnati Wheelchair Sports (GCWS) to unite the areas various wheelchair-sports groups. The wheelchair-football team is a GCWS member and now uses that name, in addition to being UWFA headquarters. The rules used by the UWFA are quite different than the Blister Bowl but they demonstrate some of the many variations of the game. While variations of wheelchair football have been played throughout the United States for over twenty years, the Universal Wheelchair Football Association (UWFA) strives to promote a version of the game that allows individuals with all types and levels of disability to actively participate.

Unlike the Blister Bowl which is portrayed as a sport that only the craziest paraplegics would play—the UWFA version can be just as wild but can also be played by quadriplegics (including ventilator dependent quads), and virtually all levels in between, including individuals who are blind, amputees, and those who have multiple sclerosis, cerebral palsy, polio, deaf, non-disabled individuals, men, women, children, adults, and seniors, making the game inclusive in nature. The game can be played indoors in a gymnasium or outdoors on a parking lot. Due to the wide range of abilities, a foam football is used.

Players who have functional use of hands, arms, and eyes must catch the ball. Individuals whose functional use is limited may be credited with a "catch" if the football hits them from the elbows up. Individuals who have no functional use of their limbs are credited with a "catch" if the ball hits them from the waist up.

Player Classifications

A three level player classification system is used with Level 1 having the most functional ability.

Level 1: Fully functioning arms, hands, and eyes (paraplegics, amputees, non-disabled, etc). Players must catch and hold onto the ball by stashing it on their lap or between their knees. A Level 1 player tackles by touching

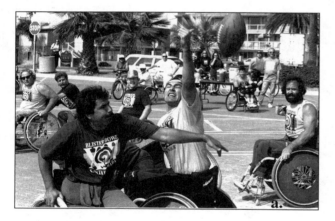

Figure 15.1 a and b. Wheelchair football action at the annual Blister Bowl, sponsored by the city of Santa Barbara, California.

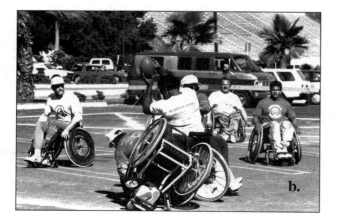

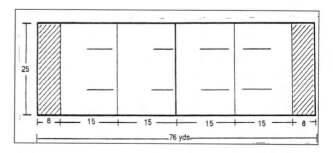

Figure 15.2. Wheelchair football field dimensions.

the person (not their chair) with one hand. Grabbing the player's chair is considered holding.

Level 2: Limited arm and hand movement (quadriplegics, etc.) or visually-impaired. Players must have the ball hit them anywhere between their hands to their elbows (with enough force that some deflection occurs in the flight of the ball) for a pass completion. In other words, a ball grazing the hair on your knuckle doesn't count. On kick-offs and punts, having the ball hit or bounce anywhere into the front of the body/chair, or running over the ball counts as a possession. After "catching" the ball or gaining possession, players proceed to "run" without the ball (defensive players need to go after them, NOT the ball). Players yell, "got it" to avoid confusion. A Level 2 player tackles by making contact with their opponent's chair. Fumbles are recovered by rolling over the ball or trapping it underneath the chair.

Level 3: Minimal or no arm movement (high quadriplegics, etc.) or blind. The same rules apply as for Level 2 players except a pass completion only requires being hit by the ball in the front or side of the body from the waist up, or in the back of the head/headrest. Noise making devices (beeping football, portable radios taped on wheelchairs, etc.) can be used to help blind players locate their targets. For example, a blind player on defense could locate the offensive quarterback if a portable radio was taped to their chair playing music. For blind players on offense, beeping foam footballs can be used. Alternatively, blind players could line up in the right direction and be told to push out 10 or 15 strokes and wait for a pass.

Suggested Modified Rules

The rules and classification levels outlined below are intended to be flexible. They are intended to be modified to adapt to various playing fields, or to accommodate players with unique disabilities.

Number of Players: Between 5 and 14 players can play the game. When the game is played with an odd number of players, a steady quarterback is used. The quarterback has 7 seconds to release the ball before the play is dead.

Equipment: Players can participate in manual chairs, power chairs, or scooters. Most contact occurs chair-to-chair so injuries are rare. Protective equipment is optional but could include a bike helmet, gloves, seatbelt, stretch cords, eyewear, boots to protect toes, etc. Spoke guards can help protect the wheels on manual chairs. A standard foam football is used.

Field:
a) Gymnasium—Boundary for a basketball court works well. Distance for a first down is from the foul line to half court or any equivalent distance as identified by other markings on the gym floor.

b) Parking Lot Field size varies on usable space available and number of players. Mark off desired boundaries with cones if available. Distance for first down should be marked (parking spaces work well).

Beginning Play: Snapping the ball is not necessary. The quarterback lines up behind the line of scrimmage and begins play by saying, "hike".

Rushing: Any number of players may rush the quarterback on any play. The game can be played with a delayed or instant rush. The delayed rush requires defensive players to count-off 3 seconds before rushing. One blitz is allowed per series of downs. The instant rush allows players to rush the quarterback at will.

Kick-offs & Punts: A "kick" in simulated by throwing the ball downfield. Balls rolling out-of-bounds before the end zone are put into play at that spot. Balls that enter the end zone can be downed and brought out to the twenty, or can be put into play (including those that bounce off the back wall of the gym).

Scoring: A touchdown equals 6 points. The game can be played with or without the extra point or field goal. Field goals are attempted from the foul line or 1.5 parking places. A passing play to the end zone equals 1 point. A running play equals 2 points.

Choosing Teams: Teams should be selected evenly to facilitate a competitive game.

Deaf Football

Traditional tackle football has a rich tradition in schools for the deaf throughout the country. Most schools offer tackle football as a part of their athletic offerings. No rule modifications are necessary to NCAA or high school rules with the exception of the use of flags to stop play rather than a whistle. The United States Flag Football for the Deaf (USFFD) is an official sport federation of the United States Deaf Sports Federation.

Blind Football

Although football is not an official competitive sport for individuals who are blind, recreational participation is possible with an auditory beeping football. This battery-operated, rechargeable, regulation size, leather football produces a continuous beeping sound for up to three hours.

ADDITIONAL RESOURCES AND WEBSITES

Football enthusiasts will find many websites related to their sport, however, few websites are available related to football for individuals with disabilities.

Santa Barbara Parks and Recreation Department
620 Laguna Street, PO Box 1990

Santa Barbara, CA 93102-1990
(805) 564-5418
Website:
http://ci.santa-barbara.ca.us/departments/
parks_and_recreation/recreation

Developmental & Adapted Programs (Blisterbowl)
Cabrillo Bathhouse
1118 East Cabrillo Boulevard
Santa Barbara, CA 93103
(805) 564-5421

United States Flag Football Federation
USA Deaf Sports Federation
3607 Washington Blvd. #4
Ogden, UT 84403-1737
(801) 393-7916 (tty)
(801) 393-2263 (fax)
Email: HomeOffice@USADSF.Org
Website: http://www.USADSF.org

Universal Wheelchair Football Association
John Kraimer
Disability Services

University of Cincinnati- Raymond Walthers College
9555 Plainfield Road
Cincinnati, OH 45236-1096.
(513) 792-8625
(513) 792-8624 (fax)
(513)743-8300 (tty)
Email: john.kraimer@uc.edu

Warm Spring Sports (Spoke Bender Bowl)
5101 Medical Drive
San Antonio, Texas 78229
(210) 592-5358
Email: sports@warmsprings.org
Website: http://www.warmsprings.org

BIBILOGRAPHY

Hamilton, B. (1990). Pigskin progress: Wheelchair football and the Blister Bowl. *Sports 'n Spokes* 15(5):32-34.
Sunderlin, A. (1999). Assault and battery: The Blister Bowl-The Superbowl of wheelchair football. *Sports 'n Spokes* 25(1):30-34.

Chapter 16

Goalball

SPORT GOVERNING BODIES:

Official Sport Of: _____DAAA   __x__USABA   _____USCPAA
                      _____DS/USA   _____USADSF   _____WS/USA
                      _____SOI

DISABLED SPORTS ORGANIZATION:
National: United States Association for Blind Athletes (USABA)
International: International Blind Sports Association (IBSA)

PRIMARY DISABILITY: Blind and Visually Impaired

SPORT OVERVIEW

Known as a quiet sport, Goalball is a unique sport developed specifically for individuals who are blind or visually impaired. The game is played on a smooth surface such as a gymnasium floor within a rectangular court that is divided into two halves by a center line (Figure 16.1). Each half is then divided into three sections. Goals are placed at either end of the court and span the width of the court. Court boundaries are generally outlined using clothesline rope taped to the floor with wide decorative high quality tape. This enables a player to determine their position on the court and the direction in which they are facing, by feeling for the markings with their feet or hands.

Two teams of 3 players are blind-folded allowing blind, visually impaired and sighted players to compete together. The game has achieved much popularity in physical education classes because of its inclusive nature.

The object of the game is for the offensive team to roll a ball containing bells past the defensive team into their goal. Teams alternate rolls, rolling the ball either fast or slow depending on the strategy utilized. The defensive team listens for the noise of the ball as it approaches and attempts to block it with their body, usually accomplished by diving horizontally with arms and legs extended, preventing it from entering their goal (Figure 16.2 a and b). For this reason, the crowd is required to remain quiet at all times. The alternate rolling by each team continues until time has expired in each half. Games generally consist of 2 halves of five or seven minutes with the team having the most goals winning. If a tie remains after this time, the two teams play two sudden-death overtime periods until one team scores a goal. Like most sports, teams can call timeouts, make substitutions, and receive penalties (Figure 16.3). Penalties may include a) a *high ball*, where a player throws the ball so that it does not land before the overthrow line, b) three throws, when a player throws more than two balls in a row, and c) eight seconds, when a team does not release the ball within the given time limit. A penalty shot is awarded where only one defensive player remains on the floor to block the shot. Refer to the IBSA web site for more detailed rules.

SPORT ORIGIN

In addition to the many sports that came about for individuals with physical disabilities after World War II, the development of Goalball is attributed to an Austrian, Hanz Lorenzen, and a German, Sepp Reindle, who used the game in the rehabilitation of blinded war veterans in 1946. The game was first played internationally at the 1976 Paralympic Games in Toronto and is now governed by the International Blind Sports Association.

EQUIPMENT

Court

The Goalball court is an indoor court (usually the floor of a gymnasium) measuring 18 meters long by 9 meters wide. Each half of the court is further divided into 3 areas, the Team Area, Landing Area, and Neutral Area.

Team Area: Comprises the first 3 meters after the goal line. The team defends the ball within this area.

Landing Area: Comprises the next 3 meters after the Team Area. When the ball is thrown, it must land before the overthrow line, otherwise a High Ball penalty will be awarded to the opposition resulting in a penalty shot.

Neutral Area: Comprises the remaining 6 meters between the opposing team's Landing Areas. The half way line runs through the center of this area.

Goalball court tactile markings:

Goalball court dimensions are as follows:

Side Lines 2 x 18m
Goal Lines 2 x 9m
Front Lines of Team Areas 2 x 9m
High Ball (Overthrow) Lines 2 x 9m
Center Line 1 x 9m
Orientation Lines 4 x 1.5m, 4 x 0.5m, 4 x 0.15m

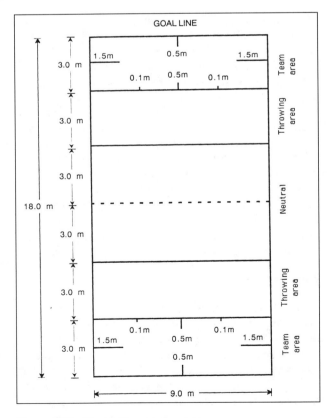

Figure 16.1. Goal ball court dimensions.

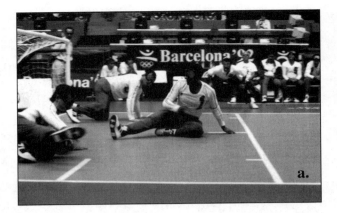

Figure 16.2 a and b. Defensively, players often use their outstretched bodies to prevent the ball from crossing the goal line. (Courtesy of Michael Paciorek and Specialized Sports Unlimited)

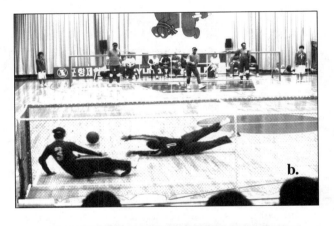

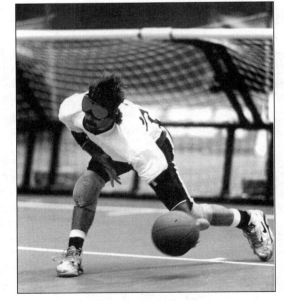

Figure 16.3. The ball must be delivered using an underhand throw. Blindfolds are worn by all players and may be adjusted only by the referee. (Courtesy of Specialized Sports Unlimited)

Goal

The official goal is 1.3 meters high by 9 meters wide. Goals are used in official tournaments but not necessary in other competitive environments. When goals are not available, a goal is scored when the ball crosses *completely* over the goal line.

Goalball

The game is played with a 1.25kg, 76cm in diameter ball which is manufactured to an IBSA specification. The essential feature of the ball is that it is audible when in motion so that players may locate the ball by listening for it.

Eyeshades

In goalball all the players have to be blindfolded, to equalize the disadvantages of poor vision and total blindness. For tournament play the quality of the shades needs to meet exacting standards, but in less formal play, the blacking out can take a less rigid form. The rules require that players must not touch their eyeshades during play; players must seek the permission of a referee to make any necessary adjustment to their eyeshades during play. During less formal play or in physical education classes, a pair of blacked out swim goggles work well as eyeshades.

Protective Padding

Protective padding is largely a matter of personal preference. Knees, elbows and hips, are vulnerable parts of the body that tend to make floor contact and should be padded. Padding in the genital area for men and breasts in women is necessary for protection when getting struck by the ball. Many players make their own padding from foam and elasticized bandaging. Commercially available padding for volleyball and skateboarding are also used. Elbow padding used in ice hockey also seems to work well. Goalball equipment can be purchased through USABA

EQUIPMENT SUPPLIERS

Handi Life
Blakke Moellevej
18B 4050
Skibby, Denmark
47 52 60 22
47 52 60 97 (fax)
Email: hls@handilifesport.com
Website: http://www.handilifesport.com/

ADDITIONAL RESOURCES AND WEBSITES

At this point the number of Goalball oriented web sites are limited to a few developed by avid Goalball players. The IBSA web site is the most comprehensive and provides links to other pages. Some of the sites that provide the most information are as follows.

USABA
Women's Head Goalball Coach
    Ken Armbruster (719) 550-1120

Men's Head Goalball Coach
    Tom Parrigin (904) 824-0260

D's Goalball Links
Website: http://www.cuug.ab.ca/~hamiltod/

Goalball New Zealand
Website:
        http://www.blindsport.org.nz

IBSA Goalball Site:
Website: http://www.ibsa.es/sports/goalball.html

Michigan Association for Competitive Goalball Homepage
Website: http://www.bestmidi.com/goalball/

Chapter 17

Golf

SPORT OVERVIEW

The two key aspects to golf for individuals with disabilities are accessibility to courses and adapted equipment. The very nature of golf, played over rolling terrain with natural and man-made obstacles, provides some unique accessibility challenges. Federal law has affirmed the responsibility of public golf course owners to make their courses as accessible as possible under Section 504 and the American's with Disabilities Act (ADA). The fundamental right of individuals with disabilities to have access to golf courses coupled with the right of golf course owners to ensure their courses are protected from damage, has been debated for the past few years. Professional golfer Casey Martin's successful discrimination suit against the PGA brought these issues into the forefront of the public's eye. Today, organizations are fighting for and designing golf courses that are accessible to all individuals. With the aging of the population, golf course designers are taking a closer look at issues regarding accessibility. Golf course owners are keenly aware of the economic impact golfer's with disabilities can have. Breakthroughs in technology and adapted equipment are now enabling golfer's with disabilities to be competitive on golf courses. Lightweight golf carts have been designed that are accessible even on putting surfaces. This chapter will describe the various golf programs and organizations for individuals with disabilities. Various types of adapted equipment and golfing techniques will be described as well.

HISTORY

The game of golf has been played and enjoyed for centuries. There are references dating back to 1457, when King James II issued his famous edict in Parliament outlawing the game. It seems his archers were spending more time playing _Golf_ than practicing their profession. This is also evidence of how addicting this game can become.

The first golf organization in the United States formed in 1894 as The Amateur Golf Association of the United States. The name was soon changed to the United States Golf Association (USGA). The USGA is the National Governing body for golf in this country. They have worked closely with disability sport organizations in the promotion of golf, and in the development of specific golf rules for individual with disabilities.

Although golf has been played by individuals with disabilities for some time, it has only been since World War II that the sport saw the development of disability specific organizations. In 1949, a group of golf enthused war veteran amputees, lead by Dale Bourisseau, formed "Possibilities Unlimited," their motto being "it doesn't matter what you've lost; it's what you do with what remains." The group held tournaments in various cities for individuals with amputations until the group was incorporated in 1954 as the National Amputee Golf Association (NAGA). NAGA now boasts more than 4,300 members while hosting two major annual tournaments, the National and National Seniors events, and supporting a number of regional and local tournaments across the country.

Golf for individuals who are blind traces it's origins back to 1925 although the first golf organization for the blind was not established until 28 years later. The idea that an individual who is blind could be a competitive golfer seems unlikely to most people. However, elite competitive blind golfers routinely shoot in the 70's and 80's. Oddly enough, the first blind golf championship was sponsored by Ripley's Believe It or Not in 1932 between Clint Russell of Duluth, Minnesota and Dr. Beach Oxenham of London, England. The publicity generated from this competition lead to an awareness of the sport by people who were blind and inclusion of the sport in Veteran's Administration rehabilitation programs. Bob Allman, a blind golfer and lawyer, formed the United States Blind Golfers Association (USBGA) in 1953. The USBGA continues to sponsor tournaments and to promote the sport for individuals who are blind.

The idea of organizing blind golfers from around the world was initiated by Haruhisa Handa. The founding of the International Blind Golf Association (IBGA) in 1998, is further evidence of the growth of this sport worldwide.

Due to the great increase in the number of new courses, and people playing golf, many of the disability sports organizations have added golf to their official lists of sports offerings. At this time the Dwarf Athletic Association of America (DAAA), Special Olympics Inc. (SOI), and the United States Deaf Sports Federation (USADSF) offer the sport. Other sport-specific organizations including the United States Blind Golf Association (USBGA) and the National Amputee Golf Association (NAGA) meet the needs of interested golfers. At one time there was a National Deaf Golfers Association, But with golf becoming an official sport of the USADSF the NDGA disbanded.

Golf for the disabled is not modified for competition except that male golfers with certain disabilities may elect to tee off from the forward tees. In most cases the medium for involving individuals with disabilities is not adapted equipment, but proper instruction by an experienced golf professional. In 1997 the United States Golf Association published a "rules decisions". It is a modification of the rules of golf for golfers with disabilities. It addresses each disability and rules that might effect the participation of the disabled golfer. The purpose is to allow the golfer with a disability to play equitably with an able-bodied individual or a golfer with another type of disability. A full transcript of the revised rules for golfers with disabilities, completely printable and downloadable, is available on the USGA web at: http://www.usga.org/rules/golfers_with_disabilities.html or contact the USGA (see Additional Resources) for a printed version.

More recently a battle was won for the rights of disabled golfers, but not on the golf course. It was won in the courtroom involving Casey Martin, a professional golfer with a rare circulatory disease, which makes walking very painful. In 1998 Martin sued the PGA Tour for the right to use a golf cart during competition (it should be noted that the PGA Tour and the PGA of America are separate entities). Martin won the initial case and it was appealed by the Tour. The PGA Tour felt that by allowing Martin to use a cart it would change the nature of the competition, in a sense giving him an unfair advantage. In March of 2000 the federal appeals court upheld the appellate courts ruling allowing Martin to ride. Yet, this issue is far from over. The day after the Martin ruling, another case heard in the Midwest involving a club-pro and the USGA on exactly the same issue and argument, was won by the USGA. These two rulings on the same argument has set-up the possibility of further litigation.

A recent interpretation by the federal government regarding the use of carts affirms the right of golfers with disabilities to use carts during professional competitions. The federal government affirms that carts do not change the fundamental nature of the game.

According to a recent document *Access for Individuals with Disabilities to the Game of Golf 2/12/98. (Section 504 of the Rehabilitation Act of 1973, as amended, and Title II of the Americans with Disabilities Act); Walking, using a caddy, or pulling a hand cart around the golf course is not considered a fundamental part of the game of recreational golf. Using a riding cart is a modification which may allow golfers to play a round in less time and exert less energy. Any damage to the turf caused by a cart, we do not believe relates to the fundamental nature of the game but to whether or not maintenance of the turf becomes an undue burden in relation to the resources of the entity and other accepted practices (i.e. walking, taking divots, use of tractors and utility carts, etc.) as previously discussed. The Casey Martin decision, which has indicated, in part, that walking in professional tournaments is not a fundamental part of the game of golf, has, perhaps, clarified this position to a greater extent.*

SPORTS ORGANIZATIONS AND RESOURCES

A variety of organizations and resources are available to assist people in accessing golf opportunities and in promoting the sport.

American Disabled Golfers Association (ADAG)

An excellent organization for resources, equipment, and accessible golf courses is the American Disabled Golfers Association (ADAG). The Association of Disabled American Golfers (ADAG), founded in 1992, is a not-for-profit (501)(C)(3) organization dedicated to ensuring that golfers with disabilities have access to the sport. ADAG serves as the clearinghouse for information regarding golfers with disabilities and the golf community, while promoting the inclusionary nature of the game. ADAG has become the nation's leading organization in promoting the inclusion of golfers with disabilities into the game and advising the major associations and individuals of the golf community of important issues.

Physically Challenged Golf Association (PCGA)

The Physically Challenged Golf Association was founded in 1995 by Brian A. Magna, and non-profit status was obtained in 1997. Since 1995, the association has conducted many workshops/seminars/clinics for physically challenged golfers, as well as healthcare and golf professionals. The Association boasts many regional adaptive sports programs and a PGA and LPGA staff of trained professionals who conducts clinics and workshops. The organization is open to anyone interested in golf (see Additional Resources).

Get a Grip

Get a Grip is a personalized golf program developed for survivors of brain injury. The program uses golf as a therapeutic vehicle to enhance an individual's quality of life by helping him or her gain self-confidence and self-esteem. The program provides such golf opportunities as personalized instructions, custom (adaptive) golf equipment, and recreational golf activities.

Walking Impaired Golfers Association (WIGA)

The Walking Impaired Golfers Association (WIGA) is another of the recently formed advocacy groups for disabled golfers. WIGA seeks to maximize opportunities for golfers with disabilities to play and to enjoy the game of golf. They actively assist golf course operators to identify and to modify operational policies that create barriers for golfers with walking impairments. For more information on WIGA use the information listed under additional resources.

National Center on Accessibility

With the aging of the general population and popularity of golf through the lifespan, golf course accessibility is a major challenge. An excellent resource on golf accessibility is provided through the National Center on Accessibility. They provide information on golf organizations, programs, instructors, assistive technology, courses designed for accessibility (in specific regards to accessibility), architects with expertise in accessibility and single rider golf cars. They list two architects currently designing courses that are accessible for golfers with disabilities, Richard Phelps and D.J. Devictor.

First Swing Program

The First Swing program is sponsored by the National Amputee Golf Association and is designed for people with a variety of disabilities including spinal cord injuries, amputations vision or hearing impairments, stroke and neurological disorders. The one or two day program provides instruction on golf and introduces the sport to individuals who may not have thought the game possible for them. The program also trains therapists and golf professionals to work with people who have disabilities.

FORE ALL!

FORE ALL! is a non-profit sports, leisure, and recreation management company with a very ambitious objective; the development of the *National Accessible Golf Course*. The course is being designed to be fully accessible by people with physical disabilities, including individuals who are blind, hearing impaired and wheelchair users. When complete, it should be the first such golf course facility in the world. The 18-hole course, located in Capitol Heights, Maryland, is part of Watkind Mill Regional Park. Unique features will include special hearing devices, carts and corridors designed to accommodate a variety of needs (see Additional Resources).

FORE HOPE

FORE HOPE is an Ohio-based non-profit organization that brings the therapeutic value of golf to persons with disabilities, their families, and those with inactive lifestyles. FORE HOPE is a chapter member of The First Tee, a national coalition of the game's leading golf organizations whose goal is to make golf accessible for people from all walks of life. FORE HOPE uses golf as an instrument to help in the rehabilitation of individuals challenged by strokes, arthritis, amputation, paraplegia or other disabilities. Residents in care centers and assisted living facilities benefit from the activity of golf as it increases mobility, endurance, concentration, and improves their outlook on life.

HandiGolf Foundation

A unique organization from Britain called the HandiGolf Foundation was established in the late 1980's to promote golfing from adapted electric carts. HandiGolf organizes tournaments, an awareness day, and a national championship for sitting golf. Tournaments involve players without disabilities who are required to play seated.

Special Olympics

In accordance with its emphasis on providing life-long sports for an aging population, Special Olympics has adopted golf as an official sport. Currently, over 6,000 athletes participate in 49 US Programs and in 14 nations around the world (SOI website). As with all Special Olympics sports, the focus is on training first and competition second. In training the first time player, the philosophy is to learn the game from the green back, this approach is consistent with many PGA instructors. Five levels of golf are played depending on the ability of the athlete.

Level 1-Individual Skills Contest

The purpose of the Individual Skills Contest is to allow athletes, especially those with lower level skills, to train and compete in basic golf skills. Six different skills are tested:

1. Short Putting

Two circles, with a radii of .5 and 1.5 meters respectively, are drawn around a selected target hole. The athlete strikes 5 balls(uphill preferred) from 2 meters and scores points based on where the ball eventually stops.

2. Long Putt

The task is identical to the short putt contest, but the athlete strikes the balls from 8 meters instead of 1.5 meters.

3. Chip Shot

Two circles, with a radii of 3 and 6 meters respectively, are drawn around the designated hole. A 3m x 3m hitting area, 14 meters from the hole is selected, and the athlete has 5 attempts to chip balls as close to the hole as possible. Points are awarded based on where the ball stops.

4. The Pitch Shot

This contest measures the athlete's ability to hit controlled pitch shots in the air and in the proper direction. A 12 meter in diameter target area is used, with a hitting area placed 10 meters from the target area (Figure 17.1). A 1 meter high x 5 meter wide barrier is placed equal distance between the hitting area and target area. The athlete receives five attempts to chip a ball over the barrier and

into the target area. Points are awarded according to where the ball lands.

5. Iron Shot

With an iron, the athlete has 5 shots to hit a ball more than 90 meters within a 35-meter-wide boundary area. Four points are awarded for a shot over 90 meters, three points for a 60-to-90 meter shot, two points for a 30-to-60 meter shot, and one point for making a stroke at and striking the ball.

6. Wood Shot

This event is similar to the iron shot contest but with different dimensions. The athlete is given 5 shots to hit a ball with a wood more than 120 meters, within a

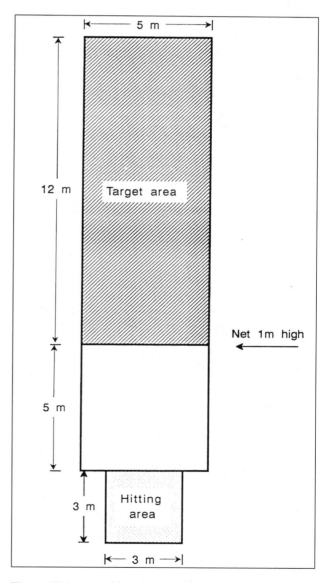

Figure 17.1. Area dimensions for the Special Olympics pitch shot event.

50-meter-wide boundary area. Points are awarded on distance.

For a complete description of the Individual Skills Competition, contact your local chapter of Special Olympics or Special Olympics Inc.

Level 2-Alternate Shot Team Play Competition

Level 2 pairs an athlete with mental retardation with an athlete without mental retardation for the purpose of transition from skill play to individual play. Using one ball, the players alternate strokes until the ball is holed.

Level 3 and 4-Individual Play

Level 3 and 4 are for players who wish to play individually in a tournament. Level 3 golfers play 9 holes while level 4 golfers play 18 holes.

Level 5-Unified Sports Team Play

In level 5 athletes with and without mental retardation are paired in teams. This provides the Special Olympics athlete an opportunity to play in a team format with teammates of similar ability.

Visually Impaired

The international slogan for Blind golf is "You don't have to see it to tee it". The members of United States Blind Golf Association (USBGA) are divided by ability levels, a BGA Member, an Associate member, and a Support member. A BGA member is anyone that plays golf and is totally Blind (B-1). An Associate membership is for visually impaired (B-2 or B-3) golfers. The support membership is for professionals, coaches, or just friends and backers of blind golf.

Only a few modifications to golf for a blind or visually impaired athlete exist, including the use of a coach. The USGA defines a coach as a person who assists a blind golfer in setting up to the ball and with alignment of the body and club prior to the playing of a stroke. Two of the primary functions of a coach are to properly align the club in the direction of the shot and to give the golfer the correct distance. This is different from the caddie whose responsibility is to track and locate the ball for the golfer. The other modification deals with grounding the club in a hazard, and where a caddie and coach should position themselves during a stroke played on the putting surface. The USBGA routinely conducts regional and national tournaments, while the IBGA focuses on international tournaments. For more information on blind golf and rules consult the USBGA or the USGA (see Additional Resources).

Amputee Golf

There are numerous associations to assist individuals with amputations seeking to play or learn to play golf. The National Amputee Golf Association(NAGA), the Eastern Amputee Golf Association, and the Western Amputee Golf

Association provide many clinics and workshops (Figure 17.2). These associations organize regional and national tournaments. At the tournaments, golfers are divided into "flights" or divisions by classification, similar to amputee athletes in other sports. As with other sports, athletes have the choice of playing with or without their prosthetic device (Figure 17.3). Improved adaptive devices have played an important role in the growth of amputee golf, especially in holding the golf club. Rotators in lower limb prostheses allow pivoting more easily, turning the body during the swing. Special gloves have rubber inserts, Velcro strips on the fingers, and longer straps than a normal golf glove to wrap around arthritic hands or those missing fingers. In many cases, these adaptations have been made by individuals working with their orthotist or prosthetist and are matter of preference by individual golfers.

EQUIPMENT

Golf Carts

In the past, individuals with spinal cord injuries and other lower extremity impairments often had to use chairs, stools, or modified stools to provide stability. Great strides have been made recently in chair design and golf carts, allowing golfers in most cases to drive right onto the putting surfaces. The *Hi-Rider* (Figure 17.4) de-

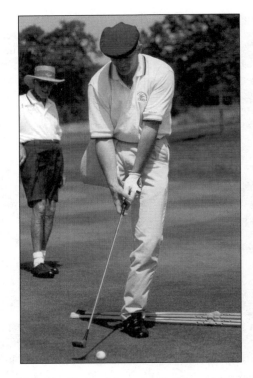

Figure 17.2. The National Amputee Golf Association (NAGA) offers more than 40 local and regional tournaments and a national championship each year. (Courtesy of the Rehabilitation Institute of Chicago's Wirtz Sports Program)

signed by Tom Houston and made by Falcon Rehabilitation (see equipment suppliers) is light enough to do just that. It also holds the golfer in a standing position to make a more natural swing.

The *Golf Xpress* (Figure 17.5) is only 1/3 the weight of a conventional golf cart, and the patented single-rider golf car goes everywhere the golfer goes—onto the tees, into the traps and even onto the greens. It can carry up to 450 pounds, including golf bag and rider. The golfer may choose to play seated two-handed or one-handed, or standing but supported.

Another innovation is the *AteeA*, by Solorider Industries, a single person golf car that can go anywhere on the course, even in sand traps. Since it is an electric car, the risk of leaking oil or gas on the greens is eliminated. This vehicle is lightweight and balanced to provide less ground pressure than a riding greens lawnmower or a walking individual.

Golf Accessories

For those who choose to play golf from a sitting position, Ortho-Kinetics Incorporated of Waukesha, Wisconsin, produces a golf accessory called the *Teestick*. The Teestick allows golfers to tee a ball up from a sitting position without bending over. The golfer can also use the device to pick up tees and balls. Another device used by golfers with back problems is the *Putter Finger*, a suction cup molded to fit on the grip end of a putter. A golfer simply turns the club around and picks the ball up without bending over.

Clubs

Clubs may be customized or shortened for short-statured individuals. Golf has been a popular competitive and recreational sport within The Little People of America organization and its sport counterpart, The Dwarf Athletic Association of America (DAAA) (Figure 17.6). The Billy Barty Golf Tournament and the National Dwarf Games provide at least two major golf competitions for short-statured individuals each year.

Golfers with physical impairments who golf from their wheelchair may find the *Clever Clubs*, by Access to Recreation suitable for their needs. These shortened clubs allow a person to hit a golf ball from their wheelchair. They can be used on carpet, grass, or hard flooring.

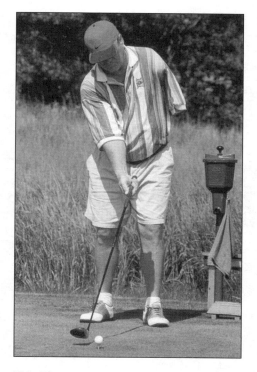

Figure 17.3. The NAGA offers separate competition for arm and leg amputees. (Courtesy of the Rehabilitation Institute of Chicago's Wirtz Sports Program)

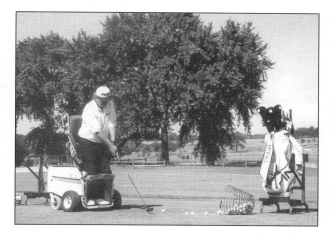

Figure 17.4. The Hi-Rider is a specially designed golf cart that allows the golfer to play from a standing position. (Courtesy of the Rehabilitation Institute of Chicago's Wirtz Sports Program)

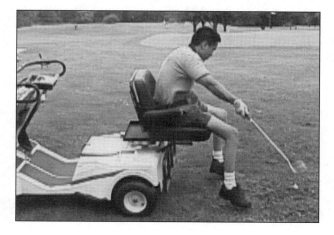

Figure 17.5. A swivel seat attached to the Golf Xpress golf cart inlcudes a seat belt to increase support to the golfer. (Courtesy of the Rehabilitation Institute of Chicago's Wirtz Sports Program)

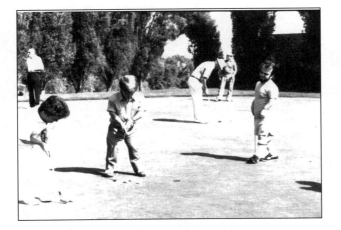

Figure 17.6. Short-statured golfers practice on the putting green prior to competition. (Courtesy of Daniel Margulies, LPA)

(800) 518-1194
Website: http://www.elitegolf.com/golfxpress/index.html

Golf Express Cart
4275 County Line Rd,#214
Chalfont, PA 18914
(877) 494-6532
Website: http://www.4golfxpress.com

Hi-rider
Tom Houston
Falcon Rehabilitation Products, Inc
4404 E. 60th Ave.
Commerce City, CO 80022
(800) 370-6808
(303) 287-6434
Website: http://www.hirider.com

U.S. Kids clubs are making clubs lighter and shorter for children, but they could they could also be used by the golfer with a disability.

Prosthetic devices

A number of commercial devices to assist in securing the clubs are available for individuals with upper extremity amputations. Specific rules have been established by the USGA regarding the use of artificial limbs. The *Amputee Golf Grip* (Figure 17.7 a and b) by TRS, Inc. and the *Robin-Aids Golfing Device* (Figure 17.8 a and b) meet these USGA regulations. Both are flexible devices that attach to the prostheses and do not require the clubs to be modified.

There are devices on the market for golfers with lower extremity amputations. A shank torque ankle rotator built in to the prosthesis, allows nearly normal body rotation by permitting the hips to rotate independently of the foot. The *Total Knee*, by Century XXII innovations, allows the above the knee amputee improved movement without the fear of collapsing. In addition to prosthetic limbs, ICEROSS comfort system minimize friction between the residual limb and the socket interface. It uses a silicone gel to provide protection and impact cushioning. The S.A.F.E. (stationary attachment flexible endoskeletal) foot helps keep a golfer's foot flat on the ground during the swing. The foot is adaptable to irregular terrain and offers a wide range of motion.

EQUIPMENT SUPPLIERS

Carts

Golf Xpress Cart
Elite Golf International

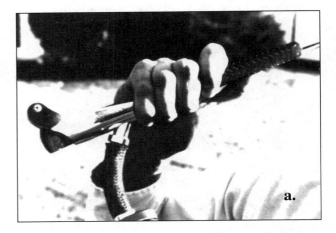

Figure 17.7 a and b. The Amputee Golf Grip is a standardized manufactured product that meets USGA requirements.

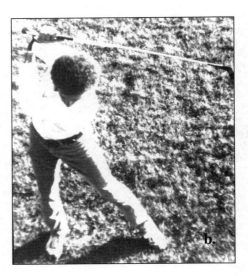

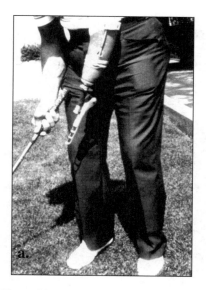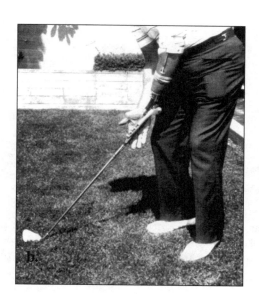

Figure 17.8 a and b. The Robin-Aids Golfing Device. (Courtesy of TRS)

Lone Rider
175-56 Toryork Dr.
Weston, Ontario
Canada
(416) 749-1461
(416) 749-5848 (fax)

Solorider
Solorider Industries Inc.
2060 S. Tucson Way
Englewood, CO 80112
(303) 858-0505
(800) 898-3353
(303) 858-0202 (fax)
Website: http://www.solorider.com

Teestick/ Fairway Golf Car
Ortho-Kinetics, Inc.
P.O. Box 1647
W220 N50 Springdale Rd.
Waukesha, WI 53187-1674
(888) 320-4850
(414) 542-4258
Website: http://www.teestick@sharpdesigns.com

Clubs

Clever Clubs
Access to Recreation, Inc.
8 Sandra Court
Newbury Park, CA 91320
(800) 634-4351
(805) 498-8186 (fax)
Email: dkrebs@gte.net
Website: http://www.accesstr.com

U.S. Kids Golf Clubs
U.S. Kids Golf
PO Box 817
Duluth, GA. 30096
(770) 495-9626
(888) 387-5437
(770) 495-9527 (fax)
Email: webmaster@uskidsgolf.com
Website: http://www.uskidsgolf.com/

Prosthetic Devices

Amputee Golf Grip
Therapeutic Recreation Systems Inc.
2450 Central Avenue, Unit D
Boulder, CO 80301-2844
(800) 279-1865
(303) 444-4720
(303) 444-5372 (FAX)
Website: www.oandp.com/trs

S.A.F.E. Foot
Campbell-Childs, Inc.
400 Industrial Circle
White City, OR 97503
(800) 446-7233
(541) 826-6511
(541) 826-6658 (fax)

Total Knee
Century XXII Innovations Inc.
PO Box 868
Jackson, MI 49204
(517) 782-1975

(800) 788-9878
(517) 780-0404 (fax)

ICEROSS
Ossur Prosthetics/ Orthotics
(354) 515-1300
(354) 515-1366

ADDITIONAL RESOURCES AND WEBSITES

Golfers will find many websites related to their sport. Because this sport is accessible for those with and without disabilities, most participants will find the following sites satisfactory for gathering information.

Accessible Golf Course Architects

Richard (Dick) Phelps
PO Box 3295
Evergreen, CO 80439
(303) 670-0470

D.J. DeVictor
DeVictor Langham, Inc.
45 West Crossville Rd. Suite 502
Roswell, GA 30075
(770) 642-1255

Golf Organizations and Other Resources

Association of Disabled American Golfers
PO Box 2647
Littleton, CO 80161-2647
(303) 922-5228
Email: adag@usga.org
Website: http://www.adag.org

Eastern Amputee Golf Association (EAGA)
2015 Amherst Dr.
Bethlehem, PA 18015-5606
(888) 868-0992
(610) 867-9295 (fax)
Email: info@eaga.org
Website: http://www. EAGA.org/

The First Tee
170 Highway A1A North
Ponte Vedra Beach, FL 32082
(904)940-4300
(904)280-9019 (fax)
Website: http://www.thefirsttee.com/
First Tee is a program to create facilities and programs that make golf more affordable and accessible, with a strong emphasis on introducing children of all races and economic backgrounds to golf.

Fore All!
PO Box 2456
Kensington, MD 20891-2456
(301) 881-1818
(301) 881-2828 (fax)
Email: fore_all@juno.com
Website: http://www.foreall.org

Fore Hope, Inc.
c/o Darby Dan Farm
925 Darby Creek Drive
Galloway, Ohio 43119
(614) 870-7299
(614) 870-7245 (fax)
Email: frhope123@aol.com

Get A Grip
552 W. Berridge Lane
Phoenix, AZ 85013
(602) 728-0218
Email: GetaGripRw@aol.com
Website: http://www.getagripgolf.com
            Video: Adaptive Golf and the Therapist

Golf 4 Fun
Bob Nelson
P.O. Box 27595
Denver, CO 80227
(303) 985-3403
Email: Brownie1925@hotmail.com
Website: http://www.golf4fun.org/
Golf 4 Fun offers group lessons by PGA professionals to all interested people with physical disabilities.

HandiGolf Foundation
c/o Andrew Greasley
Stone Cottage, Lanton Road
Stratton Audley, Oxen
England OX6 9BW
Tel: 01869 277369

International Blind Golf Association
Derrick Sheridan - President
25 Langhams Way, Wargrave, Berks,
RG10 8AX, England
E-mail: Derrick@Sheridan25.freeserve.co.uk
Website:
    http://www.blindgolf.com/International/about_us.htm

National Amputee Golf Association (NAGA)
(800) 633-NAGA
Email: info@nagagolf.org
Website: http://www.nagagolf.org

National Center on Accessibility
Gary Robb, Director
5040 State Road 6/ N.
Martinville, IN 46151
(765) 349-9240
(765) 349-1086 (fax)
Email: nca@indiana.edu
Website: http://www.indiana.edu/~nca

National Golf Foundation
1150 U.S. Highway One
Jupiter, FL 33477
(800) 733-6006
Website: http://www.ngf.org/

Physically Challenged Golfers Association, Inc.
Brian Magna, Exec. Dir.
Avondale Medical Center
34 Dale Rd - Suite 001
Avon, CT 06001
(860) 676-2035
(860) 676-2041
Email: pcga@townusa.com
Website: http://www.townusa.com/pcga/index.html

The Professional Golfers' Association of America (PGA)
100 Avenue of the Champions
P.O. Box 109601
Palm Beach Gardens, FL 33410-9601
(407) 624-8400
(407) 624-8439 (fax)
Website: http://www.PGA.com/

United States Blind Golf Association (USBGA)
Bob Andrews, President
3094 Shamrock St. North
Tallahassee, FL 32308-2735
(850) 893-4511 (tel./fax)
Email: USBGA@blindgolf.com
Website: http://www.blindgolf.com

United States Golf Association (USGA)
P.O. Box 708
Far Hills, NJ 07931

(908) 234-2300
(908) 234-9687 (fax)
Email: usga@usga.org
Website: http://www.usga.org/

Walking Impaired Golfers of America
Fred L. Montgomery, Director
PO Box 1058
Los Altos, CA 94022
(877) 480-9442
E-mail: wiga@mindspring.com
Website: http://www.wiga.org

Western Amputee Golf Association (WAGA)
5980 Sun Valley Way
Sacramento, CA 95823
(800) 592-WAGA

BIBLIOGRAPHY

Access for Individuals with Disabilities to the Game of Golf 2/12/98 (1998). (Section 504 of the Rehabilitation Act of 1973, as amended, and Title II of the Americans with Disabilities Act). National Park Service: Equal Opportunity Program.

Avery, B. (1995). Disabled-But Not Disqualified. *Golf Journal* (Sept.) pp. 40-42.

Chamalian, D. (2000, June). Tee Time For All. *Exceptional Parent Magazine*.

Cunneff, T. (1998). *Walk a mile in my shoes: The Casey Martin Story*. Nashville, TN: Rutledge Hill Press

Jones, G. (April, 1998). Golf Course Accessibility. *Arizona Golf Magazine*.

Longo, P. (1988). Challenge golf: A game for everyone. *Amputee Golfer 6*(4):22-24.

Official Special Olympics Summer Sports Rules. Special Olympics Inc: Washington, D.C.

Parker, S. & Williams, J. (1999). Back on Course. *Park & Recreation 34*(6)60-63.

Wolohan, J. (1998). Casey at the Tee. *Athletic Business 22*(4)22, 24

Chapter 18

Hockey

SPORT GOVERNING BODIES:
National: USA Hockey
International: International Ice Hockey Federation (IIHF)

Official Sport Of: _____DAAA   _____USABA   _____USCPAA
                           _____DS/USA   __x__USADSF   _____WS/USA
                           __x__SOI

DISABLED SPORTS ORGANIZATION:
National: United States Sled Hockey Association (USSHA)
International:

PRIMARY DISABILITY: Individuals with physical disabilities

SPORT OVERVIEW

Hockey is played in various forms within the realm of disability sport and the sport is not always played on the ice. Variations include playing the game on ice skates, sleds, in wheelchairs, or by running up and down a court. This chapter will focus mainly on sled hockey but other variations of the sport will be discussed as well.

SLED HOCKEY

Sled (or sledge) hockey is an exciting sitting equivalent of ice hockey for individuals with permanent lower extremity physical disabilities, with the sled used in place of ice skates. The game is known as sledge hockey in many parts of the world (sledge being Norwegian for sled). The game is physical and fast-paced and includes as much body checking as the standing game. Penalties, face-offs, and changing on the fly are consistent with the standing version of the game. Some infractions are specific to sled hockey due to the use of the sled and picks. Official rules may be found on the United States Sled Hockey Association website. With six players per team including the goalie, sled hockey is played on a regulation size ice rink and is based on slightly modified International Ice Hockey Federation rules. Three 15-minute periods are played as opposed to 20 minute periods in the standing game. Players sit on their sled and use two sticks to pass, stick-handle, shoot the puck, and to propel and maneuver their sledge. The game is played with a regulation hockey puck. Standard hockey equipment such as helmets, gloves and elbow pads are used. Goalies must wear face shields and all players must wear neck guards.

HISTORY OF SLED HOCKEY

Sled hockey is a relatively new sport originating in Norway in the 1960's where it quickly spread to Canada and throughout Europe. Sled Hockey made its Paralympic debut in Lillehammer in 1994, with five international teams competing. John Schatzlien is credited with bringing sled hockey to the United States in 1989. He established a program in the Minneapolis area and later in Wisconsin, and was the founder and first President of the American Sledge Hockey Association (ASHA). The ASHA grew into The United States Sled Hockey Association Inc. which is currently the National Governing Body for Sled Hockey in the United States (Figure 18.1). Their mission is to promote the sport of sled hockey nationally and internationally for athletes with disabilities. They develop rules and regulations, equipment specifications, and organize regional and national championships. The United States Sled Hockey Association is recognized by Wheelchair Sports USA and USA Hockey Inc. and conducts trials for international competitions and Winter Paralympic Games. The association also conducts developmental camps and clinics to promote the sport and to encourage its expansion throughout the United States. There are currently more than a dozen affiliated sled hockey programs throughout the United States.

EQUIPMENT

Sled

The primary piece of equipment is the sled itself with costs ranging from $300-$1,300. The 2-4' sled is an oval-shaped metal frame that has three points of contact with the ice: two skate-like blades and a small runner (Figure 18.2). The blades used in sled hockey are shorter than the type used in ice sled racing and are about one-third the length of the sled. The blades can be placed wider apart for a beginning player who needs more balance or closer together for an advanced player who wants better maneuverability. Seat size and backrest height vary according to disability and individual needs. Strapping is used to keep legs in position and stable. Sleds are often custom-made to individual player specifications.

Sticks/Picks

Specially designed hockey sticks (about 29" long) made of wood, aluminum or carbon fiber are used by sled hockey players. A typical pair of sticks costs about $40. Since the sled hockey player sits much closer to the ice, standard hockey sticks cut in half are not satisfactory. Each stick has a "Pick" attached to the end. Picks are metal pieces with teeth on the end (Figure 18.3 a and b).

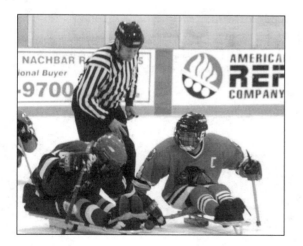

Figure 18.1. Sled hockey developed greatly in the United States due in part to support from various NHL teams, such as the Chicago Blackhawks. (Courtesy of the Rehabilitation Institute of Chicago's Wirtz Sports Program)

Each pick must have a minimum of three teeth, and teeth must measure no longer than four millimeters. Each stick must have two picks (a minimum of six teeth). The goalie may use one stick or two. If using two sticks, only one stick may be a larger stick with the other one being the same size as the other team members. If using one stick the goalie is allowed to use a blocker and trapper.

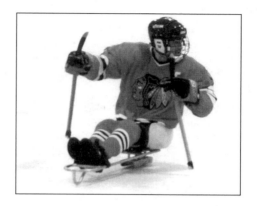

Figure 18.2. The sledge is the wheelchair athlete's answer to ice skates. (Courtesy of the Rehabilitation Institute of Chicago's Wirtz Sports Program)

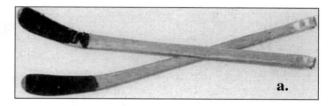

Figure 18.3 a and b. (a) Sled hockey sticks are designed for pushing the sled and handling the puck. (b) Pics must have at least three teeth and be no wider than the shaft of the stick. (Courtesy of the Rehabilitation Institute of Chicago's Wirtz Sports Program)

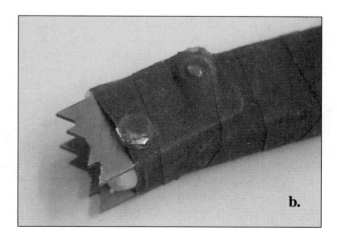

The player propels him or herself down the ice very much like a cross-country skier digging the picks into the ice, providing traction. When he or she gets near the puck, the player slides a hand down the shaft of the stick where the picks are attached. This gives the player the leverage to shoot the puck with the blade end of the stick. A player's hands can be taped or attached with Velcro to the glove and stick if grasping is difficult.

Prosthetic Devices

Given the high level of interest in hockey, it is not surprising that prosthetic devices specific to hockey have been developed. A Canadian Prosthetic Company has had success with developing a "skating leg" (see Additional Resources) (Reilly, 1998).

The Slap-shot Tds. is a production-made hockey device designed specifically for arm amputees available from TRS. It comes in two versions, one designed for the "end stick-ES" handling (donut shape), the other for "shaft stick-SS" handling (tuning fork shape). Slap Shots offer versatility in handedness and style of play. They are built rugged to withstand the rigors of ice or street hockey. One model will be preferred over the other based upon the player's hand dominance and stick handling style. The ES model uses a strong flexible coupling and slips over the end of the stick. The SS model has a jointed construction and snap on and off anywhere along the shaft.

OTHER HOCKEY VARIATIONS

Hearing Impaired Hockey

Hockey for individuals with hearing impairments is available through the American Hearing Impaired Hockey Association (AHIHA), an affiliate of the United States Deaf Sports Federation. Founded in 1974 by Hall of Fame Chicago Black Hawk great Stan Mikita, the AHIHA is dedicated to assisting individuals with hearing impairments in all aspects of life through the sport of hockey.

Visually Impaired Hockey

Hockey is played by individuals who have visual impairments through the Vancouver Blind Hockey Team affiliated with the Western Association of Persons with Vision Impairment. The Vancouver Blind Ice Hockey Program is a recreational ice hockey program for blind and visually impaired individuals. Standard hockey rules apply although a specially designed puck with ball bearings inside allow the player to hear the puck as it moves across the ice. It is also about twice the size of a regular puck to help those with partial vision to locate it. A beeping puck has yet to be developed. The Vancouver program uses volunteer sighted players whose job is to get the puck to the blind players. The program only utilizes a few modified rules:

- The goalie must be totally blind.
- Only two sighted players are allowed on the ice at a time.
- Since the puck is silent as it travels through the air, the puck cannot be raised more than the height of the goalies stacked pads.
- When playing another visually impaired team, only the blind can score.

Wheelchair Hockey

A variation of hockey for individuals with physical disabilities who do not desire, or who do not have access to sled hockey is wheelchair hockey (Figure 18.4 a and b). Since official rules are still being developed, flexibility in the number of players is allowed based on the area to be covered and skill of the players. The game can be played on ice or a hard surface. When played on a hardcourt surface, a plastic ball is used in place of a puck. The Disabled Athletes Floor Hockey League, The Michigan Wheelchair Hockey League and Sports on Wheels of Anaheim, CA are excellent sources of information for interested players.

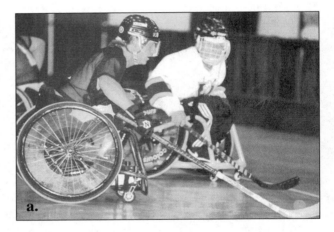

Figure 18.4 a and b. Wheelchair hockey can be played indoors and outdoors. Either way, protective equipment is recommended. (Courtesy of Sports 'n Spokes 1997 23/6; 39, and 1998 24/2: 13)

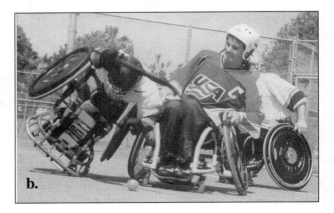

Electric Wheelchair Hockey

Electric or power wheelchair hockey began in Canada more than a decade ago with the formation of the Canadian Electric Wheelchair Hockey Association (CEWHA). The CEWHA sponsors a number of events and a hosts a national championship on an annual basis. Electric Wheelchair Hockey is for individuals with disabilities who have limited upper body strength and/or mobility, who could significantly benefit from the use of an electric wheelchair in competitive sport (Figure 18.5). The United States Electric Wheelchair Hockey Association (U.S.EWHA) is dedicated to the development of this sport within the United States. Electric wheelchair hockey is played using standard hockey rules with minor adaptations made to allow all power wheelchair users to play. The game is played with 5 players per side using light-weight plastic sticks and a plastic ball. Individuals with severe arm and hand disabilities are allowed to tape the stick to their wheelchair. The United States Electric Wheelchair Hockey Association (USEWHA) promotes the game primarily in Minnesota but they are attempting to develop leagues throughout the country. A complete set of official rules and the Power Hockey Report Newsletter are available through the USEWHA.

Special Olympics Floor Hockey

Three versions of hockey are offered through Special Olympics. The officially recognized sport of floor hockey is played by the majority of Special Olympics programs and in international competition, while a variation of the game called Poly Hockey is played by some chapters (Figure 18.6). Both of these variations include competition in team play, individual skills (a version of lead-up floor hockey), a 10-meter puck dribble, target shot, and Unified team competition. Additionally, the sport of ice hockey is played by some chapters within SOI's "Nationally Popular Sport" category.

Floor hockey is played with 6 players per side including the goalie. Players are rotated into the game through a similar line shift rotation an in ice hockey. The puck is a circular felt disc with a center hole. It is directed around the court by floor hockey sticks which are wood or fiberglass rods or dowels. The goaltender uses a regulation goaltender's stick.

The concept of poly hockey is very similar to floor hockey and to wheelchair hockey without the wheelchair. Poly hockey is played in many physical education classes throughout the United States and Canada. The puck, instead of being a felt disc, is made of hard plastic similar (but lighter) than a standard ice hockey puck. Sticks are small plastic versions of conventional hockey sticks and are available through most physical education equipment suppliers (Flaghouse, Wolverine Sports, Sportime, etc.). In international competition, the sport of floor hockey is played, rather than poly hockey.

EQUIPMENT SUPPLIERS

Prosthetic Devices

Reilly, James
Hamilton Health Sciences Corporation
Chedoke Prosthetics and Orthotics Dept.
Box 2000
Hamilton, Ontario
Canada L8N 3Z5

Therapeutic Recreation Systems Inc. (Slap Shot Hockey Tds)
2450 Central Avenue, Unit D
Boulder, CO 80301-2844

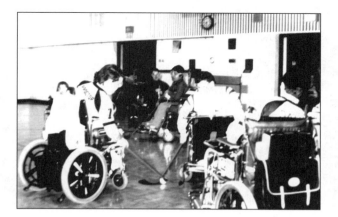

Figure 18.5. Wheelchair floor hockey can be played by individuals in manual or power wheelchairs. (Courtesy of the Canadian Electric Wheelchair Hockey Association)

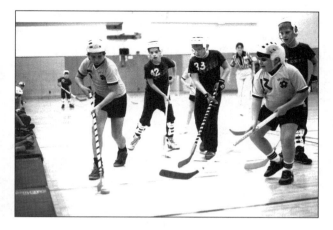

Figure 18.6. Poly Hockey, a growing sport in physical education classes, intramurals, recreation programs, and Special Olympics, combines teamwork, strategy, and a variety of physical skills. (Courtesy of Special Olympics Michigan)

(800) 279-1865
(303) 444-4720
(303) 444-5372 (fax)
Website: www.oandp.com/trs

Sleds

Access to Recreation, Inc.
8 Sandra Court
Newbury Park, CA 91320 .
(800) 634-4351
(805) 498-7535
Fax (805) 498-8186
Email: krebs@westworld.com
Website: http://www.accesstr.com

Advanced Mobility Products Ltd.
Unit # 111-2323 Boundary Rd.,
Vancouver, B.C., V5M 4V8
Canada
(604) 293-0002
(800) 665-4442
(604) 293-0005 (fax)
Email: mobility@mobilityproducts.com
Website: http://www.mobilityproducts.com

Canwin Sports
46 McFarlane Rd.
Nepean, Ontario
Canada K2E6V5
(613) 723-7428

Gopher Medical
2550 Delaware Street, SE
Minneapolis, MN 55414
(612) 623-7706

Invacare Corporation
One Invacare Way
P.O. Box 4028
Elyria, OH 44036-2125
440-329-6000
Email: info@invacare.com
Website: http://www.invacare.com

New Hall's Wheels
P.O. Box 380784
Cambridge, MA 02238
(617) 628-7955
(617) 628-6546 (fax)
Email: newhalls@tiac.net
Website: http://www.newhalls.com/

PennSled
Olympic Wheelchair Sales & Service
25 Rothsay Ave.

Kitchener, Ontario
Canada N2B3A2
(519) 741-0795
(519) 741-9771 (fax)

Spokes N Motion
2225 S Platte River Drive W
Denver, CO 80223
(303) 922-0605
(303) 922-7943 (fax)
Email: info@spokenmotion.com
Website: http://www.spokesnmotion.com/

Unique Inventions
559 Chamberlain Street
Peterborough, Ontario
Canada K9J4L6
(888) 886-0881 (toll free)
(705) 743-6544
(705) 743-1740 (fax)
Email: unique@pipcom.com
Website: http://www.pipcom.com/~unique

Zebra Sports
Phoenix AZ
(602)765-1848

Jentsch and Company Inc.
290 South Park Ave.
Buffalo NY 14204
(716-852-4111
(716) 852-4270 (fax)

Stick Manufacturers

Gary Ludwig
NY Rte.78
Strykersville, NY 14145
(716) 457-3082

Floor Hockey

Flaghouse, Inc.
601 Flaghouse Drive
Hasbrouck Heights, NJ 07604-3116
(800) 793-7900
(800) 793-7922 (fax)
Email: info@flaghouse.com
Website: http://www.flaghouse.com/

Sportime
One Sportime Way
Atlanta, GA 30340
(770) 449-5700
(800) 845-1535 (fax)
(800) 444-5700

Email: customer.service@sportime.com
Website: http://www.flaghouse.com

Wolverine Sports
School-Tech Inc.
745 State Circle Box 1941
Ann Arbor, MI 48106
(734)761-5072
(734)761-8711 (fax)
Email: wolverine@school-tech.com
Website: http://www.wolverinesports.com/

ADDITIONAL RESOURCES AND WEBSITES

At this time, the number of websites related to disability hockey is growing. Various sites are available throughout the world. By accessing the following sites, readers will have links to most other sites. Most participants will find the following sites satisfactory for gathering information.

Electric Wheelchair Hockey

Canadian Electric Wheelchair Hockey Association (CEWHA) (Calgary Division)
Email: info@wheelchairhockey.com
Website: http://www.wheelchairhockey.com

United States Electric Wheelchair Hockey Association (U.S.EWHA)
7216 39th Ave. No.
Minneapolis, MN 55427
(612) 535-4736
Email: hockey@usewha.org
Website: http://www.powerhockey.com

Floor Hockey

Special Olympics
1325 G Street, NW, Suite 500
Washington, DC 20005-3104
(202) 628-3630
(202) 824-0200 (fax)
Email: SOImail@aol.com
Website: www.specialolympics.org

Hearing Impaired Hockey

American Hearing Impaired Hockey Association
1143 West Lake Street
Chicago, IL 60607
(312) 829-2250
Website: http://www.ahiha.org/

Sled Hockey

International Paralympic Committee Sledge Hockey Page
Website: http://www.paralympic.org/
            sports/sections/sledge-hockey.asp

Ottawa-Carleton Sledge Hockey & Ice Picking Association
46 Nestow Dr.
Nepean, Ontario
K2G 3X8, Canada
Designed for those who have some upper body movement, O.C.S.H.I.P. organizes ice picking races in mid-February attracting individuals and teams from across Canada, the U.S. and Europe.

Sledge Hockey of Canada
P.O. Box 20063
Ottawa, Ontario
K1N 5W0 Canada
(888) 857-8555 (toll free)
(613) 723-5799
(613) 226-2050 (fax)
Email: shoc@shoc.ca
Website: http:// www.shoc.ca/

United States Sled Hockey Association
21 Summerwood Court
Buffalo, NY 14223
(716) 876) 7390
Email: Info@sledhockey.org
Website: http://www.sledhockey.org/

Visually Impaired Hockey

Western Association of Persons with Vision Impairment (WAPVI)
The Vancouver Blind Hockey Program
110 - 5055 Joyce St.
Vancouver, B.C.
V5R 4G7 Canada
Email: office@wapvi.bc.ca
Website: http://www.wapvi.bc.ca

Wheelchair Hockey

Disabled Athletes Floor Hockey League
Southeast Association for Special Parks & Recreation
6000 S. Main St.
Downers Grove, IL 60516

Michigan Wheelchair Hockey League
Email: andyice@aol.com
Website: http://www.scorezone.com/wchl/
This league is located in Southfield, Michigan and can supply information on the development of similar wheelchair hockey leagues.

Sports on Wheels
1591 South Sinclair St.
Anaheim, CA 92806
(714) 939-8727
(714) 978-2891 (fax)

Other

International Ice Hockey Federation
Parkring 11
8002 Zurich
Switzerland
+41-1-289 86 00
+41-1-289 86 22 (fax)
Email: iihf@iihf.com
Website: http://www.iihf.com/

USA Hockey
1775 Bob Johnson Drive
Colorado Springs, CO 80906-4090
(719) 576-USAH
(719) 538-1160 (fax)
Website: http://www.usahockey.com/

BIBLIOGRAPHY

Davis, B. (1998). Face Off. *Sports 'n Spokes 24*(2)10-14.

Davis, B. (1997). The Iceman Cometh. *Sports 'n Spokes 23*(7)25-27.

Pedersen, L. (2000). Power Hockey All-Stars. *Sports 'n Spokes 26*(3)32.

Reilly, J. (1998) Winter-wear: Cool Prosthetic Gear for Cold Weather Activity. *Active Living 8*(1)34-36.

Riley, C.A. (1999). The Ice Pack. *We Magazine 3*(2)55-56.

Chapter 19

Hunting

SPORT GOVERNING BODIES:
National: National Rifle Association (NRA)

DISABLED SPORTS ORGANIZATION:
National: Buckmaster Quadriplegic Hunters Association (BQHA),
                     Disabled Hunters of North American (DHNA),
                     Physically Challenged Bowhunters Association (PCBA),
                     United Foundation For Disabled Archers (UFFDA)

RECREATIONAL ACTIVITY ONLY

PRIMARY DISABILITY: All

SPORT OVERVIEW

It has been said that for those that hunt, no explanation is necessary, and for those who don't, no explanation is sufficient (Jones, 1993). The ability of a person with disabilities to hunt depends on two variables: Safe handling of a gun and accessible hunting locations. Advances in technology and the expanding availability of accessible areas, along with increased awareness, have created many opportunities for the disabled hunter.

This chapter will discuss information on various forms of adaptive equipment, State laws and regulations, hunting opportunities available for people with disabilities, and list equipment suppliers. Evidence for the popularity of the sport for people with disabilities is provided due to the many exceptional resources that are now available. A list and description of these resources will also be provided. This chapter will focus on general hunting with no specific reference to the type of game. However, bow hunting involves large game (deer, elk) rather than small game (birds).

EQUIPMENT

Selection of Gun

The ability to control a gun is dependent on four elements; holding the gun, windage movement, elevation movement, and operation of the trigger. Varying difficulties will be encountered with each element (Sullivan, Buckmasters Disabled Hunters, 1999, p. 5). Gun selection is usually based on the type of game being hunted, and the physical abilities of the individual. Since each person has unique characteristics, there are no special gun manufacturers for people with disabilities. Any gun specialist can assist with selection, however, those with upper extremity impairments may wish to select lightweight rifles, rifles with thumbstocks (Figure 19.1) and, where permissible by law, using handguns rather than rifles.

Adaptations

The variety of guns available allows the disabled hunter to pick what best fits his/her need, thus requiring adaptations in many cases. For the most part any adaptive alterations are done after the guns are purchased. There are several adaptations available commercially but most are created with the ingenuity of the person who would be shooting the gun, in combination with a machinist or someone mechanically inclined (Lucas, BQHA). Persons interested in hunting with the use of adapted equipment should seek all available options, considering, safety, function, and performance from a qualified person knowledgeable in this area.

121

Gun Mounts and Shooting Rests

Some of the most common adaptations used in hunting are shooting rests or gun mounts. Depending on the needs of the hunter and willingness to spend money, there are many different kinds of rigs available from home made to very sophisticated commercially manufactured. Trap suspension systems and tripod devices support the barrel end of the rifle while allowing the hunter to follow game for sighting purposes. All equipment is intended to assist in ease of operation, allowing for maneuverability, stable gun positioning, and accurate firing. Most equipment such as the Blackberry Technologies Uni-Mount System, Levellok Tripod & Monopods, the Universal Arm and Accuizer 1 are easily mounted to wheelchairs and tree stands, while devices such as the Body Pod and Steady Arm (Figure 19.2) are attached to the individual. These devices typically allow for full range of motion while maintaining the ability to lock in any position. Horizontal and vertical positions are attained quickly and efficiently. Simple stationary supports may be mounted to car windows, golf carts and ATVs as well (Figure 19.3). The use of homemade gun rests meet the needs of many hunters who have disabilities (Figure 19.4), while a body harness gun rest is an ideal solution for the hemiplegic hunter (Figure 19.5). This device allows the hunter to perform all functions with just one hand.

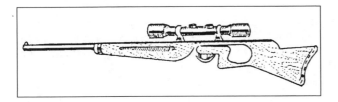

Figure 19.1. The use of a rifle with a thumbhole stock will add stability for hunters with slight grasp problems.

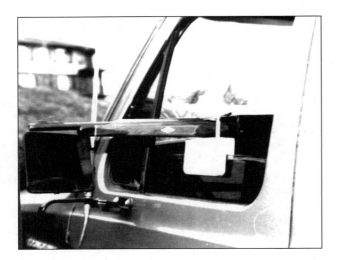

Figure 19.3. Shooting rest by IDEA. (Courtesy of IDEA)

The SR-77 Shooting Rest (Figure 19.6) is another excellent device for the hunter with quadriplegia since it is totally hands-free. With practice and by using a mouth piece or a joy-stick, the hunter controls the movement left and right, up and down, and when zeroed in on target a sip on a vacuum tube will touch it off.

Gun Attachments and Trigger Devices

The ability to aim and support a gun, even with adapted equipment, does not always include the ability to pull the trigger. Gun attachments, such as specialized pistol grips (Figure 19.7), and trigger devices make this possible for hunters with limited or no hand use (Figure 19.8). Schulz (1984) documented the successful use of a shoelace as a trigger activating device (Figure 19.9). The

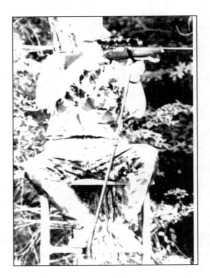

Figure 19.2. The Steady-Arm Gun rest is also adapted for mounting on the footrest of a wheelchair. (Courtesy of H&O Manufacturing Co.)

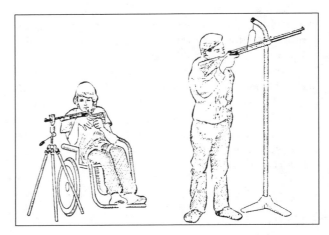

Figure 19.4. Homemade gun rests meet the individual needs of shooters.

hunter used his teeth to pull the string, activating the trigger. Although standard terminal devices can usually operate the trigger devices of most guns (Radocy, 1987, p. 144), the gun itself can be modified safely to make operation by individuals with upper extremity impairments much easier. Modifications made to commercial triggers, and guns are most common, and easily done. The solenoid sip and puff trigger, The Trigger Activator, Blackberry Technologies Gun Mount with power options, and the Bite Trigger, are all devices that can be attached to any gun or rifle, and can be adapted to work for most any physical disability of the hands (Figure 19.10). All products are available commercially.

Bows and Crossbows

Many hunting purists will only hunt with a bow. An alternative for those individuals who cannot safely shoot or choose not to use a gun is the use of a bow or crossbow. Compared to hunting with a gun, bow hunting is considered by most the ultimate challenge, as it is a pure form of hunting. The same elements and considerations described for guns (above) are applicable for bow hunt-

ing. A variety of adaptations are used to successfully shoot with a bow. The "Ground Stake Hunt-N-Buddy" is one product that allows the hunter to stand the bow upright with an arrow knocked in a ready-to-shoot position for hands-free comfort and motionless hunting.

Another alternative to bow hunting is the use of a crossbow. This accommodates those persons without sufficient upper-body strength that makes it difficult, or impossible to draw a conventional or compound bow. Some crossbows (such as those by Hunter's Manufacturing Company) have automatic cocking devices that allows a person with a hand or arm dysfunction to operate it easily. Special crossbow hunting permits are available for persons with disabilities, depending on the State. There are approximately 20 states that offer crossbow permits. Each state is different, but the overall requirement is a Physician's certification of disability completed and signed by a licensed Doctor in the particular state in which you are hunting. This has been a controversial issue but laws are being continually modified to meet the needs of hunters with disabilities and to comply with the American's with Disabilities Act (ADA). Buckmasters.com and Todd Albaugh's Handicapped Hunting Resource Guide (see the following) offers a State-by-State list of laws and requirements and links to appropriate State agencies. For those persons who are not connected to the Internet contact your local Department of Natural Resources for further information.

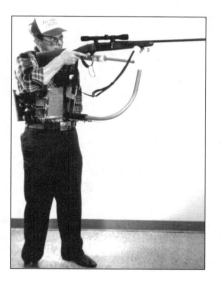

Figure 19.5. Body Harness gun rest for the hemiplegic hunter. (Courtesy of FreeHanderson Co.)

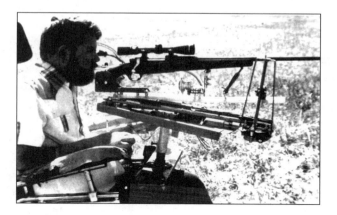

Figure 19.6. The SR-77 quad shooting rest is solenoid activated. (Courtesy of SR-77 Enterprises)

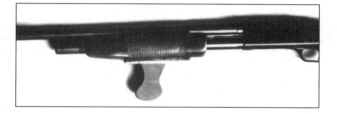

Figure 19.7. Additional stability can be gained by adding a modified pistol grip. (Courtesy of TRS)

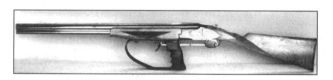

Figure 19.8. Modified over-and-under shotgun. (Courtesy of TRS)

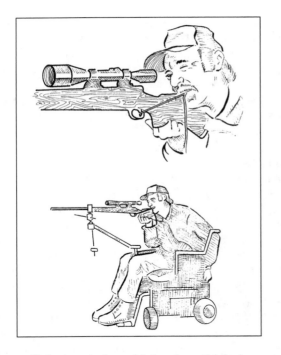

Figure 19.9. A spinal cord-injured quadriplegic uses a shoelace to pull the trigger.

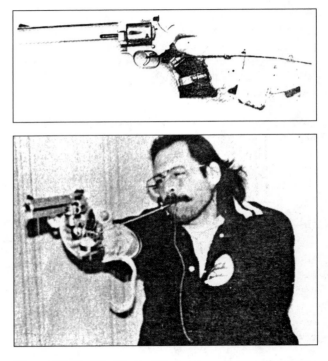

Figure 19.10. The Bjorke Rig incorporates a splint strong enough to support the recoil action of a .357 magnum revolver. (Courtesy of *Disabled Outdoors* Magazine)

Adaptive Hunting Blinds

There are a variety of hunting blinds specifically designed for people with disabilities (Figure 19.11 a-d). An all in one ATV/Deer Blind by Wolf Den Hunting Products is a unique design that allows the hunter to take their blind with them as they move in their ATV or wheelchair. Many deer blinds are also easily adjustable and allow the hunter with a physical disability to elevate themselves into trees or well above the ground. Examples of these types are the Limited Mobility Deer Blind, the Wright Stand and Deer Master (see Equipment Resources).

Shooting for Individuals with Visual Impairments

It may be assumed that a person who is a totally blind person could not safely shoot a rifle, much less hunt whitetail deer or other game. But with slight equipment modifications, and help from a sighted assistant, a vision-impaired hunter can be just as successful as he or she was before the loss of sight. Most fabrication and machine shops across the country will be delighted to offer assistance to a vision-impaired hunter. A simple mounting bracket can be constructed to extend a sight bar or scope out to the side of a firearm, compound bow, or crossbow. A sighted hunting partner can then aim over the shoulder of the vision-impaired shooter. The two can work together in developing touch and whisper signals to raise, aim, and shoot the weapon safely and effectively.

In the case of a rifle for deer hunting, it is most com-mon to mount a pistol scope four inches off of the center of the barrel. A variable-powered pistol scope works exceptionally well and offers extended eye relief for the sighted partner. The bracket can be made of 1-inch, thin-walled, stainless steel tubing or machined aluminum, and designed to fit into existing scope rings on the rifle. The bracket will have its own second set of rings to accept the pistol scope. All scope rings and bases should be quality products made of steel. To avoid interference between the scope bracket and the bolt-action rifle, it will be necessary for right-handed hunters to shoot left-handed guns and visa versa.

An additional method for hunting involves the use of a laser light for sighting (Veine, M. 1998). This controversial method has been legalized in some states for hunters with visual impairments.

WILDERNESS ACCESS

Finding an adequate place to hunt and getting there can present a major obstacle for the hunter with a disability. However, laws requiring handicap accessible sites are becoming mandatory, making normally hard to hunt places easily accessible. More than 20 states offer special permits to hunters with disabilities to shoot from standing vehicles. These permits have led to the use of all-terrain vehicles (see Chapter 1), cars & trucks, and even custom made hunting blinds. Many new organizations such as Disabled Hunters of North America, Buckmas-

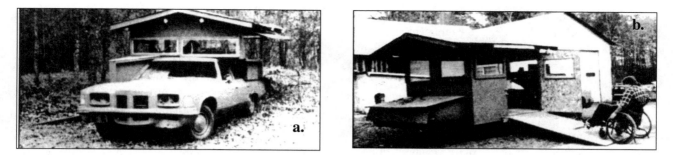

Figure 19.11 a-d. A homemade hunting blind mounted on a 1972 Pontiac allows access to the woods by a hunter with a disability. (Courtesy of *Outdoors Forever*)

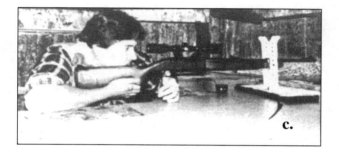

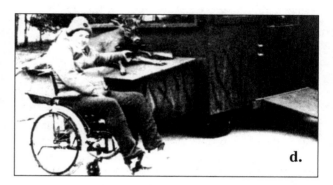

ters Quadriplegic Hunter Association, Capable Partners, and Outdoor Buddies are just a few of the organizations and resources assisting hunters with disabilities (see the following for descriptions).

RESOURCES AND ORGANIZATIONS

The resources that have become available for the hunter with a disability have grown in proportion to the popularity of the sport. Gun manufacturers and outfitters have realized that there is a profit to be made by providing equipment and opportunities for hunters with disabilities. The following are just a few of the excellent resources and organizations available to the person with a disability who wishes to hunt.

Buckmasters.com

The most comprehensive resource for hunters with disabilities on the internet (or anywhere else) is Buckmasters.com. It is Buckmasters' goal to create the most comprehensive, extensive and helpful resource for disabled hunters and outdoors enthusiasts on the internet. This site includes information on adaptive equipment, accessible places to hunt, fish and camp, outfitter listings, scholarships, grant opportunities for adaptive equipment, and many other useful resources. Buckmasters also provides a list of disabled hunts scheduled for each year. Some hunts are organized at commercial hunting lodges, called Commercial Lodge Disabled Hunts. These offer accessibility, experience with disabled clients and a discounted price for participants. No Fee Disabled Hunts are

planned on private properties across the country, where there is no cost for the event.

One of the more useful resources provided by Buckmasters is a listing of ADA laws and DNR regulations for all states regarding special permits including hunting from a standing vehicle, hunting with a modified bow, hunting with a crossbow, off road vehicle use, fishing license exemption for persons with mental disabilities, senior citizen fishing licenses for legally blind individuals and senior citizen hunting/fishing license for veterans with 100% disability. These regulations vary from state to state.

Buckmasters Whitetail Magazine features regular columns for disabled hunters and includes periodic feature articles on the subject. The Buckmasters Television Series on TNN includes episodes dedicated to disabled hunters. These special shows are seen by millions, increasing awareness and creating opportunities for disabled hunters nationwide.

Buckmasters Quadriplegic Hunters Association (BQHA)

In 1999 Buckmasters formed a special niche for quad hunters, the Buckmasters Quadriplegic Hunters Association (BQHA). This organization is made up of new and experienced hunters with quadriplegia, as well as volunteers who assist them. Through the Buckmasters web site and periodical mailings, the BQHA communicates with one another offering help, advice, fellowship, opportunities and information. The BQHA will help newly injured individuals with quadriplegia to assess their level of injury to better decide what adaptive equipment and hunting techniques are needed. It is common for a recently injured individual, as well as friends and family, to underestimate the ability needed to operate a gun or bow.

Disabled Hunters of North America (DHNA)

The Disabled Hunters of North America (DHNA), is a non-profit organization, dedicated to helping the disabled hunter connect to reputable outfitters and manufacturers to help them get into the woods for a great hunt. The DHNA evaluates and assists outfitters and manufacturers to better their products to accommodate disabled hunters. DHNA also assists the disabled hunter with organizing their hunts.

Physically Challenged Bowhunters Association (PCBA)

Founded in 1993 in Indian Bluffs, Lexington, MS, the Physically Challenged Bowhunters Association (PCBA) is a non-profit organization to help disabled persons realize the therapeutic value of bowhunting. A major emphasis is placed on reaching people with disabilities who have never been exposed to bowhunting.

Newly injured and inexperienced sportsmen with disabilities are provided critical information and services through PCBA and its members. Information and instruction is provided to learn to shoot a bow and hunt, regardless of the impairment.

PCBA serves as a national clearing house for techniques, opportunities and adaptive equipment for challenged archers. As with able-bodied bowhunters, fellowship is emphasized and promoted through special social events and hunting opportunities. Members develop a great bond among one another.

PCBA continuously seeks the help of manufacturers, archery and hunting organizations, research facilities and experienced hunters to improve the quality of life for others through bowhunting and advocates for changes in State regulations. PCBA works closely with hospitals and rehabilitation facilities to introduce bowhunting to individuals who may not have considered the idea.

United Foundation For Disabled Archers (UFFDA)

The United Foundation for Disabled Archers (UFFDA) promotes and provides a means to practice all forms of archery for any physically challenged person. The UFFDA has been in existence since the fall of 1994. It currently has nearly 400 members throughout the United States, and hunts are sponsored throughout the country. The goal of the organization is to increase the number of hunts and eventually have an UFFDA sponsored hunt in every state of the Union.

The hunters are selected each year by a drawing and then assigned their own personal guides. The guides contact the hunters to discover what their exact circumstances and personal needs are. By the time the hunters arrive at camp, their guides have prepared the hunting sites and have met all of the hunters' special needs. The entire event is provided at no cost to the hunters, less travel expenses. The lodging, meals, hunters' hospitality package, awards, door prizes, and programs are provided by the all-volunteer fund-raising efforts of the hunt committee. Similarly to the Physical Challenged Bowhunters of America, the UFFDA works with rehabilitation institutions to identify and recruit new members who may enjoy the experience of hunting. UFFDA is also working toward becoming a clearinghouse of information for archers with disabilities. Data on products and equipment that will be of assistance to these special people in the field and on the target range are being assembled. Accessible outfitters and private landowners who are providing additional hunting opportunities for disabled members are being identified as well.

Wheelin' Sportsmen of America, Inc.

Wheelin' Sportsmen of America, Inc., provides the disabled a variety of outdoor events for individuals, small and large groups. On individual outings, the disabled and non-disabled are paired through the WSA database matching common interests, locations, schedules and abilities. Small and large group activities are held at many locations annually. There is no charge to the individual to participate.

Laws and Regulations

Special provisions are designed to assist hunters with disabilities. Approximately 34 states offer special permit to better accommodate those who wish to hunt but are limited. Some examples are: free lifetime permits or reduced fees for Veterans, hunting with an all-terrain vehicle (ATV), use of cross-bows, and a variety of adapted equipment.

Special Hunts, Camps, Lodges, and Outfitters

There are a number of states, which offer special hunts for the disabled. Most hunts take place on private land and during regular hunting seasons. Buckmasters offers a variety of hunts through their club, and strive to accommodate all persons with disabilities. You do not have to be a member to participate in their programs. The only requirement is that applicants have substantial impairment(s) that prohibit their ability to hunt in a normal fashion. A list is provided at the end of this chapter of Buckmasters- sponsored hunts and events along with various other hunts.

There is no question that the population of hunters with disabilities has grown, and along with the interest is an increasing amount of camps, lodges, and outfitters that specialize in services to assist individuals with disabilities. Because there is such a large selection only a portion is listed at the end of this section. These references are all links to a variety of services available.

EQUIPMENT SUPPLIERS

The following is a list of suppliers that specialize in adapted equipment for persons with disabilities: Gun rests, gun mounts, trigger devices, hunting blinds and motorized equipment.

ATV and Vehicle Conversions

(see Chapter 1 for additional of-road options)

Beamer Ltd. (Tramper)
Email: info@tramper.co.uk/
Website: http://www.tramper.co.uk/

BC Wheels (Six-Wheeled All-Terrain Vehicles)
Hwy 22 PO Box 914
Wyocena, WI 53969
(800) 279-4335
Email: bobc@bcwheels.com
Website: http://www.bcwheels.com

6wheeldrive.com
Website: http://www.6wheeldrive.com/

Tomco Conversions (All-Terrain Motorized Wheelchair and TARA All-Terrain Vehicle)
P.O. Box 30
Rte. #321
Wilcox, PA 15870
(888) 516-4814
(814) 929-5284 (fax)
Email: info@tomcoconversions.com
Website: http://www.tomcoconversions.com

Bow Supports

The Bow Brace
20-9th Ave., NE
Glenwood, MN 56334
(320) 634-3660
Designed for amputees, The Bow Brace allows for easy loading and firing.

Cross-Bows

Barnett International, Inc.
Post Office Box 934 13447 Byrd Drive
Odessa, Florida 33556
(800) 237-4507
Email: Barnett@BarnettCrossbows.com
Website: http://www.barnettcrossbows.com

Bow-Pro Archery Equipment
1605 Treanor St.
Saginaw, Michigan 48601
(517) 752-8859
Email: BowPro123@aol.com
Website: http://www.bow-pro-archery.com/

Excalibur Crossbow Inc.
45 Hollinger Cres.
Kitchener ON, Canada
N2K 2Z1
(519) 743-6890
(519) 743-6964 (fax)
Email: service@excaliburcrossbow.com
Website: http://www.excaliburcrossbow.com/

Hickory Creek, Inc. (The Draw-Loc)
21595 Yankeetown Road
Saucier, MS 39574
(228) 832-2649
(228) 539-0225 (fax)
Website: http://www.drawloc.com/

Horton Manufacturing
484 Tacoma Avenue
Tallmadge, Ohio 44278
(330) 633-0305
(330) 633-7751 (fax)
Website: http://www.crossbow.com/

Hunter's Manufacturing Company, Inc.
1325 Waterloo Road
Suffield, OH 44260-9608
(330) 628-9245
(330) 628-0999 (fax)
Features the ACU-Draw automated cocking device.

Tenpoint Crossbow Technologies
Website: http://www.tenpoint.net/
Converted Tenpoint Crossbow for People with Disabilities
Email: bluff@wavefront.com
Website: http://www.visi.com/%7Ebluff/crossbow/

Gun Mounts and Shooting Rests

The Accurizer 1
2440 North Beckley
Lancaster, Texas 75134
(972) 224-0077
(877) 220-0077
(972) 224-8726 (fax)

Blackberry Uni-Mount System
Blackberry Technologies Inc.
3813 Conventryville Road

Pottstown, PA 19465
(800) 413-4824
(610) 469-9268 (fax)
Email: blkberry@bellatlantic.net
Website: http://www.blackberrytech.com/

Blackberry Uni-Mount System
Access To Recreation
8 Sandra Court
Newbury Park CA 91320
(800) 634-4351
(805) 498-7535
(805) 498-8186 (fax)
Email: dkrebs@gte.net
Website: http://www.accesstr.com

Body Pod MFG.
PO Box 224
Bernie, MO 63822-0224
(573) 293-4270
Email: mcgowan@sheltonbbs.com
Website: http://www.bodypod.com/

Level-lok
Brutis Enterprises
105 South 12th Street
Pittsburgh, Pennsylvania 15203
(888) In-1-shot
(412) 431-1569 (fax)
Email: levellok@levellok.com
Website: http://www.levellok.com/

Sharp Shooter Wheelchair Kit (mount for gun)
Narvaez Enterprises
301 West Saunders
Laredo, TX 78040
(956) 722-4819
(956) 725-8571 (fax)

    The Sharp Shooter Wheelchair Kit is adjustable to a variety of wheelchair arm rest lengths. It is made of steel and may be used by left-handed and right-handed hunters.

SR 77- Shooting Rest
SR-77 Enterprises
Bob Bowen
363 Maple St.
Chadron, NE 69337
(308) 432-2894
Email: bob@sr77.com
Website: http://www.sr77.com/

Steady Arm
JLB Innovations Inc.
ATT- Jerry Brown

P.O. Box 65
Pinckney, MI 48169
(734) 878-5610
(734) 878-5610 (fax)
Email: jbrown@steadyarm.com
Website: http://www.steadyarm.com/

SureShot Premium Shooting Rest
Rugged Gear
32588 477th Avenue
Elk Point, SD 57025
(800) 784-4331
(605) 356-2491
(800) 784-3268 (fax)
(605) 356-3135 (fax)
Email: webmaster@ruggedgear.com
Website: http://www.ruggedgear.com/

TGS-10 The Turret Rifle/Gun System
Taylor's Alternative Therapeutic Devices
33933 Madera De Playa
Temecula, CA 92592
(909) 676-3269
    Wheelchair attachable mount.

The Wheelchair Accessory Stand
C/o David Helman
11965 West Van Buran Rd.
Riverdale, MI 48877
(517) 833-7221

Universal Arm
Enable, Inc.
5436 North Dean Road
Orlando, Florida 32817
(407) 678-1729

Hunting Blinds/Stands

Huntmaster
New Heights, Inc.
P.O. Box 942553
Atlanta, GA 31141
(800) 826-2844
Email: dennis-hm@remote-ability.com
Website: http://www.new-heightsinc.com
    Battery powered hunting blind that can be raised from ground level to 20' in seconds.

Limited Mobility Deer Blind
Richter Hunting Innovations, Ltd.
P.O. box 389
Sabinal, TX 78881
(210) 988-2440
(210) 988-2566
    Self-propelled elevator deer blind.

The Wright Stand (Portable Deer Stand for Disabled)
T&M Enterprises
10286 Hwy 566
Clayton, LA 71326
(318) 757-2499
(318) 757-7556
Manual or electric tree stand that is easily raised and lowered.

Wolf Den Hunting Products
3000 NW 46th
Oklahoma City, OK 73112
(405) 947-7583
(405) 478-8826 (fax)
Email: Wolfdenpro@aol.com
Offers an all in one ATV/Hunting blind. Take your blind with you as you move.

Trigger Systems

Access to Recreation
(see address above)

Trigger Activator
Leisure Company
4189 Chatford Cove
Tucker, GA 30084
(770) 496-5948

Mechanical Releases

Tru-Fire Corporation
N7355 State Street
North Fond du Lac, WI 54937-1572
(920) 923-6866
(920) 923=4051 (fax)
Email: info@trufire.com
Website: http://www.trufire.com/

Assorted Hunting Equipment

Follow Me Outdoors
Email: chada@ev1.net
Website: http://www.angelfire.com/tx/followmeout-doors
Provides information to hunters on the latest adaptive equipment and hunting guides. Equipment and information includes accessible blinds, accessible shooting devices, accessible outfitters,

Broken Arrow Hunting Specialties
H.C. 4 Box 90
Blanco, Texas 78606
(800) 370-8452
(210) 833-5764
(210) 833-5386 (fax)
Email: brokenarrow@huntinginfo.com

ACCESSIBLE OUTFITTERS, CAMPS, LODGES & RESORTS

The following camps and lodges accommodate the disabled hunter, depending on the type of hunting you will do, the state in which you would like to hunt, and the specific accommodations you will need. Some will offer special hunts catering to specific disabilities, while others are handicap accessible (wheelchair accessible, use of ATV's). A complete list of outfitters can be found on the Buckmasters website (see below).

T&D Hunting Corporation
7184 Dryburg Road
Scottsburg, Virginia, 24589
(804) 572-3592

Billingsley Ranch Outfitters
PO Box 768
Glasgow, MT 59230
(406) 367-5377
Email: billingsley@recworld.com
Website:
   http://www.montanahuntingfishing.com/hunting.html

Buckmasters online
Website: http://buckmasters.rivals.com
This sight from Buckmasters lists dozens of outfitters serving hunters with disabilities.

Cactus Hunting Service
RR 3
304 Seminole Road
Roswell, New Mexico 88201
(505) 623-7208

Flying W Outfitters
Bart Schmidthuber
PO Box 251
Conner, MT 59827
(406) 821-4900
Email: flying@cybernetl.com

HandiCAPABLE Guide Services, Inc.
PO Box 222
Gilbertsville, KY 42044-0970
(270) 362-0970
Website: http://www.handicapable.net

The Minnesota Broken Wing Connection
HC 76 Box 105
Backus, MN 56435
(888) 752-9373
(218) 947-3044
A national resources center on hunting for individuals with disabilities.

Milliron 2 Outfitters
Billy L. Sinclair
1513 Culbertson
Worland, WY 82401
(307) 347-2574

Bear Paw
345 Highway 20 East # A
Colville, WA 99114-9007
(509) 684-6294
(509) 669-6294 (cell)
Email: bearpaw@huntinfo.com

SPECIAL HUNTS

Buckmasters Disabled Hunts
  The ultimate goal for Buckmasters is to create accessible hunting opportunities for all interested hunters with disabilities. A list of many special hunts offered by Buckmasters can be found on their website.
Website: http://buckmasters.rivals.com/

Helluva Hunt
1562 Esterbrook Road
Douglas, WY 82633
(307) 358-6580
  The annual Helluva Hunt (antelope) takes place during the first week in October in Douglas, WY.

One-Arm Dove Hunters Association
PO Box 582
Olney, TX 76374
(904) 564-2102
(940) 564-5496 (fax)
Email: 1armjack@brazosnet.com
Website: http://www.amp-info.net/hunt.htm

Georgia Hunt for the Disabled
Michael Eyer or David Barr
(706) 645-2937

ADDITIONAL RESOURCES AND WEBSITES

Bowhunting Net
Website: http://www.bowhunting.net/
  Provides complete information for the bowhunter.

Buckmasters On-Line
David Sullivan
Director, Disabled Sportsman Resources
11802 Creighton Avenue
Northport, Alabama 35475
Email: dsullivan@buckmasters.com
Website: http://buckmasters.rivals.com/
  Buckmasters disabled hunter keeps current hunting

opportunities, laws, and equipment and is a complete on-line resource for hunters

Outdoor Buddies, Inc.
PO Box 37283
Denver, Colorado 80273
(303) 771-8216
Email: outbud@juno.com
Website: http://www.outbud.freeservers.com/
  Provides outdoor opportunities for people with physical disabilities and underprivileged youths.

Capable Partners
P.O. Box 28543
St. Paul, MN 55128
(612) 542-8156
Email: comunications@capablepartners.org
  A volunteer organization that provides hunting, fishing, and related opportunities for the physically challenged.

Buckmasters Quadriplegic Hunters Association (BQHA)
Jeff Lucas
P.O. Box 117
Hyde Park, NY 12538
(914) 229-4131
Email: lucan1776@aol.com
Website: http://residents.bowhunting.net/Disabled Hunters/
  New and experienced hunters with quadriplegia, along with volunteers who offer help, advice, fellowship, hunting opportunities and information. This webpage contains adaptive ideas for disabled sportsmen and women. Also includes a message board, bow and crossbow rigs, hunting blinds, and ATV accessories.

Disabled Hunters of North America Inc. (DHNA)
Email: normdhna@charter.net
Website: http://www.dhna.org
  Evaluates and assists outfitters and manufactures to better their products to accommodate the disabled hunters. It also assists the disabled hunter with organizing their hunts. This website also provides links to many outfitters and gun dealers.

National Rifle Association (NRA)
NRA Disabled Shooting Services
C/o David Baskin
11250 Waples Mill Road
Fairfax, VA 22030
703-267-1495
703-267-3941 (fax)
Website: http://www.nra.org/
            http://www.nrahq.org/shooting/compete/disabled.asp

North American Bowhunter
P.O. Box 251
Glenwood, MN 56334
(320) 634-3660
Email: dhendricks@hunting.net
Website: http://www.hunting.net/nab/

Physically Challenged Bowhunters of America (PCBA)
Karen Vought
RD#1, Box 470
New Alexandria, PA 15670-9240
(724) 668-7439
Website: http://www.pcba-inc.org
A non-profit organization founded to assist persons with physical disabilities through active participation in bow hunting and archery sports.

Todd Albaugh's Handicapped Hunting Resource Guide
Website: http://www.ismi.net/handicapinfo/
This internet resource by a private citizen is a very complete website providing information on al aspects of hunting for individuals with disabilities.

United Foundation For Disabled Archers (UFFDA)
Dan Hendricks
P.O. Box 250,
29th Ave
Glenwood, MN 65334
(320) 634-3660
Email: dhendricks@hunting.net
Website: http://www.hunting.net/uffda/

Yahoo Disabled Hunting & Fishing Club
Website: http://clubs.yahoo.com/clubs/huntingand-fishingdisabled?s/
Provides an opportunity to chat with others who have similar interests.

Wheelin' Sportsmen Of America, Inc.
5510 Wares Ferry Rd., Suite G
Montgomery, AL 36117
(888) 832-6967
(334) 395-6300
(334) 395-6311 (fax)
Email: mail@wheelin-sportsmen.org
Website: http://www.wheelin-sportsmen.org/

VIDEOS

"The Incredible PCBA Story"
"Overcoming The Challenge, Adaptive Equipment Guide"
PCBA, Inc. Videos
RR 1 Box 470
New Alexandria, PA 15670-9240
The preceding videos are available for $15.00 each or 2/$25.00.

BIBLIOGRAPHY

Jones, W. (1993). Special licenses for handicapped hunters. *Conservationist* 48(2)20.
Lucas, J. (2000). Adaptations for guns and rifles. *Disabled Outdoorsman*
Sullivan, D. (1999). New Quadriplegic Hunters Association. *Buckmasters Magazine* p5.
Veine, M. (1998). Laser Sight Puts Blind on Target. *Michigan Out-of Doors*, September.

Chapter 20

Ice Skating/Sledding

SPORT GOVERNING BODIES:
National: United States Figure Skating Association (USFSA)
United States Speed Skating Association (USSSA)
International: International Skating Union (ISU)

Official Sport Of:	____DAAA	__x__USABA	____USCPAA
	____DS/USA	____USADSF	____WS/USA
	__x__SOI		

DISABLED SPORTS ORGANIZATION:
National: Skating Association for the Blind and Handicapped (SABAH)
International:

PRIMARY DISABILITY: All

SPORT OVERVIEW

The great success of American figure and speed skaters in recent Winter Olympics has helped to make ice skating a popular year-round sport in most areas of the country. The therapeutic value of ice skating for individuals with physical disabilities has been noted throughout the literature. Ice skating can benefit lower leg amputees by helping them develop prosthetic awareness skills and overcome gait deviations. Various forms of ice skating are possible for people with disabilities including competitive figure skating, speed skating and ice sledding for individuals with spinal cord injuries or amputations.

Although ice skating is very popular with many individuals who have disabilities as a recreational activity only USABA and Special Olympics offer the activity in their programming. Special Olympics is the only disability sports organization that offers competitive skating programs in both figure and speed skating while USABA offers speed skating as one of their official sports.

SPORT ORIGIN

Although the art of figure skating is relatively young, speed skating events have been contested for hundreds of years and references can be found well back into ancient times. The sport has remained essentially unchanged since that time. The origin of skating occurred in Scandinavia as a matter of functional use. People used crude skates fastening the bones of various animals to the bottoms of their boots to maneuver across frozen lakes. It is only reasonable to assume that this functional transportation system evolved quickly into a competitive sport. The use of runners without edges made it difficult to maneuver and poles had to be used to assist in gliding across the ice. The Dutch are credited with taking skating to the next level with the introduction of metal runners with edges. Originally used for the transportation of goods in Holland, skating quickly evolved into a recreational activity with organized speed skating starting in the 1500's. The first speed skating club was started in the United States in 1849 with the first world championships being held in 1889. The United States International Speed Skating Association, now known as U.S. Speed Skating was formed in 1966 and remains the national governing body for speed skating in the United States.

Although originally started in Europe, American Jackson Haines is credited with making figure skating what it is today by combining skating with dance just prior to 1860. The United States Figure Skating Association (USFSA), an outgrowth of the International Skating Union of America, was formed in 1921 to govern the sport and promote its growth on a nationwide basis. The USFSA is the National Governing Body for the sport of figure skating in the United States Competitive figure skaters must pass a series of progressively more difficult proficiency tests. The highest test level in singles skating is the USFSA gold (or eighth) test. Special Olympics uses a system similar to the USFSA in its competition

SPECIAL OLYMPICS

Figure Skating

Special Olympics competition in figure skating consists of singles, pairs and ice dancing events for both men and women (Figure 20.1). Unified Sports™ figure skating events that pairs an athlete with mental retardation and a partner without mental retardation as a team, is also offered in pairs and ice dancing. Figure skating events were first held at the 1977 International Winter Games. International Skating Union rules are followed, except when they are in conflict with Special Olympics rules. Only minor modifications, primarily in the placement of athletes within divisions, are necessary. Special Olympics figure skating competition is offered in five ability levels, determined by the number of skill assessment badges the athletes have earned. This allows for a consistent progression and reward system to encourage the athlete and is based upon the United States Figure Skating Association Badge Program. Special Olympics maintains an affiliation with the USFSA and has had athletes skate exhibitions in USFSA Championships since 1986.

Speed Skating

Similar to the introduction of figure skating, speed skating was first offered at the 1977 Special Olympics

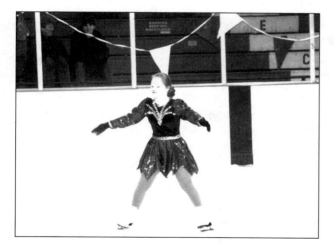

Figure 20.1. Figure skating is a competitive sport within Special Olympics. (Photo by Michael Paciorek)

World Games. Special Olympics athletes compete in speed skating events covering distances from 25-1,500 meters although some chapters offer events as short as 10 meters. Unified events and team relays are held as well. International Skating Union rules are followed, except when they are in conflict with Special Olympics rules. Specific modifications to ISU rules are listed in the Official Special Olympics Winter Sports Rules book. Individuals interested in Special Olympics competitive figure and speed skating should consult the rule book and local Special Olympics area directors.

UNITED STATES ASSOCIATION FOR BLIND ATHLETES

Skating for Individuals with Visual Impairments

The rules and policies for USABA speed skating events are unique to this organization. Speed skating for the blind consists of races of 500 and 1,000 meters for men and women of all classes. The course is a 100-meter oval laid out with bright. A variety of guide systems are including sighted guides, callers, audio cones, or a combination of sighted guides and callers. Courses are laid out with bright cones.

SKATING FOR INDIVIDUALS WITH PHYSICAL DISABILITIES

Short Track Racing (Sled Racing)

Sled racing or ice sledding is the seated equivalent of speed skating in its competitive form and ice skating in its recreational form. Originating in Norway around the mid-19th century, it is enjoyed as "ice-picking" by Canadians. The sport requires excellent technique for success and is usually done on a speed skating oval, propelled by the use of 2 picking sticks or shortened ski poles. Lightweight sledges are used in place of skates. Competitors may use straps to fasten themselves to the sledge and steering is done by shifting of body weight. Short track racing is the Paralympic version of short track speed skating, making its debut in the Salt Lake City 2002 Paralympic Games, replacing ice sledge racing (long track) that was introduced as a Paralympic event at the 1994 Paralympic Winter Games in Lillehammer, Norway. Both men and women compete in 100-meter, 500-meter, and 1,000-meter races and relay. Short track racing is the event with the fewest competitors.

Sled Racing Classification

Sled racing is divided into two functional classifications based on medical documentation of the disability.

- Class LW10 is comprised of athletes with disabilities in the lower limbs, who have no functional sitting balance.

- Class LW11 is comprised of athletes with disabilities in the lower limbs with a fair sitting balance.

A complete list of rules of specifications for classification can be found on the International Paralympic Committee website for sled racing (see Additional Resources).

Skating Association for the Blind and Handicapped, Inc. (SABAH)

The Skating Association for the Blind and Handicapped, Inc. (SABAH) out of Buffalo, N.Y. is perhaps the premier organization in this sport for individuals with disabilities. With over 20 years of experience teaching people with physical, emotional, sensory and cognitive disabilities to ice skate, SABAH has perfected the technique and equipment needed to help people with disabilities access ice skating. Starting at 16 months of age through adulthood, more than 8,000 people have learned to skate successfully. Trained volunteers work one-on-one or two-on-one with skaters to develop skills, and skaters progress to higher skill levels. All skaters participate and perform in an annual ice show spectacular, which is seen by more than 12,000 spectators. SABAH's assistive equipment includes walkers, its own line of adaptive ice skates and harnesses, functionally extending traditional concepts of assistive technology to the recreation arena. SABAH is attempting to expand its sphere of influence and expertise by developing local chapters in various regions of the country. Information on starting a SABAH Chapter can be found on their website.

ADAPTED EQUIPMENT

There is no estimate of the number of disabled recreational ice skaters but we can assume that the number is large. SABAH has developed its own line of adaptive equipment for recreational ice skating. Some of their products are described in the following pages. Further information on purchasing this equipment can be found on the SABAH website. There are several ways to assist skaters in overcoming the challenges of the ice.

Adaptive Skates

Ankle support concerns most ice skaters. Add the problems associated with some disabilities, and ankle stability can become a prohibiting factor for numerous potential skaters. Modified and specially designed adaptive skates allows the person with various physical disabilities to overcome this problem. SABAH describes three designs of adaptive skates.

- Model 1 is specially designed for people with Down Syndrome or surgically corrected clubbed feet. It is cut wider than the normal figure skate and is built with no arch to accommodate the typically wider, flatter foot of a person with Down Syndrome, clubbed feet, or other structural abnormalities.
- Model 2 is designed for skaters who wear ankle foot orthoses (AFOs) or supra-malleolar orthoses (SMOs), or reciprocating gait orthoses (RGOs). These include people with cerebral palsy or spina bifida. It is designed with 21 design modifications from a normal figure skate, mostly a widened heel pocket and extra ankle wrap to reach around the orthoses. The heel has been substantially reduced to enhance the Achilles tendon stretch during skating and match the right angle of the orthotic.
- Model 3 is designed for all skaters with disabilities who would benefit from a skate with the greater comfort provided by softer leather and increased ankle padding. The skates are cut wider to accommodate a range of differences in width of feet. Skaters who may benefit from this skate include people with mental retardation or hypersensitivity.

Walkers

The most popular piece of equipment used by individuals with low extremity impairments, balance, and/or stability problems is a support walker (Figure 20.2). Before the introduction of this skating aid, many people with lower extremity impairments used chairs for stability. Various walker models may be ordered from the Skating Association for the Blind and Handicapped, Inc. (SABAH). These walkers come in three models ranging for use by people who can bear full weight to people who can bear weight for a limited amount of time, to a walker where skaters are supported by a sling seat with adjustable straps, which assist them in remaining upright on their skates.

Harnesses

Harnesses have long been used in teaching beginning skiers, allowing them to gain the independence and confidence needed to ski. Harnesses for ice skaters allows the instructor to support the torsos of skaters with severe balance problems and those unable to bear their own weight, thus protecting the person from injury due to falls. SABAH uses a variety of harnesses but since each is custom made, they are not available at this time to the general public

Outriggers

Adams and McCubbin (1991, p.255) and Kegel (1985, p.27) describe the use of an outrigger device similar to the outriggers used in adapted skiing. The difference in skating is the skate blade is mounted to the end of the crutch. Like a walking crutch, the outrigger provides support and propulsion power.

Wheelchair Runners

If an individual's disability is too severe to make the previously mentioned devices feasible, wheelchair runners invented by the Parks Public Activities Department of the National Capitol Commission of Ottawa, Canada, allows passive participation. Adapted from standard snowmobile steering skis, the runners can be used on hard packed snow (Figure 20.3 and 20.4).

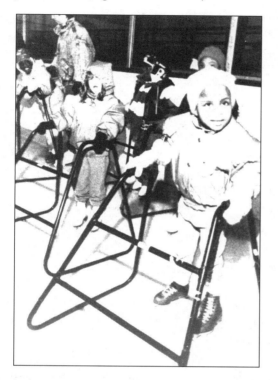

Figure 20.2. Skating aids, available through SABAH, provide support for independent skating, as well as close one-to-one instruction. (Courtesy of SABAH)

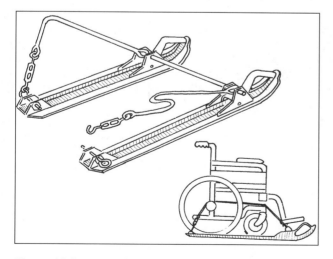

Figure 20.3. Wheelchair runners are functional on ice and snow.

Ice Sledge

The sled (or sledge) for ice sledding or sledge racing is slightly different for the sledge hockey model. The short blades that give the hockey version more maneuverability are replaced with longer steel runners for speed. The small front runner is also eliminated.

EQUIPMENT SUPPLIERS

Sled Suppliers

Access to Recreation, Inc.
8 Sandra Court
Newbury Park CA 91320
(800) 634-4351
(805) 498-7535
(805) 498-8186 (fax)
Email: dkrebs@gte.net
Website: http://www.accesstr.com

Advanced Mobility Products Ltd.
Unit # 111-2323 Boundary Rd.,
Vancouver, B.C., V5M 4V8
Canada

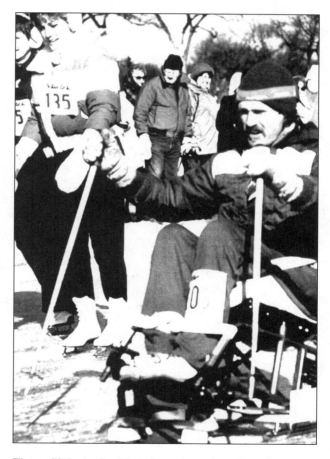

Figure 20.4. A wheelchair frame is used as the main component of a homemade ice sled.

(604) 293-0002
(800) 665-4442
(604) 293-0005 (fax)
Email: mobility@mobilityproducts.com
Website: http://www.mobilityproducts.com

Can Win Sports
621-2446 Bank Street
Ottawa, Ontario
Canada K1V1A8
(613) 247-7041

Gopher Medical
2550 Delaware Street, SE
Minneapolis, MN 55414
(612) 623-7706

Jentsch and Company Inc.
290 South Park Ave.
Buffalo NY 14204
(716-852-4111
(716) 852-4270 (fax)

Midwest Skate Co.
Website: http://www.midwestskate.com/

New Hall's Wheels
P.O. Box 380784
Cambridge, MA 02238
(617) 628-7955
Website: http://www.newhalls.com/

PennSled
Olympic Wheelchair Sales & Service
25 Rothsay Ave.
Kitchener, Ontario, Canada
(519) 741–0795
Email: jpenner@pennsled.com
Website: http://www.pennsled.com/

Spokes N Motion
2225 S Platte River Drive W
Denver, CO 80223
(303) 922-0605
(303) 922-7943 (fax)
Website: http://www.spokesnmotion.com/

Unique Inventions
559 Chamberlain Street
Peterborough, Ontario
Canada K9J4L6
(705) 743-6544
Email: unique@pipcom.com
Website: http://www.pipcom.com/~unique/
(705) 743-6544

Zebra Sports
Phoenix AZ
(602)765-1848

Stick/Pic Suppliers

Dave Conklin
2931 Hamilton Street
LaCrosse, WI 54603
(608) 781-0616
Email: Dpconklin@aol.com

Rehabiliation Institute of Chicago
Wirtz Sports Program
710 North Lakeshore Dr. 3rd Floor
Chicago, IL 60611
(312) 908-4292
Website: http://www.richealthfit.org

Dale Wise
20 Oakland Ave.
Needham, MA 02492-3150
Email: ctwise@mediaone.net
(781) 444-1019
Gary Ludwig
NY Rte.78
Strykersville, NY 14145
(716) 457-3082

ADDITIONAL RESOURCES AND WEBSITES

Ice skaters, figure skaters, speed skaters, and sledge racers will find many websites related to their sport. Because this sport is accessible for those with and without disabilities, most participants will find the following sites satisfactory for gathering information.

Amateur Speedskating Union National Office:
1033 Shady Lane, Glen Ellyn, IL 60137
(630) 790-3230
(630) 790-3235 (fax)
Email: ASUYates@aol.com
Website: http://speedskating.org/

International Paralympic Committee Sledge Racing Page
Website:
     http://www.paralympic.org/sports/sections/sledge-racing/general.htm

International Skating Union (ISU)
Chemin de Primerose 2
CH 1007 Lausanne, Switzerland
(+41) 21 612 66 66
(+41) 21 612 66 77 (fax)

Email: info@isu.ch
Website: http://www.isu.org/
The ISU is the international governing body for both figure and speed skating.

Ottawa-Carleton Sledge Hockey & Ice Picking Association
46 Nestow Dr.
Nepean, Ontario
K2G 3X8, Canada
Designed for those who have some upper body movement, O.C.S.H.I.P. organizes ice picking races in mid-February attracting individuals and teams from across Canada, the U.S. and Europe.

Skating Association for the Blind and Handicapped, Inc. (SABAH)
120 East and West Road
West Seneca, NY 14224
(716) 675-7222
Email: sabah@sabahinc.org
website: http://www.sabahinc.org/

United States Figure Skating Association
20 First Street
Colorado Springs, CO 80906-3697
(719) 635-5200
(719) 635-9548 (fax)
Email: usfsa@usfsa.org
Website: http://www.usfsa.org
This is the national governing body for figure skating in the United States

United States Figure Skating Association
Special Olympic Committee
Website:
        http://hometown.aol.com/socommittee/index.htm
This group provides information on therapeutic ice skating.

United States Speed Skating Association
P.O. Box 450639
Westlake, OH 44145
(440) 899-0128
Email: usskate@ix.netcom.com
Website: http://www.usspeedskating.org
The organization was founded in 1966 when a small group of speedskating enthusiasts broke away from the Amateur Skating Union (ASU) to form the United States International Speedskating Association (USISA). U.S. Speedskating is a member of the U.S. Olympic Committee and International Skating Union.

Chapter 21

Lawn Bowls

SPORT GOVERNING BODIES:
National: American Lawn Bowls Association (ALBA)
International: World Bowls Board (WBB)

Official Sport Of: _____DAAA   _x__USABA   _x__USCPAA
                                    _x__DS/USA   _____USADSF   _x__WS/USA
                                    _____SOI

x = international play only

DISABLED SPORTS ORGANIZATION:
National:
International:

PRIMARY DISABILITY: All

SPORT OVERVIEW

Lawn bowls, lawn bowling, or bowling on the green as it is historically known, is a highly competitive sport played throughout the world, but is most popular in the British Commonwealth. Although the game is not highly publicized in the United States, hundreds of clubs are located throughout the country. Links to many of these clubs may be found in the Additional Resources and Websites at the end of the chapter.

Boccia and curling are sports that are very similar to lawn bowls. The object of the game is to get your bowls (a large wooden ball) closer to the jack (a smaller target ball) than your opponent. The jack is usually located 70-120 feet from where the bowl is rolled (mat). This is achieved by players from each team taking turns rolling four bowls down the green toward the jack. Play alternates from one side of the rink to the other. After all the bowls have been rolled, points are awarded to the person based upon how many bowls are closest to the jack. Although there are different versions of scoring rules, the game proceeds until the predetermined number of rolls has been achieved, or until 25 points has been scored. The person with the most points is declared the winner of the match. The game is as complex as boccia in that the jack may be moved at any time during the game after being struck by a bowl. The game may be played by singles, pairs, triples, or fours.

Although the game has been perceived by many as being a game for seniors, the charm of the game is that it can be played by people of all ages, and genders. People with and without disabilities can play side by side. It is a game that is increasingly being played by younger people especially in elite international level play.

The Cerebral Palsy International Sports and Recreation Association, International Stoke Mandeville Wheelchair Sports Federation, International Blind Sports Association, and the International Sports Organization for the Disabled international competitions are conducted in strict accordance with the Laws of the Game of Lawn Bowls as specified by the World Bowls Board (WBB). Athletes with disabilities do not require rule modifications, and unlike the cerebral palsy game of boccia, ramps and/or chutes are not allowed.

SPORT ORIGIN

A form of Lawn Bowls is thought to have originated with the Egyptians due to the finding of artifacts in tombs circa 5,000 BC. The sport spread across the world with the modern version of the game originating in England in the 12th century. The game naturally found its way across the seas with the colonization of America in the early 1600's. Lawn Bowls lost popularity after the revolutionary war due to its attachment with the British Empire, but was revived in the late 19th century as clubs began to form on the east coast. The American Lawn Bowling Association was founded in 1915 to develop and promote the game throughout the United States. Today hundreds of clubs exist in the United States.

The World Bowling Board (WBB) is responsible for the standardization of rules across the world, and is charged with the task of encouraging the growth of the game worldwide.

Paralympic Lawn Bowls

Lawn Bowls is an official Paralympic event played by athletes with physical disabilities (Figure 21.1 a and b). Athletes are grouped into one of the following 8 classification categories according to functional ability, so that the players compete against others of equal playing abilities. Although Lawn Bowling has been a Paralympic Sport for years, Lawn bowling for individuals who are blind was first introduced in the 1996 Atlanta Paralympic Games.

Paralympic Lawn Bowls Classifications

- LB1 Wheelchair User: Unable to bowl from a standing position, and with reduced strength in the bowling arm to a degree that they cannot compete with standard size bowls.
- LB2 Wheelchair User: Unable to bowl from a standing position.
- LB3 Ambulatory Class-Combination of Lower and Upper Limb Disability: More than 10 points reduction in each effected limb.
- LB4 Ambulatory Class-Lower Limb Disability: More than 10 points reduction in each effected limb.
- LB5 Ambulatory Class-Upper Limb Disability:

More than 10 points reduction in each effected limb.
- LB6 Totally Blind: No light perception in either eye, up to light perception but inability to recognize the shape of a hand at any distance or in any direction.
- LB7 Partially Sighted: From ability to recognize the shape of a hand up to a visual acuity of 2/60 and/or a visual field of less than 5 degrees.
- LB8 Partially Sighted: From visual acuity above 2/60 up to visual acuity of 6/60 and/or a visual field of more than 5 degrees and less than 20 degrees.

Paralympic events include men's, women's, mixed singles, pairs, triples and fours events. As in all international competitions, the World Bowls Board Rules govern the competitions, amended so as to accommodate bowlers with a disability (see the following).

Selected Amended Rules (a complete set of amended rules can be found on the IPC web site).

- For class LB1 the minimum length of the rink shall be 40' and the minimum Jack length shall be 18' from the back edge of the rink.
- All LB1 bowlers shall bowl from a fixed mat position one on each side of the center line.
- LB1 Bowlers may use gloves.
- Competitors may play with or without prosthesis or orthosis as they wish.
- No visual aids or mechanical aids which are solely used as an extension to the body, other than wheelchairs, walking sticks, or crutches for mobility shall be allowed.
- Each bowler in classes LB6, LB7 and LB8 will be allowed a sighted assistant whom shall be referred to as the Bowls Guide. Each bowls guide shall coach, guide, and assist the bowler as requested, but shall not in any way indicate visually the line of aim, green/grass to be taken, center line or any other instruction which could be construed as a visual aid.

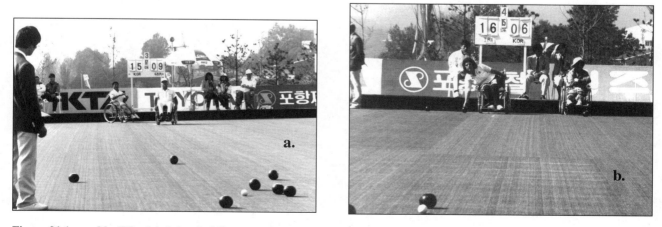

Figure 21.1 a and b. Wheelchair bowls follows standard international rules.

Blind Bowls

Blind Bowls began in 1977 in South Africa and now boasts 10 member countries with 5,000 bowlers. The International Blind Bowls Association (IBBA) has worked for years to integrate blind bowlers into sighted bowls clubs. IBBA sponsors a world tournament every four years. All sighted rules apply to IBBA competition, except that a coach or director may pass on information about the distance between the jack and the blind player's bowls.

EQUIPMENT AND FIELD OF PLAY

The game is played on a field called a green, measuring 37 meters by 37 meters and it is divided into rinks. The bowl is a wooden ball weighing about 3 lbs. and is biased. A biased bowl is manufactured as a spherical ball that is not perfectly balanced. When a bowl is rolled, there is sufficient momentum to keep it running straight along its course. As the bowl slows down, it attempts to find its true balance. When this occurs, the bias is imparted on the direction of the bowl, forcing it to curve (bend) in the desired direction.

Prosthetic Devices

Athletes with amputations may select to bowl with or without a prosthesis (Figure 21.2 a and b). Prostheses are generally custom designed and made with the individual's prosthetist.

Bowling Ball Arm

The Original Bowling Bowl Arm, available from Achievable Concepts, allows the bowler to deliver the bowl without bending down. This device is ideal for people with back problems, poor balance or decreased strength. The Bowling Arm also has the option of a special hand grip for bowlers with arthritis. The arm is produced in standard and wheelchair size with thumb or palm release, which is suitable for bowlers with arthritis.

Bowls Pick Up

The Bowls Pick Up available from Achievable Concepts, allows the bowler to easily pick up the bowls from the turf without bending down. It can be easily adapted for indoor bowls.

EQUIPMENT SUPPLIERS

Lawn Bowls equipment can be purchased through many athletic vendors. The following websites offer lawn bowls equipment online.

Achievable Concepts
P.O. Box 361 Moonee Ponds
Victoria 3039 Australia
613 9752 5958
613 9754 4798 (fax)
Email: sales@achievableconcepts.com.au
Website: http://www.achievableconcepts.com.au/

Bowls-Centre Shop Online
Email: nfo@bowls-centre-shop.co.uk
Website: http://www.bowls-centre-shop.co.uk/

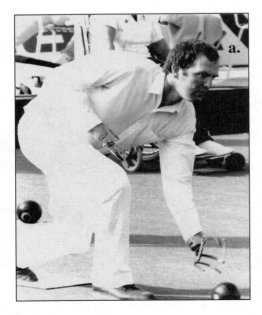 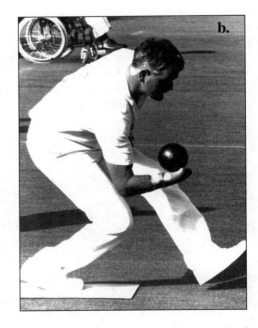

Figure 21.2 a and b. A customized terminal device was designed specifically for bowls, while a competitor chooses to bowl without one. (Courtesy of Specialized Sports Unlimited)

The full service site provides information on the purchasing of any equipment related to Bowling.

Drakes Pride
128 Richmond Row
Liverpool L3 3BC, England
Website: http://www.drakespride.co.uk

ADDITIONAL RESOURCES AND WEBSITES

Lawn Bowlers will find many websites related to their sport. Because this sport is accessible for those with and without disabilities, most participants will find the following sites satisfactory for gathering information.

American Lawn Bowls Association
Email: woodyo@aol.com
Website: http://www.bowlsamerica.org/
This website lists many of the Lawn Bowl Clubs in the United States.

Bowls Canada Boulingrin
1600 James Naismith Drive
Gloucester, Ontario
K1B 5N4 Canada
Phone: (613) 748-5643
Fax: (613) 748-5796
Email: office@bowlscanada.com
Website: http://www.bowlscanada.com/
Bowls Canada Boulingrin is the Canadian sport association overseeing bowls, which includes the promotion and development of lawn bowls, lawn bowling, indoor bowls, short mat bowls and carpet bowls. An extensive program of adaptive lawn bowls is provided by this group.

International Paralympic Committee Lawn Bowl Section
Chairperson
Bob Tinker
2a First Avenue
Forestville 5035, Australia
Tel & Fax: + 618 829 38139

Lawn Bowls International
Website: http://www.lawnbowls.com.au
This website claims to be the most comprehensive site for lawn bowls on the web. It provides a list of lawn bowl clubs world wide.

Ontario Lawn Bowls Association
1185 Eglinton Avenue East
Suite 205
North York, Ontario M3C 3C6
Phone: 416.426.7161
Email: olba@interlog.com

Interlog.com
Website: http://www.interlog.com/~olba/index.html
This site provides many links and features related to the sport.

The Unofficial Lawn Bowl Homepage
Website: http://www.tcn.net/~jdevons/test1.htm
Another page with many links and features related to the sport.

World Bowls Board (WBB)
Secretary/Treasurer: David W Johnson.
Lyndhurst Road
Worthing, West Sussex
BN11 2AZ, England
National (01903) 820222
International +44 903 820222
International +44 903 820444
The website for this international governing organization can be accessed through the International Paralympic Website http://www.paralympic.org

Chapter 22

Martial Arts

SPORT GOVERNING BODIES:
National: USA Judo, USA National Karate-do Federations, U.S. Taekwondo Union
International: International Judo Federation (IJF), Federation Mondaile de Karate
                    (FMK/WKF), World Taekwondo Federation (WTF)

Official Sport Of: _____DAAA   x USABA   _____USCPAA
                            _____DS/USA   _____USADSF   _____WS/USA
                            _____SOI

DISABLED SPORTS ORGANIZATION:
National:
International: International Disabled Self-Defense Association (IDSA)

PRIMARY DISABILITY: All

SPORT OVERVIEW

With its origins embedded in the Asian cultures over many centuries, martial arts is an umbrella term that covers many sports such Karate, Judo, Ju-Jutsu, Chinese Wushu, Aikido, Kendo, Tai-Chi Chuan, Iaido and Taekwondo, to name a few. The popularity of these activities have become more popular by people with disabilities as opportunities have grown and benefits have become more well known (Figure 22.1 a and b). With information about the benefits of martial arts for people with physical disabilities becoming widely available, martial art therapy programs have gained wide acceptance in many communities.

As instructors become more comfortable with integrated classes, people with disabilities who are ambulatory, and wheelchair users are being fully integrated into programs with individuals who do not have disabilities. Presently, only the United States Association for Blind Athletes offers any form of martial arts as a competitive activity. USABA athletes in Judo are well-known for their skill and prominence throughout the world.

LOCAL PROGRAMS AND RESOURCES

The number of local programs offering programs specifically for individuals with disabilities is not as great as one might think. This is due to the fact that generally, no adaptations are needed to allow a person with a disability to participate, and most martial arts programs readily welcome individuals with disabilities (Figure 22.2). Some local programs have gained national exposure due to their inclusionary philosophy including the following clubs.

Challenge Karate Club

The Challenge Karate Club of Conoga Park, California, is a prime example of this inclusion philosophy. Wheelchairs and crutches have become familiar sights as karate students with disabilities endure the disciplined rigors of training along nondisabled teammates.

Encino Judo Club

The Encino Judo Club in California has offered extensive Judo programs for individuals with visual impairments for more than 20 years. Under the guidance of Neil

Ohlenkamp, the Club has worked with the Braille Institute Youth Center of Los Angeles to teach the principles of Judo to visually impaired children and adults.

International Disabled Self-Defense Association (IDSA)

The International Disabled Self-Defense Association (IDSA) was founded in 1996 by Master Instructor Jurgen Schmidt in response to the need for a new kind of Disabled Association. A Worldwide Membership Organization, the IDSA is dedicated to providing all people with and without disabilities, with a dynamic and supportive forum where members can fraternize, explore, exchange, review and discover new and exciting activities as well as find products and services that increase the overall quality of life. The group promotes the most practical, realistic and effective science of Self-Defense for individuals with disabilities. The difference between defense-ability and martial arts is that defense-ability is a technically modified self-defense system based on the ICHF Combat Hapkido Martial Art style and is designed to be suitable for use by individuals with varying types of disabilities.

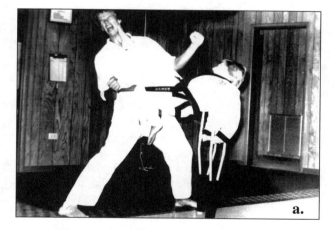

Figure 22.1 a and b. Karate instructor Nancy Stewart (4 feet tall) executes a flying front snapkick to student Frank Lee, Jr. (6 feet 2 inches tall). Nancy teaches the art of karate to a class of eager students. (Courtesy of Nancy Stewart)

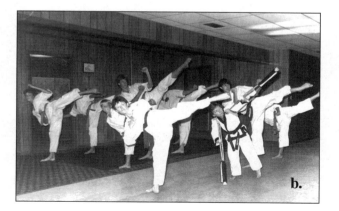

The Combat Hapkido system is a new and modern style of Hapkido. Defense-Ability and Combat Hapkido both differ from other Hapkido styles philosophically, as well as technically.

Martial Arts For The Handicapable Inc. (MAH Inc.)

The Martial Arts For The Handicapable Inc. is a nonprofit organization, founded in 1971 by a US Marine Korean War veteran, Ted Vollrath, that provides individuals with disabilities a sense of independence and empowerment through the medium of martial arts. Grand Master Ted Vollrath, of Harrisburg, Pennsylvania, is the first person in the world to have earned a black belt in karate while training from a wheelchair. The program is open to all students regardless of the nature or the degree of disability. Additionally, the program offers an instructor training program in all legitimate styles of martial arts to work with students in their own locations, and in their own field of expertise. Upon completion of training, the MAH, Inc. issues teaching certification and affiliation credentials to instructors desirous of assisting students with disabilities within the MAH organizational network.

Ron Scanlon's Kung Fu San Soo Academy

Further evidence for involving people with physical disabilities in martial arts is demonstrated by Ron Scanlon's mastery of the ancient art of Kung Fu San Soo. Since the art has been practiced from a sitting position for thousands of years, Scanlon, a paraplegic, realized he was not doing anything new by being seated. An eighth-degree black belt, Scanlon was the coordinator of self-defense activities for the Casa Colina Wheelchair Sports, Recreation and Outdoors Program before opening his own studio in Marina Del Rey in 1991.

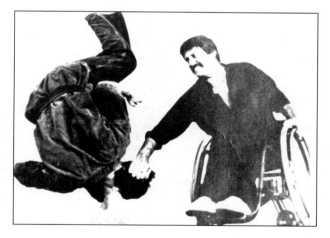

Figure 22.2. A growing number of martial arts programs are including instruction for wheelchair users. (Courtesy of *Sports 'n Spokes* 1/92:72)

MARTIAL ARTS DISCIPLINES

Dozens of variations and types of martial arts exist. It would be impossible to review all of the forms in this chapter. We have chosen to describe the four forms of martial arts, three of which are included within the Olympic family (Judo, Karate, and Taekwondo). All four have been very popular with individuals with disabilities and Judo is an official Paralympic sport. Kung Fu San Soo is also reviewed due to its popularity as a form of self-defense.

Karate

Karate is a Japanese word meaning "empty hand." It is the martial art of unarmed self-defense in which focused blows of the feet and hands are dealt from poised positions. Often, these blows are accompanied by shouts. The three elements of speed, strength and technique are vital to Karate. Lethal kicks and punches are taught, rather than wrestling and throwing maneuvers as in judo and jujitsu. Karate (as well as many other forms of martial arts) emphasizes self-discipline, positive attitude and high moral purpose. It is taught professionally at different levels, and under different Asian names, as a self-defense skill, a competitive sport and a free-style exercise.

Karate has long been recognized as a medium for the development of self-discipline, self-esteem, and self defense. More options have become available for wheelchair users interested in karate. The sport of wheelchair karate was demonstrated at the 1992 Paralympic Games and is included in Breath of Nature Outdoor Karate Championships.

Karate requires only that a person have some mobility. The student does need to hear, or see, and the sport can be practiced from a chair or the floor. Wheelchair users can be taught how to use various maneuvers to position themselves to apply devastating blows to aggressive attackers. Karate is an excellent activity for cross-training. It can increase cardiovascular endurance, concentration and focus. The sport may also increase balance, coordination, and attention span in people with head injuries. It has also been recognized as an activity that increase range of motion in people with cerebral palsy.

Kung Fu San Soo

Buddhist monks in China perfected this effective fighting art many centuries ago. The combinations of kicks, punches, strikes and leverages are based on the scientific principles of physics. When these combinations are directed to vital parts of the body, using balance, coordination, and timing, they are extremely powerful and effective.

The techniques can be changed to fit any given situation and do not follow a set pattern. These natural, circular movements of San Soo make it a common sense self-defense fighting art. Since the art was developed and used for protection of life, rules of fighting can not apply. Therefore, San Soo is not a sport and not used in tournaments or competition. Though there are many principles and applications of the art that can take years of study to master, a person can defend their life with one technique when it is executed correctly.

The physical exercise, coordination, mental awareness and self-defense ability gained through participation are all benefits available to the San Soo student.

Judo

The sport of judo traces back to the brutal hand-to-hand combat of the ancient Japanese samurai warriors. Literally meaning "soft way," judo was developed by Dr. Jigoro Kano in 1882 as a gentler alternative to the more dangerous martial arts. The sport preaches strict training to produce a mind and body in a state of harmony and balance. USA Judo is the National Governing Body for the sport of Judo in the United States and coordinates with the United States Association of Blind Athletes on the conduct of blind judo (Figure 22.3 a and b). USA Judo also trains referees to conduct the blind contest. They are also the only disability sports organization that offers any of the martial arts as an official sport.

Judo is a competitive sport, very similar to wrestling, contested by two players from the same classifications. Matches generally range in length from two to five minutes or as quickly as the time it takes to score a pin. The match is started with the contestants gripping or holding the shirt of the opponent. In Judo, the competitors or "judokas" employ specialized principles of movement, balance and leverage to score points. Points may be scored by throwing the opponent to the mat, pinning the opponent to the mat, choking the opponent while avoiding any action which might injure the neck or the spine of the opponent, or through holds like arm bars which makes the opponent plea submission. Judo has been an official Paralympic sport since 1988 following International Blind Sports Association and International Judo Federation rules.

Taekwondo

Taekwondo originated in Korea and is a free-fighting combat sport in which an individual uses bare hands and feet to repel an opponent. Taekwondo literally means the "way of kicking and punching." It consists of sharp, strong angular movements with free flowing circular movements to produce a balance of beauty and power. With the addition of Taekwondo's trademark kicking techniques it is a complete system of self-defense and personal improvement, thus gaining great popularity throughout the United States. All of its activities are based on the defensive attitude that originally developed

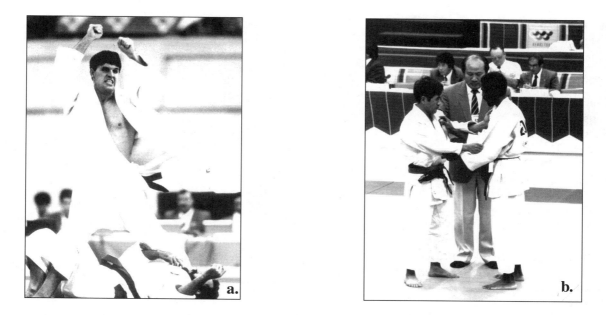

Figure 22.3 a and b. Judo for blind athletes follows the same rules as for sighted athletes. However, if competitors are separated during a match, they are restarted by the official with each athlete grasping their opponent. (Photo by USABA)

for protection against enemy attacks. Taekwondo offers a total fitness program integrating mind, body and spirit.

EQUIPMENT SUPPLIERS

Allblackbelt.com
Website: http://www.allblackbelt.com/
AllBlackBelt.com is the Web's largest source for martial arts supplies.

ADDITIONAL RESOURCES AND WEBSITES

Individuals interested in martial arts will find many websites related to their sport. Because people with disabilities are easily included in most martial arts programs few organizations have been developed specifically for people with disabilities. Because this sport is accessible for those with and without disabilities, most participants will find the following sites satisfactory for gathering information.

Cat Ching Do Enterprise
4817 West Farmington Rd.
Peoria, IL 61604
(309) 674-0350
Program run by amputee Ray Couch III, specializes in teaching individuals with disabilities.

Encino Judo Club
Email: JudoSensei@aol.com

Website: http://JudoInfo.com/ejc.htm
Offer programs specifically for individuals who are blind.

Federation Mondaile de Karate (FMK/WKF)
122 Rue de la Tombe Issoire
75014 Paris, France
Email: support@wkf.net
Website: http://www.wkf.net

International Judo Federation (IJF)
101-1, Ulchi-Ro, 21st Floor Doosan Bldg., I-KA
Chung-Ku, Seoul, Korea
(82+2) 3398 1017
Email: yspark@ijf.org
Website: http:// www.ijf.org

International Disabled Self-Defense Association (IDSA)
22-C New Leicester Hwy., #259
Asheville, North Carolina 28806
(828)683-5528
(828)683-4691 (fax)
Email: info@defenseability.com
Website: http://www.defenseability.com/
IDSA offers a Defense-Ability video series and links to a number of websites.

Judo information site
Website: http://JudoInfo.com/
This is a complete website featuring all aspects of Judo.

Kenpo Karate: Wheelchair Self-defense Studio
562 Monterey Blvd.
San Francisco, CA 94127
(415) 586-8566

Martial Arts for the Handicapable, Inc.
22 Knight Rd.
Harrisburg, Pa. 17111
(717) 583-2150
Email: Yudncha@aol.com
Website: http://mahinc.net/

Martial Arts Net
Website: http://www.martialarts.net
    This is a complete Martial Arts Resource Site providing information on 39 forms of martial arts.

National Handicapable Martial Arts Association (NHMAA)
C/o D. Richard Eunice
112 East Gay Street
Lancaster, SC 29270
(803) 286-5155

Paradise Karate Academy
927A Skyway
Paradise, CA 95969
(53)) 876-9520
Email: musmly@yahoo.com
Website: http://www.paradisekarateacad.bigstep.com

Ron Scanlon's Kung Fu San Soo Academy
12740 Culver Blvd, Unit E.
Marina Del Rey, CA 90066
(310) 305-4144
Website: http://home.sprynet.com/~syzygy/Ron.htm

U.S. Taekwondo Union
One Olympic Plaza, Suite 405
Colorado Springs, CO 80909-5792
(719) 578-4632 (719) 578-4642
Email: USTUTKD1@aol.com
Website: http://www.ustu.org

USA Judo
One Olympic Plaza
Colorado Springs, CO 80909
Email: usjudoexdr@aol.com
Website: http://www.usjudo.org

USA National Karate-do Federation
P.O. Box 77083 Seattle, WA 98177-7083
(206) 440-8386
(206) 367-7557 (fax)
Email: karate@usankf.org
Website: http://www.usankf.org/

United States Judo Association
21 North Union Blvd.
Colorado Springs, CO USA 80909
(719) 633-7750
(719) 633-4041 (fax)

United States Judo Federation
P. O. Box 338
Ontario, OR 97914
(541) 889-8753
(541) 889-5836 (fax)
Email: natofc@usjf.com
    The USJF is a national non-profit corporation dedicated to the development of judo. The USJF regularly forms committees and events at the local, regional and national level for these purposes.

United States Martial Arts Association
8011 Mariposa Avenue
Citrus Heights, CA 95610
(916) 727-1486
(916) 727-7236 (fax)
Email: psp4@flash.net
Website: http://www.mararts.org/

World Taekwondo Federation (WTF)
635 Yuksam-Dong, Kangnam-ku
Seoul 135-081 Korea
Email: wft@unitel.co.kr

BIBILIOGRAPHY

Couch, R. (1997). Disability Doesn't Mean Vulnerability. *In-Motion* 7(2)41-43.

Himmelstein, L. (1992). Karate-Wheelchair Style. *Sports 'n Spokes* 18(3)55-56.

Thomas, C. (1998). Blind Ambition: Kevin Szott's Olympic Vision is Crystal Clear. *Active Living* 7(4)10,12.

Chapter 23

Powerlifting

SPORT GOVERNING BODIES:
National: USA Powerlifting (USAPL)
International: International Powerlifting Federation (IPF)

Official Sport Of: __x__DAAA   __x__USABA   __x__USCPAA
                            __x__DS/USA   ____USADSF   __x__WS/USA
                            __x__SOI

DISABLED SPORTS ORGANIZATION:
National:
International:

PRIMARY DISABILITY: All

SPORT OVERVIEW

Powerlifting and weightlifting are terms that confuse many people. Weightlifting, however, includes only the competitive events of the clean and jerk and the snatch. Both are Olympic events and governed by USA Weightlifting (USAW) and the International Weightlifting Federation (IWF). Weightlifting is not a sport traditionally competed in by athletes with disabilities. The use of modified equipment is rare and generally consists of the use of a prosthesis or a wide bench for the bench press.

Powerlifting is a true indicator of brute strength and is a sport open to both men and women. The object of traditional powerlifting is to lift the most weight by adding up the totals from the events of the squat, bench press, and deadlift in that order. There are also competitions, especially in disability sport, where each event is done separately. The bench press is the most popular of all events for athletes with disabilities. Although these are not Olympic events, all three powerlifting events are performed in Special Olympics whereas only the bench press is done in the Paralympic Games (Figure 23.1). These non-Olympic events are overseen by USA Powerlifting (USAPL) and the International Powerlifting Federation (IPF). Although we have listed them as such due to their inclusion in disability sports, they are not true national governing bodies since they do not belong to the Olympic family. Weight Training is another related, but different activity that is discussed later in this book.

SPORT ORIGIN

The idea of lifting weights (usually stones) to prove ones strength and manhood has been documented for centuries from ancient China and Greece. Weightlifting was a part of the first modern Olympic Games in 1896 and continues today as a popular competitive and recreational activity. As mentioned above, weightlifting is an official Olympic event, but not a Paralympic event, whereas powerlifting, with different events, is not an Olympic event but is an event in Paralympic and Special Olympics competitions.

The history of powerlifting for athletes with disabilities is very thin due to the past divergence among the different disability groups. Each disability group has its own history concerning the evolution of the sport. The oldest lifting events for wheelchair athletes began around 1950-1955. These competitions, governed by the International

Stoke Mandeville Wheelchair Sports Federation were first offered at the 1964 Paralympic Games in Tokyo for male athletes with spinal cord injuries. The event was later opened to athletes from other disabilities categories. The 2000 Paralympic Games in Sydney were the first time women competed in the event. Today, Paralympic Powerlifting encompasses a multi-disability register of athletes competing in 10 weight classes for both men and women.

Competitions for blind powerlifters began in the early 1980's in the United States, Australia, Canada and Great Britain. In 1988, the first World Cup of Powerlifting (for blind athletes only) was held in Canada under IPF rules. When Special Olympics began in 1968, the dead lift was the only event offered. Eventually the bench press, and squat were added. Most disability sports organizations organize their competitions around disability classification, age, weight and gender to ensure equitable competition. The United States Powerlifting Federation has included athletes with disabilities in their organization through the development of the Disabled Athletes Committee.

POWERLIFTING EVENTS

Bench Press

All disability sport organizations offering powerlifting competition include the bench press. As indicated above, the bench press event is run under the auspices of USA Powerlifting and International Powerlifting Federation. Weight divisions and age categories differ among organizations, as does access by female competitors. The bench press event for spinal cord-injured competitors is referred to as "wheelchair weightlifting" although it is technically a powerlifting event (Figure 23.2). Differences in techniques and types of benches used distin-

guish powerlifting of the United States Cerebral Palsy Athletic Association, United States Association for Blind Athletes, and Disabled Sports USA, from the weightlifting of Wheelchair Sports USA. Generally in this event, the athlete lays on a bench in a supine position. The bar is then handed to the lifter by spotters. Once receiving the bar the lifter keeps the bar at arms length with elbows locked waiting for the referee's signal. After receiving the signal, the lifter lowers the bar to the chest, holds it motionless on the chest and then presses it upward, after a referees second signal, with an even extension of the arms to arms length where it is then held motionless.

Squat and Deadlift

The United States Association for Blind Athletes and Special Olympics offers the squat and deadlift in addition to the bench press (Figure 23.3). Both are run in accordance with IPF rules. The squat consists of placing the bar behind the head resting on the shoulders. The lifter squats down, and then rises again to a standing position. The deadlift is performed by a lifter raising a weighted bar from the floor to hip level with straight arms from a standing position.

Special Olympics

In addition to the events mentioned above, Special Olympics offers competition in Unified events consisting of the squat bench press, deadlift, and combination (total weight of bench press and deadlift). Unified powerlifting is where athletes with and without mental retardation compete together. A combined score of each team determines the winner. Other official weightlifting events that promote fitness for athletes with lower ability levels, including modified push-ups, sit-ups, and exercycle are also offered.

Although powerlifting has been a Special Olympic event only since 1987, the sport has enjoyed tremendous

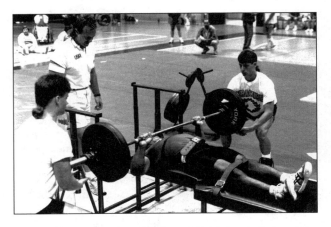

Figure 23.1. USCPAA, NHS, and DAAA are three of the DSO's who offer powerlifting under the rules of the International Powerlifting Federation. (Photo by Oscar Izquierdo)

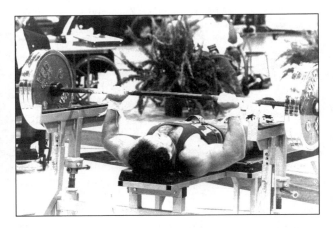

Figure 23.2. Wheelchair weightlifting is actually an adapted version of the powerlifting event bench press. (Courtesy of Specialized Sports Unlimited)

success and growth. The sport is especially popular by athletes with Down Syndrome. Aerobic activity may prove difficult for these individuals due to circulatory system immaturity, but their short and stocky body type and physical characteristics are well-suited for success in powerlifting.

Modifications to Rules

Athletes competing in Special Olympics or Paralympics must abide by the same technical rules of the IPF regarding the performance of the lift(s) themselves. However, the International Paralympic Committee has made the following adaptations to IPF rules to accommodate lifters with disabilities in the Paralympic Games.

- Lifters are allowed two minutes to complete a lift. IPF rules allow only one minute.
- Lifters are allowed to use a thumbless grip. IPF rules do not permit thumbless grips.
- Lifters are not allowed to use a bench shirt. IPF rules allow lifters to wear bench shirts.
- Lifters are required to keep their feet off the floor during the bench press (SOI also). IPF rules require both feet to be flat on the floor during the bench press.
- Amputee lifters have the option to use a prosthesis during the lift. IPF rules consider a prosthesis as an illegal piece of equipment. *Note: Amputees body weight is adjusted to account for the lost limb.
- Lifters with Cerebral Palsy may use a personal wedge or cushion. IPF rules consider wedges as illegal pieces of equipment.
- Lifters have the option to use a modified bench. IPF rules require a standard bench. The modified bench is longer (2.1m) and higher (45-50cm) than a standard IPF bench. The modified bench is wider at he bottom (61cm) and tapered near the top (30.5cm) to

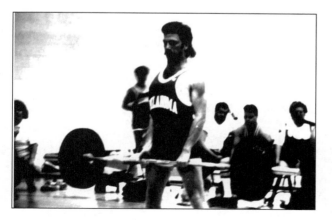

Figure 23.3. Blind powerlifting competes in the deadlift. (Courtesy of USABA)

approximately standard width. The modified bench also has two optional belts (10cm thick) to strap the lifter down for stability.

ADDITIONAL RESOURCES AND WEBSITES

Powerlifters and weightlifters will find many websites related to their sports. Disabled powerlifting websites outside of the disability sports organizations are rare, but because this sport is accessible for those with and without disabilities, most participants will find the following sites satisfactory for gathering information.

International Powerlifting Federation
Email: mike@ipf.com
Website: http://www.ipf.com

International Weightlifting Federation (IWF)
Hold u.1
1374 Budapest, P.O.Box 614 Hungary
Email: iwf@iwf.net
Website: http://www.powerlifting-ipf.com

Powerlifting.com
Website: http://www.powerlifting.com/
Powerlifting.com is an online resource intended to provide athletes, fans and the world's media with a definitive source of Powerlifting information. It contains hundreds of links to Powerlifting related sites across the globe. Powerlifting.com is an independent service and is officially approved by the International Powerlifting Federation.

USA Powerlifting/American Drug Free Powerlifting Association, Inc.
124 West Van Buren Street
Columbia City, IN 46725
(219) 248-4889
(219) 248-4879 (fax)
Website: http://www.usapowerlifting.com/

USA Powerlifting Disabled Athletes Committee
Fran Haley
12101 Reagan St.
Los Alamitos, CA 90720
(562) 596-6866

USA Weightlifting
One Olympic Plaza
Colorado Springs, CO 80909-5764
Email: usaw@worldnet.att.net
Website: http://www.usaweightlifting.org

USCPAA Sport Technical Officer (Powerlifting)
Michael McDevitt
8420 West Chester Pike
Upper Darby, PA 19082
(610) 356-1910
Website: http://www.uscpaa.org/

US Wheelchair Weightlifting Federation
Bill Hens (Director)
39 Michael Place
Levittown, PA 19057
(215) 945-1964
(215) 946-2574 (fax)
Website: http://www.wsusa.org/weightrule.htm (rules)

Chapter 24

Quad Rugby

SPORT GOVERNING BODIES:

Official Sport Of: _____ DAAA _____ USABA _____ USCPAA
_____ DS/USA _____ USADSF __x__ WS/USA
_____ SOI

DISABLED SPORTS ORGANIZATION:
National: United States Quad Rugby Association (USQRA)
International: International Wheelchair Rugby Federation (IWRF)

PRIMARY DISABILITY: Spinal Cord Injured Quadriplegics

SPORT OVERVIEW

Combining aspects of basketball and soccer and a penalty system similar to hockey, wheelchair rugby (known as quad rugby in the United States, provides an exciting team sport for quadriplegics left out of the game of wheelchair basketball. Wheelchair rugby is played in four (4) eight (8) minute periods, on a regulation basketball court with restricted areas designated by pylons and tape. A goal line at each end of the court measures eight meters (26' 3"). A key area extends from the goal line and is 1.75 meters deep (Figure 24.1).

Two teams consist of four players apiece. The game begins with a center toss similar to basketball. The object of the game is for the offensive team to touch or carry a regulation volleyball over the defensive team's goal line (Figure 24.2). A variety of offensive strategies have been developed to maximize defensive weaknesses. The defensive team attempts to force turnovers by blocking, intercepting, or batting the volleyball away from the offensive players.

The ball may be passed, thrown, batted, rolled, dribbled, or carried in any direction subject to the restrictions laid down in the rules. Certain restrictions apply in the key area. One restriction is that only three defensive play-ers are allowed in the key, and if a fourth enters, a penalty can be assessed or a goal awarded. Another restriction is that an offensive player can only stay in the key area for ten seconds. Otherwise a turnover will be assessed.

A player with the ball may take an unlimited number of pushes but must bounce or pass the ball within 10 seconds. The offensive team must get the ball into the front court within 15 seconds of possession. Generally, offensive penalties result in the loss of possession while defensive penalties and major infractions result in banishment to the penalty box. A complete set of the international rules of the game can be found on the USQRA website.

SPORT ORIGIN

Wheelchair rugby was developed as an alternative to wheelchair basketball by athletes with quadriplegia. Originally developed as a game called murderball, due to the aggressive nature of the game, wheelchair rugby has enjoyed unparalleled growth in recent years. Created in the mid-1970s by three Canadians, Duncan Campbell, Ben Harnish, and Jerry Terwin, the game is a cross between wheelchair basketball and ice hockey. It was introduced into the United States in 1981 by Brad Mikkelsen, and the name changed to quad rugby. Over the years the game has evolved with standardized rules and equipment being adopted.

The United States Quad Rugby Association (USQRA) was formed in 1988 to promote the sport on a national and international basis, and now boasts teams in over 27 states and in 20 foreign countries. Competition culminates in an annual national championship tournament. Eventually with the formation of the International Wheelchair Rugby Federation to oversee the games development, the name of Wheelchair Rugby was formally adopted.

The International Wheelchair Rugby Tournament has been hosted in Toronto since 1989. Quad rugby was recognized at the 1990 Stoke Mandeville Games during exhibition play and now enjoys status as a medal sport at the Stoke games. In the fall of 1992 USQRA became an official member of Wheelchair Sports-USA, and became a full medal event in the 2000 Paralympic Games.

CLASSIFICATION SYSTEM

A classification point system similar to that used in wheelchair basketball ensures that players with varying disability levels have the same opportunities to play. Based on a variety of functional tests, players are given point values for arm, hand, and trunk function. Players are given a classification number from one of seven classifications ranging from 0.5-3.5 (half-point intervals). The 0.5 player has the greatest impairment and is comparable to a C5 quadriplegic. Of those eligible to participate, the 3.5 player has the least impairment and is similar to a C7-8 incomplete quadriplegic. Both male and females are encouraged to play, and because of the classification process gender advantages don't exist. Team totals may not exceed 8.0 for the four players on the court at one time. A complete description of the classifications may be found on the USQRA website.

EQUIPMENT

The use of equipment in wheelchair rugby is limited to the official ball (volleyball) available from the USQRA, a good rugby chair with protective bumpers, and gloves. Gloves are seen more often in wheelchair rugby than in wheelchair basketball primarily because upper extremity and hand dysfunction is so severe in quadriplegics. Depending on individual needs, the use of trunk, waist, leg, and foot strapping is also allowed. Many wheelchair manufacturers now provide wheelchairs designed specifically for wheelchair rugby (see appendix). See the resources listed below and in the appendix.

ADDITIONAL RESOURCES AND WEBSITES

Many individual team websites exist for the sport, however, the United States Quad Rugby Website is the most extensive and the only one needed to access information. The USQRA website lists official rules, classification system, and current teams.

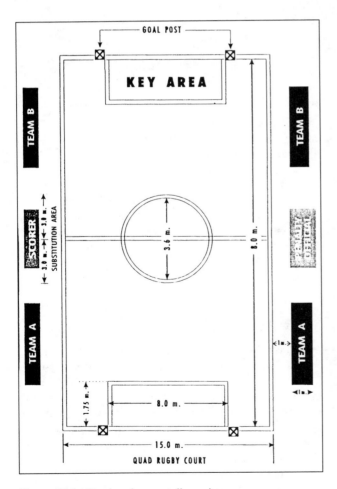

Figure 24.1. Quad rugby court dimensions.

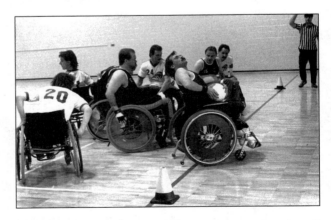

Figure 24.2. The purpose of quad rugby is to carry the ball across the opponent's goal line. (Courtesy of Rehabilitation Institute of Chicago's Wirtz Sports Program)

International Wheelchair Rugby Federation
Pawel Zbieranowski
67 Riverside Blvd.
Thornhill Ontario L4J 1H8 Canada
(905) 886-1252 (Res)
(416) 396-6765 (Bus)
(416) 396-6770 (fax)

Canadian Wheelchair Rugby Association
Marco DisPaltro – Chairman
1155 Monte Ste-Therese, # C
Bellefeuille, QC
JOR 1A0, Canada
 (514) 585-5300
 (514) 585-5300 (fax)

United States Quad Rugby Association
Kevin Orr
101 Park Place Circle
Alabaster, Alabama 35007
(205) 868-2281
(205) 868-2283 (fax)
Email: supersports@mindspring.com
Website: http://www.quadrugby.com

Chapter 25

Racquetball

SPORT ORIGIN

The invention of racquetball is credited to Joe Sobek, in Connecticut in 1949, when he combined the basic concepts of handball and squash while using a short strung paddle. The game became extremely popular in the 1970's as people saw the fitness benefits that could be derived from playing. The game could be played indoors which made it a perfect activity in colder climates. Athletic clubs soon began making courts available. The sport is already fully integrated in that wheelchair players can get 2 or more bounces before they hit the ball while ambulatory players get only one bounce (Figure 25.1).

SPORT OVERVIEW

Founded in 1968, The United States Racquetball Association (USRA) is the national governing body to promote the development of competitive and recreational racquetball in the United States. With over seven million individuals playing racquetball in the United States, the USRA has incorporated the interests of players with disabilities by endorsing the establishment of affiliated organizations. Current active affiliates include the National Wheelchair Racquetball Association (NWRA) and the National Racquetball Association of the Deaf (NRAD). The USRA official rule book includes rules governing play by wheelchair users and players who are deaf or blind.

To provide services and support, the USRA has established a standing commission for wheelchair racquetball. Its main function is to review and recommend rule modifications that will accommodate competition for players with disabilities. In addition, the USRA's committee offers promotional, professional, and technical support for competitions and special events.

Wheelchair Racquetball

The National Wheelchair Racquetball Association (NWRA) reorganized in 1991 under the auspices of the United States Racquetball Associations Committee for the Disabled. What makes the collaboration of these two organizations so successful is that racquetball is one of the few sports in which players can compete side-by-side with ambulatory players. In general, the USRA's standard rules governing racquetball play for wheelchair users are followed with a few modifications.

Two bounces (instead of one) are used in wheelchair racquetball in all divisions except the Multi-Bounce Division (see the following). The ball may hit the floor twice, if needed, before being returned. The player may not come out of their seat when hitting the ball or serving, and the player must have their <u>rear wheels</u> behind the service line when serving (international rules require all 4 wheels to be behind the service line).

In order to protect playing surfaces, players must have non-marking tires and it is suggested (mandated in international rules) that wheelchairs be equipped with roller bars or wheels under the platforms. Sharp edges should be removed or covered for additional protection.

Multi-Bounce Division

The Multi-Bounce Division is for individuals whose mobility is such that wheelchair racquetball would be impossible if not for the Multi-Bounce Division. The ball may bounce as many times as the receiver wants, though the player may swing only once to return the ball to the front wall. The ball must be hit before it crosses the short line on its way back to the front wall, and the receiver cannot cross the short line after the ball contacts the back wall.

A complete list of rules for wheelchair play is available by contacting the USRA or by accessing their website.

Deaf Racquetball

The National Racquetball Association of the Deaf (NRAD) follows specific USRA rules without the need for adaptations. Eligibility rules are based on hearing loss of 55db or greater in the better ear for any NRAD tournament.

Visually Impaired Racquetball

The USRA official rule book includes modifications for players with visual impairments.
Eligibility standards follow the USABA classification system. A player's visual acuity must not be better than 20/200 with the best practical eye correction or else the player's field of vision must not be better than 20 degrees. The three classifications of blindness are B1 (totally blind to light perception), B2 (able to see hand movement up to 20/600 corrected), and B3 (from 20/600 to 20/200 corrected).

On the return of serve and on every return thereafter, the player may make multiple attempts to strike the ball until the ball has been touched, the ball has stopped bouncing, or the ball has passed the short line after touching the back wall. The only exception is if the ball (other than on the serve) caroms from the front wall to the back wall on the fly, the player may retrieve the ball from any place on the court (including in front of the short line) so long as the ball has not been touched and is still bouncing.

Other Disabilities

Individuals with lower extremity disabilities, amputations (Figure 25.2), or mental impairment can make rule changes based on needs and skill levels. As players become more skillful, decisions to advance to competitive racquetball are made on an individual basis.

EQUIPMENT

Standard racquets and balls are used by wheelchair players. Most competitive players use lightweight sport wheelchairs similar to those used in wheelchair basketball and tennis. USRA rules stipulate that officials can prohibit use of chairs with black tires or anything else that may mark or damage the court. Readers should refer

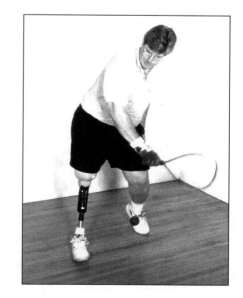

Figure 25.2. The technology of the QSA Single Axis Knee and the Ducpaco Hydraulic Unit allows an above the knee amputee to successfully participate in racquetball. (Courtesy of Hosmer-Dorrance)

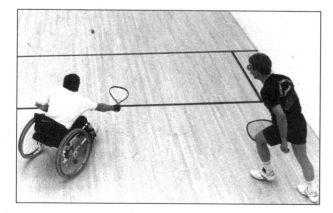

Figure 25.1. Racquetball is one of the many sports that easily incorporates ambulatory and wheelchair players into joint competition. (Courtesy of Rehabilitation Institute of Chicago's Wirtz Sports Program and Oscar Izquierdo)

to the equipment appendix for additional information on appropriate wheelchairs.

ADDITIONAL RESOURCES AND WEBSITES

United States Racquetball Association
1685 West Uintah
Colorado Springs, CO 80904-2921
(719) 635-5396
(719) 635-0685 (fax)
Email: racquetball@usra.org
Website: http://www.usra.org

International Racquetball Federation (IRF)
1685 West Uintah
Colorado Springs, CO 80904-2921
(719) 635-5396
(719) 635-0685 (fax)
Website: http://www.worldsport.com/worldsport/
            sports/racquetball/home.html

Morris Adams, USRA Commissioner for Wheelchair
8644 Portola Circle, #12-A
Huntington Beach, CA 92645
714/969-5786 (H)

Chapter 26

Road Racing

SPORT GOVERNING BODIES:
National: USA Track and Field
International: International Amateur Athletic Federation

Official Sport Of: _____DAAA   _x__USABA   _____USCPAA
                             _____DS/USA   _x__USADSF   _____WS/USA
                             _x__SOI

DISABLED SPORTS ORGANIZATION:
National:
International:

PRIMARY DISABILITY: All

SPORT OVERVIEW

The marathon is one of the worlds oldest organized sporting events being traced back to the Ancient Olympic Games in Greece. The race is the climax of the Olympic and Paralympic Games and to the winner goes the title of the greatest runner in the world. The number of people involved in road racing has continued to grow since its explosion on the scene in the early 1970's. The number of one-mile fun runs, 5k and 10k runs, marathons, and triathlons provides evidence of the popularity of long-distance running. Most large road races now typically offer competition in wheelchair categories and many provide prize money. Recently, many of these runs have been organized for the benefit of various charities. Millions of people have turned to running and road racing to maintain physical and mental health and to develop closer family ties. According to the USATF Road Running Information Center, in 1999, there were an estimated 7.1 million finishers from a total of more than 12,000 U.S. running events. Just fifteen years ago the world of organized U.S. road racing was much smaller with less than 3 million participants and only 1361 certified courses (i.e., accurately measured and documented by the governing body). At that time the most popular

distances were 10Ks (38% of the total), 5Ks (11%), 8Ks (11%) and marathons (8%). In 1994, the number of USA Track & Field certified courses had grown to 12,918 with the 5K replacing the 10K as the most common distance (4002 compared to 3384 10Ks).

In the United States, USA Track & Field (USATF) is the National Governing Body for long distance running, race walking and cross country, as well as track and field. On the international level, the sport is governed by the International Amateur Athletic Federation (IAAF) through its Cross Country and Road Running Committee.

The Road Runners Club of America is the largest grass roots national running organization of over 670 Chapter Clubs located in 48 states and Guam, and representing over 190,000 members. They assist with various events related to road racing for individuals with disabilities.

Individuals who wish to run longer (ultrarunning) races will find The American Ultrarunning Association (AUA) a useful resource. The AUA is a non-profit organization whose sole purpose is to promote the sport of ultrarunning (foot racing at distances beyond the standard marathon) in the United States of America. The AUA is an affiliate of USA Track and Field.

Only three of the major disability sport organizations

offer long-distance road-racing as an option in their athletics program. Blind runners in USABA run distances of 3000 meter (F), 5000 meter (M), 10k road race (M&F), and marathons (M&F) while Special Olympians compete in all of the above plus the 15k and half-marathon. Deaf runners compete in 5K, 10k and marathons.

Many local disability sport clubs have formed running clubs and begun using community road races to provide competitive opportunities for their athletes, and increase the visibility of their organizations. One notable example is The Achilles Track Club of New York City.

The Achilles Track Club

The Road Racers Club of America supports running for the disabled through the Achilles Track Club, which was founded by an RRCA chapter, the New York Road Runners Club. The Achilles Track Club (ATC) is a worldwide cross-disability running program with almost 40 national and 20 international chapters. People with disabilities as varied as blindness, stroke, cerebral palsy, arthritis, epilepsy, amputation, MS, and polio are members of the ATC. There are several chapters affiliated with RRCA clubs around the country.

Hundreds of similar programs across the country have expanded opportunities for individuals with disabilities including cerebral palsy, visual impairments, amputations, mental impairments, and various les autres conditions (Figure 26.1). The longest distance run at the 1968 inaugural Special Olympics Games in Chicago was 100 yards. Today, many Special Olympians compete in the marathon and half-marathon.

Road racing is very different from competition on a 400-meter track, especially in half and full marathons. Athletes need to consider differences in training methods, diet, and the potential for increased contraindications for specific disabilities.

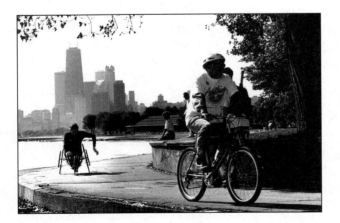

Figure 26.1. Chicago's lakefront provides an ideal location for a late summer training run. (Courtesy of Rehabilitation Institute of Chicago's Wirtz Sports Program and Oscar Izquierdo)

WHEELCHAIR ROAD RACING

Wheelchair road racing for athletes with disabilities was highlighted when wheelchair road racer Deanna Sodoma was featured in television ads for Northwest Airlines. The ads, focusing on her road racing prowess, stated that she would not get to the start line unless the airline got her and her wheelchair to her destination. Without question, the largest increases in disabled athlete participation have been in wheelchair road racing. Many races are attracting more than 100 wheelchair competitors while providing prize money for winners in several divisions as well as for new course and world records. Major marathons such as the Boston Marathon have provided greater exposure and opportunities for the wheelchair athlete (Figure 26.2 a and b). For management reasons, international event organizers are seeking to reduce the number of classes within each race. This presents a challenge to fair but meaningful competition. Athletes should not be at an advantage simply because their disabilities are not as severe as those of other competitors.

Continued technological advances in wheelchair design and better training have improved marathon times. Bob Hall completed the first wheelchair marathon in 1974 in 2:54:5 but times under 1:25 have been recorded in recent years.

Wheelchair racers have taken the sport to its limits in such races as the Midnite Sun Wheelchair Marathon hosted by Access Alaska and Challenge Alaska. Promoted as the world's longest wheelchair race, the nine day race stretches 367 miles from Fairbanks to Anchorage.

Illinois Wheelchair Classic

One of the best sources in the country for wheelchair road-racing is an annual workshop held at the University of Illinois, Urbana-Champaign. The Illinois Wheelchair Classic is a weekend wheelchair track meet held in conjunction with an educational workshop. Each year the U of I Wheelchair Track & Field staff publishes a manual which covers training and competitive issues of wheelchair track and road-racing

EQUIPMENT

Wheelchairs

Most serious road racers will want to consider expensive but essential customized chairs. Several manufacturers should be contacted in order to compare information on warranties, guarantees, and cost. A list of many lightweight wheelchair suppliers can be found in the Track & Field Chapter.

A wider variety of equipment is being manufactured to meet more specific training demands. Odometer computers, racing gloves, and wheelchair rollers are training

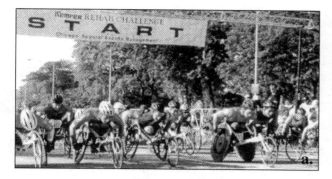
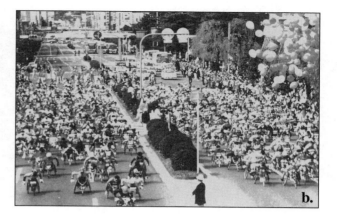

Figure 26.2 a and b. (a) Many local road races have added wheelchair divisions in the past ten years. **(b)** The start of the Japan Marathon also illustrates the popularity of wheelchair road racing. (Courtesy of the Rehabilitation Institute of Chicago's Wirtz Sports Program and *Sports 'n Spokes* 5/91:26)

devices and equipment that may help to improve performance.

ADDITIONAL RESOURCES AND WEBSITES

Individuals interested in road racing will find many websites related to their sport. Because people with disabilities are easily included in most running clubs few organizations have been developed specifically for people with disabilities. Because this sport is accessible for those with and without disabilities, most participants will find the following sites satisfactory for gathering information.

Achilles Track Club International
42 West 38th Street
New York, NY 10018
(212) 354-3978
(212) 354-3978
Email: AchillesClub@aol.com
Website: http://www.achillestrackclub.org/

All American Trail Running Association
PO Box 9175
Colorado Springs, CO 80932
This is a comprehensive source for trail running. Seasoned mountain and trail runners as well as the road runner considering a break from the pavement will find timely information from product reviews to event listings.

American Ultrarunning Association (AUA)
Email: aua@americanultra.org
The American Ultrarunning Association (AUA) is a non-profit organization whose sole purpose is to promote

the sport of ultrarunning (foot racing at distances beyond the standard marathon) in the United States of America.

Access to Recreation
How to Race (video)
8 Sandra Court
Newbury Park CA 91320
(800) 634-4351
(805) 498-7535
(805) 498-8186 (fax)
Email: dkrebs@gte.net
Website: http://www.accesstr.com

Challenge Alaska
Midnite Sun Ultra Challenge
P.O. Box 110065
Anchorage, AK 99511
(907) 344-7399
(907) 344-7349
Email: challenge@artic.net

International Amateur Athletic Federation
17 rue Princesse Florestine
BP 359
MC 98007 Monaco Cedex
(377) 93 10 88 88
(377) 93 15 95 15 (fax)
Email: headquarters@iaaf.org
Website: http://www.iaaf.org/

Road Runners Club of America (RRCA)
1150 South Washington, Suite 250
Alexandria, VA 22314
(703) 836-0558
(703) 836-4430 (fax)
Email: execdir@rrca.org
Website: http://www.rrca.org/

The Running Page
Website: http://www.runningpage.com/

The Running Page is a complete source for information about running on the Web. The Running Page contains information about upcoming races, running clubs, places to run, running related products, magazines, and other information.

University of Illinois
Wheelchair Track & Field Program
Diviison of Rehabilitation and Education Services
Champaign, IL
(217) 244-5869
Website:
http://www.rehab.uiuc.edu/campuslife/sports/trackhist.html

United States of America Deaf Track and Field
Website: http://members.tripod.com/~usadtf/

USA Track & Field
P.O. Box 120 (One RCA Dome, Suite 140)
Indianapolis, IN 46206-0120 (46225)

Email: USATFprogs@aol.com
Website: http://www.usatf.org
Website: http://www.usaldr.org/ (USATF Road Running Information Center)

Wheelchair Racing Resource Page
Email: birzer@execpc.com
Website: http://www.execpc.com/~birzer/

This website provide updated links related to wheelchair road racing including associations, equipment, and race announcements.

Wheelchair Athletics of the USA
Barry Ewing
2351 Parkwood Road
Snellville, GA 30278
(770) 972-0763
(770) 985-4885 (fax)
Email: bewing@beilesouth.net

Chapter 27

Roller Skating

SPORT GOVERNING BODIES:
National: USA Roller Skating (USACRS)
International: Federation Internationale de Roller Skating (FIRS)

Official Sport Of: _____DAAA   _____USABA   _____USCPAA
                        _____DS/USA   _____USADSF   _____WS/USA
                        __x__SOI

DISABLED SPORTS ORGANIZATION:
National:
International:

PRIMARY DISABILITY: Individuals with mental retardation, amputees, deaf, blind, les autres

SPORT OVERVIEW

Roller skating has been a popular recreational sport for many years and has increased in popularity with the development of in-line skates. Its inclusion in the Pan American Games and the United States Olympic Festival has highlighted its competitive aspect. Participation by individuals with disabilities has been primarily recreational, however, Special Olympics offers roller skating as an official competitive sport. Depending on their individual strengths, athletes may choose to use in-line or quad skates. Speed skating, artistic skating, roller and in-line hockey are all popular events. Competitive roller skating is governed nationally by USA Roller Skating (USACRS) and internationally by the Federation Internationale de Roller Skating (FIRS).

SPORT ORIGIN

With the exception of Special Olympics, information and organized programs of roller skating for individuals with disabilities is relatively scarce. With its origins in Europe, roller skating has existed for over 200 years with numerous people being given credit for developing innovative designs for roller skates. Joseph Merlin, a Belgian

inventor is credited with developing the first roller skate with metal wheels in 1760. The first patent ever taken out on a roller skate was for an in-line skate in 1819 developed by Monsieur Petitbled. Pettibled's design made turning just about impossible however. In 1867 an earlier design of Jean Garcin was picked up by industrial engineers and demonstrated at the World Fair in Paris. Modifying this design, James Plimpton of New York designed roller skates, which were sold under the trade name "Rocking Skate". Although still not perfect, the skater could turn merely by shifting his weight to one side meaning that he could perform elegant curves and figures. Once suitable skates were developed that allowed people to move and turn freely, many roller skating halls soon opened. Artistic and speed skating and roller hockey became very popular sports soon after.

The National Governing Body of roller skating in the United States is USA Roller Hockey. USA Roller Skating was founded in 1937 to oversee the development of amateur competitive roller skating programs. Today USA Roller Skating membership exceeds 32,000 skaters in the three branches of the sport-speed skating, artistic skating and roller hockey. USA Roller Skating also works closely with Special Olympics in the development of their competitive program. Roller hockey was actually a demonstration event at the 1992 Barcelona Olympics. Pan American competition and World championships are now routinely held in all roller skating events.

SPECIAL OYLMPICS COMPETITION

Special Olympics roller skating competition was first introduced at the 1987 World Special Olympics Summer Games. Competition is offered in both speed and artistic events and is based on FIRS official rules. Five-on-five roller hockey is also offered as a demonstration event. Speed skating events are conducted on a 100-meter track and include the following: 100, 300, 500 and 1,000 meters; 2x100-meter relay, 2x200-meter relay and 4x100-meter relay (Figure 27.1). All relays are also offered in the Unified Sports format where athletes without mental retardation are paired with athletes who have mental retardation. Events for lower ability athletes include the 30-meter straight line race and the 30-meter slalom. Artistic roller skating (a version of figure skating) includes competition at 4 levels of ability and includes school figures, freestyle (single, pair, Unified Sports pair), and dance (solo, team, and Unified Sports team).

Visually Impaired

Modifications for individuals with visual impairments are similar to those used for running. Tethers and sighted guides help people with visual impairments to enjoy roller skating. Likewise, the change in floor patterns at the end of many rinks provide tactile clues for the visually impaired participant when turning.

Physical Education Implications

Roller skating can be successfully taught in physical education classes for students with disabilities including those with severe mental impairments (Hussion, Silliman, & French, 1989). The authors suggest a progressive six-step teaching method beginning with assistance while the skater is on skates, moving to independent skating on both feet. As with all skating, helmet use should be mandatory.

EQUIPMENT

Walkers

The most popular piece of equipment used by individuals with low extremity impairments, balance, and/or stability problems is a support walker (Figure 27.2). Before the introduction of this skating aid, many people with lower extremity impairments used chairs for stability. Various walkers models may be ordered from the Skating Association for the Blind and Handicapped, Inc. (SABAH). Although SABAH is concerned primarily with ice skating, some of these walkers can be easily modified for roller skaters. These walkers come in three models ranging for use by people who can bear full weight to people who can bear weight for a limited amount of time, to a walker where skaters are supported by a sling seat with adjustable straps, which assists them in remaining upright on their skates.

Harnesses

Harnesses have long been used in teaching beginning skiers, allowing them to gain the independence and confidence needed to ski. Harnesses for roller skaters allows the instructor to support the torsos of skaters with severe balance problems and those unable to bear their own weight, thus protecting the person from injury due to falls. SABAH uses a variety of harnesses but since each is custom made, they are not available at this time to the general public

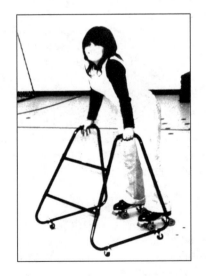

Figure 27.2. Roller skating support is easily maintained through this adapted walker. (Photo by Kelly Dean)

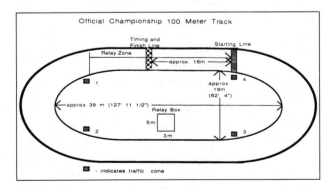

Figure 27.1. Official roller skating track dimensions for Special Olympics speed roller skating. (Courtesy of SOI)

EQUIPMENT SUPPLIERS

SABAH
548 Elmwood Avenue
Buffalo, NY 14222
(716) 883-9728
(716) 883-9735 (fax)
Email: sabah@sabahinc.org
Website: http://www.sabahinc.org/

ADDITIONAL RESOURCES AND WEBSITES

At this time, the number of websites related to roller skating for individuals with disabilities is limited. By accessing the following sites, readers will have links to most other roller skating-related sites.

Federation Internationale de Roller-Skating (FIRS)
Rambla Cataluna 80, piso 1
08008 Barcelona, Spain
Email: firs@idgrup.ibernet.com
Website: http://www.rollersports.org

Roller Skating Association International
6905 Corporate Drive
Indianapolis, IN 46278
(317) 347-2626
(317) 347-2636 (fax)
Website: http://www.rollerskating.org/
The Roller Skating Association International, is a trade association representing skating center owners and operators; teachers, coaches and judges of roller skating; and manufacturers and suppliers of roller skating equipment.

USA Roller Skating
P.O. Box 6579 (4730 South Street)
Lincoln, NE 68506
Email: usacrs@usacrs.com
Website: http://www.usarollerskating.com/

Special Olympics Director of Roller Skating
1325 G Street, NW, Suite 500
Washington, DC 20005-3104
(202) 628-3630
(202) 824-0200 (fax)
Email: SOImail@aol.com
Website: http://www.specialolympics.org
A copy of the *Roller Skating Sports Skills Program Guide* is available for purchase through SOI. This guide provides a developmental approach to teaching roller skating.

BIBLIOGRAPHY

Graham, C. (1999). Sudden Impact. *Active Living* 8(1)31, 33.

Hussion, P., Silliman, L., and French, R. (1989). Roller skating for severely and profoundly mentally retarded individuals. *Palaestra* 5(2):13-15, 46.

Official Special Olympic Summer Rules. Washington, D.C.: Special Olympics.

Chapter 28

Rugball

SPORT GOVERNING BODIES:
National:

DISABLED SPORTS ORGANIZATION:
National: Variety Village (Canada)

RECREATIONAL ACTIVITY ONLY

PRIMARY DISABILITY: All

SPORT OVERVIEW

Rugball was developed by the Variety Village of Scarborough, Ontario, as a cooperative team sport game. Similar in concept to the more widely played games of quad rugby and team handball, rugball distinguishes itself by eliminating the mobility of the player while he or she is in possession of the ball. This reinforces the primary focus of the game, which is team cooperation. Since each participant must contribute for the team to be successful, players can improve their own self-confidence by fulfilling their roles (Millage & Longmuir, 1987). Although not an official sport of any disability sport organization, the game utilizes all team members, particularly individuals with more severe disabilities or less skilled players. While minimal catching and throwing skills are important, modifications may be made for individuals who do not possess these skills.

VARIETY VILLAGE

The sport and fitness center at Variety Village, was built in the 1980s, and is one of North America's finest indoor sports facilities for children with physical disabilities. The program at Variety Village offers the choice of many types of recreational sports such a volleyball, fencing, swimming, canoeing and kayaking, etc. At this time Rugball is not listed as a program offering.

TEAMS AND EQUIPMENT

The game is played with five players per side on a regulation basketball court. Specialized markings are required on the court (Figure 28.1).

The only required equipment consists of a standard volleyball. A soft nerf type ball may be used to assist with grasping. All players, including individuals without disabilities, use wheelchairs during play, unless all players are ambulatory.

SCORING

Points are scored in two ways. A 'try' (four points) is scored when a player catches a ball in the end zone or a player crosses the goal line with possession of the ball. A two-point conversion attempt is given to a team after a "try" has been scored. Conversions are similar to free throws in basketball and are attempted from the standard free throw line.

PLAY

The game consists of two 25-minute halves started by a kickoff, with a five-minute halftime period. Once the ball is in play, the player with the ball may only stop or pivot his wheelchair and must pass the ball within five seconds or lose possession (Figure 28.2).

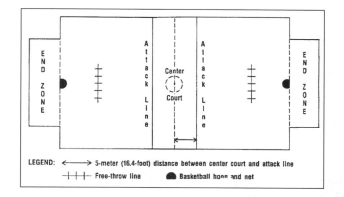

Figure 28.1. Rugball court dimensions.

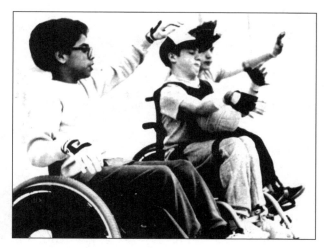

Figure 28.2. Rugball emphasizes teamwork and restricts players' mobility when in possession of the ball.

ADDITIONAL RESOURCES AND WEBSITES

Variety Village
3701 Danforth Ave.
Scarborough, Ontario M1N 2G2
Canada
(416) 699-7167
(416) 699-5752 (fax)
Website: http://www.varietyontario.com/village/

BIBLIOGRAPHY

Millage, J.G. & Longmuir, P.E. (1987). Rugball-A sport foe everyone. Sports 'n Spokes 13(2):63-64.

Mathesius, P., & Starnd, B. (1994). Touch rugby: An alternative activity in physical education. Journal of Physical Education, Recreation, and Dance 65(4):55-59.

Chapter 29

Scuba Diving

SPORT GOVERNING BODIES:
National: Professional Association of Diving Instructors (PADI)
International:

DISABLED SPORTS ORGANIZATION:
National: Handicapped Scuba Association International (HSAI)
International: International Association for Handicapped Divers (IAHD)

PRIMARY DISABILITY: Individuals with physical/sensory disabilities

SPORT OVERVIEW

Attempts have been made for over a thousand years to enable people to breathe under water. Reference have even been found to Alexander the Great making a descent in a primitive diving bell. It was until 1717 that British astronomer, Edmund Halley, devised the first diving bell. The first self-contained underwater breathing apparatus (SCUBA) was developed in France during World War II by Jacques Cousteau. Today it is widely accepted that swimming or other water exercise is very beneficial for people with or without disabilities. Many dry land mobility problems are either substantially diminished or eliminated once a swimmer with a disability is in the water. As a consequence, scuba diving can be taught to a person with a disability with virtually no modifications. Even those who never progress beyond the swimming pool may benefit from the physical activity of scuba diving. Individuals with disabilities should not be made to feel they cannot participate or that they need to wait for special classes or facilities. The focus should be on inclusion with people who do not have disabilities. In many instances no special requirements other than assistance in and out of a boat and/or selection of a wheelchair-accessible dive site are necessary (Figure 29.1). As with all divers, the emphasis on safety and selection of proper equipment and instruction is essential.

Accessibility Issues

One of the biggest obstacles faced by divers with disabilities is inaccessibility to dive boats, pools, and dive shops. Fortunately, due to recent federal legislation and the increasing numbers of divers with disabilities accessibility issues are being addressed. Fully accessible liveaboard dive boats are now available when planning your adventure. In planning any trip however, questions about accessibility should be addressed. The Handicapped Scuba Association International and other local organiza-

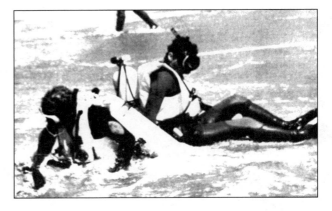

Figure 29.1. Dive site selection must involve accessibility when divers with mobility impairments are involved. (Courtesy of *Sports 'n Spokes* 7/82:24)

tions provides lists of accessible resorts and can even plan trips to accessible locations.

HANDICAPPED SCUBA ASSOCIATION INTERNATIONAL (HSAI)

The Handicapped Scuba Association International (HSAI) founded in 1981 by Jim Gatacre is the world's premier authority on diving for individuals with disabilities. Headquartered in California, HSAI conducts a full range of educational programs in conjunction with two major certifying agencies, the Professional Association of Diving Instructors (PADI) and the National Association of Underwater Instructors (NAUI), and is an independent diver training and certifying agency. Instructor trainers simulate a variety of disabilities in their training to try to understand some of the challenges faced by disabled divers. HSAI also provides information on traveling to accessible dive resorts throughout the world. Most major dive resorts throughout the world are likely to have a HSAI trained instructor on staff. In addition to their Instructor Training Course (ITC), HSAI also offers open water certification for individuals with a wide range of disabilities such as paraplegia, quadriplegia, high functioning brain injury, mild mental retardation, and people with visual impairments. Information on course content, various services offered by HSAI and available instructional materials can be found by accessing their web site.

Local Disabled Scuba Organizations

Local dive clubs for individuals with disabilities may be found throughout the United States, however many divers will find their local able-bodied club just as convenient and accommodating. Clubs for divers with disabilities however, typically provide instruction and offer opportunities for travel to accessible dive resorts. One of the more publicized disabled diving organizations is the Moray Wheels located in Boston, MA. Founded in 1982, The Moray Wheels is a non-profit SCUBA club made up of able-bodied and physically disabled divers. The club offers such services as certification classes, adventure trips, and tropical dive vacations.

Divers Unlimbited located in Pomona, CA, offers instructional classes to persons with disabilities, kids at risk and able bodied persons. Alpha One in Maine offers similar programs in independent living, while Underwater Safari's in Chicago also offers adapted scuba classes

National Instructors Association for Divers with Disabilities (NIADD)

The National Instructors Association for Divers with Disabilities (NIADD) promotes scuba diving and snorkeling as a means of recreation and therapy for individuals with disabilities. NIADD focuses on training divers in their own area.

Professional Association of Diving Instructors

The Professional Association of Diving Instructors (PADI) is the world's largest recreational diving membership organization. The membership includes dive businesses, resort facilities, academic institutions, instructor trainers, dive educators, divers, snorkelers and other watersports enthusiasts. Professional PADI Members (dive centers, resorts, educational facilities, instructors, assistant instructors and dive masters) teach the vast majority of the world's recreational divers, issuing nearly 946,000 certifications each year. PADI Professionals make underwater exploration and adventure accessible to the public while maintaining the highest industry standards for dive training, safety, and customer service.

International Association of Handicapped Divers (IAHD)

Since 1993 The International Association for Handicapped Divers (IAHD), located in Sweden, has focused on providing instruction to individuals with physical disabilities who wish to become scuba divers. Besides conducting workshops and symposiums, they have promoted diving as a sport for individuals with disabilities, and have developed standards for training. The IAHD consults with, and provides information to rehabilitation centers, diving organizations, diving instructors and the media.

VISUALLY IMPAIRED DIVERS

Divers with visual impairments will need assistance in navigation and avoiding obstacles. A possible solution is to use a five-foot tether rope attached to a sighted buddy diver. The tether keeps divers in touch and helps determine relative swimming speed. A system of tugging signals can communicate a diver's preference, location, and intentions. Powerful flashlights can also enhance lighting conditions under water for diver's with visual impairments. The use of underwater voice communication gear may allow for the sighted guide diver to describe colors, coral reefs, and fishes. Computers and gauges that have audible alarms could make it easier for the visually impaired diver to function in the water.

HEARING IMPAIRED DIVERS

A person with a hearing impairment from nerve damage should have no problems with equalization and might have an advantage with underwater communication because of sign language. A diver who is partially deaf or deaf in one ear should be warned and willing to accept the risks of damage to the inner ear due to pressure changes during diving, and the risk of damage to the other ear resulting in total loss of hearing.

SCUBA IN REHABILITATION HOSPITAL PROGRAMS

A growing number of rehabilitation hospitals and centers continue to use scuba as a part of their rehabilitation process. Because scuba is a high adventure activity, patients in rehabilitation programs can gain self-confidence and strength through participation in this sport. Rehabilitation hospitals such as St. David's of Austin Texas, have pioneered the inclusion of HSAI scuba diving classes as part of their out-patient program while the Dis-A-Dive Program of Cleveland uses scuba as in-patient therapy. These progressive rehabilitation specialists are using scuba diving as a method of transition from the rehabilitation setting into community life.

SAFETY CONCERNS

Safety concerns for scuba divers with physical disabilities are divided into two main categories. The first and most important are the standard issues of safety stressed in every scuba certification class. All divers with and without disabilities, must learn about dangers and related safety techniques in scuba classes. Communication is essential for all divers. The use of hand signals is standard operating procedure for all divers but can be an even bigger advantage for a person with hearing loss who uses sign language. For individuals with physical disabilities communication often times is achieved without the use of hands but by nods or blinks or eye rolls. Certification programs that are recognized worldwide provide anyone interested in learning the proper techniques with a number of opportunities. As mentioned above, the Handicapped Scuba Association International (HSAI) has developed a special training program for both instructors and divers, as have the professional Association of Diving Instructors (PADI) and the National Association of Underwater Instructors (NAUI). The number of PADI- and NAUI-certified dive shops that are also certifying their instructors under HSAI certification standards is increasing annually. Contact the HSAI for a recommendations regarding community dive shops offering classes to individuals with disabilities.

The second category, personal safety issue for disabled divers includes four areas of concern: use of medication, skin protection, pulmonary conditions and temperature regulation. The Divers Alert Network (DAN) provides excellent medical advice for various conditions, however, individuals with specific disabilities such as epilepsy, diabetes and exercise induced asthma should get full medical clearance from their personal physician before diving.

Medications

The use of medication may exclude certain people with and without disabilities from participation. The depth of the water and increase in pressure can cause an increase in the effects of some medications. Concerns over medication are usually addressed in the first class when medical histories are taken. Individuals with questions should consult their personal physicians.

Skin Protection

Reduced circulation, lack of sensation, and lack of movement can lead to skin breakdown unless protective steps are taken. Using carpet remnants on pool decks or rocky shorelines and wearing diving boots or other feet coverings will help protect the sensitive skin of the lower extremities (Brabant, 1983) (Figure 29.2). Individualized skin protection should supplement these suggestions.

Pulmonary Conditions

Before beginning a scuba certification program, a full medical exam with chest x-rays is in order. Contraindications do exist for some types of disabilities. Depending on the disability, certain pulmonary conditions could affect air trapping, heart conditions, and even convulsive disorders (Allen, 1991).

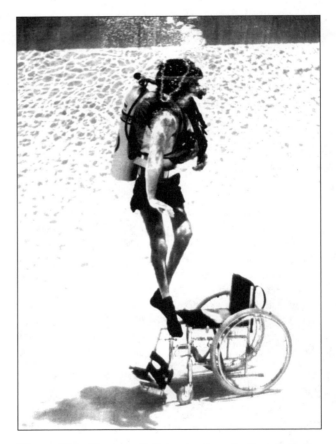

Figure 29.2. The use of diving boots and other protective equipment should be considered for skin protection. (Courtesy of *Sports 'n Spokes* 7/82:24)

Temperature Regulation

Temperature regulation is often a problem for people with quadriplegia, some paraplegics, and individuals with cerebral palsy or les autres disabilities. Cold water diving can make temperature regulation a serious health concern. The obvious solution is to use a wet suit whenever water temperature presents a problem. An individual who wishes to dive in extremely cold water may choose to use a dry suit, which is a more expensive version of a wet suit that maintains a higher temperature and does not allow water between the suit and the diver's skin, as does a conventional wet suit.

EQUIPMENT

There is not a great deal of specialized equipment needed for a diver with a disability; regulators, tanks, buoyancy compensators (BC's) are virtually the same used by all divers. However, new designs in equipment make it much easier for diving with disabilities. Power inflators on buoyancy compensators, larger buttons on inflators, and "pull to dump" features make diving more accessible to people with disabilities or reduced mobility. Equipment selections for divers with physical disabilities should be guided by careful choices rather than possible modifications in equipment. Selecting individualized equipment should be done with the assistance of a certified diving instructor. Due to the potential dangers involved, modifications to regulation equipment should be limited. The use of smaller and lighter tanks make putting on gear easier. Some general suggestions follow.

Mask

Low-volume masks with purge valves allow for easy clearing, especially for individuals with reduced respiratory ability (Figure 29.3).

Snorkel

Most snorkels come with purge valves that make the clearing process much easier than it is with non-purge snorkel. Divers with disabilities should opt for the snorkel with purge valves.

Regulator

The use of lightweight regulators makes it easier and more comfortable for a person with weak facial muscles to put it in the mouth. The use of an octopus regulator (an additional regulator that comes off the tank) is suggested to facilitate the buddy breathing system. The use of this second regulator eliminates the need to transfer a single regulator back and forth between partners, ands allows the divers to use their hands for propulsion or for carrying objects.

Buoyancy Compensator

Buoyancy compensators, or BC's as they are known in the diving world, come in several different varieties. Jacket types are preferred over the horse collar versions for divers with disabilities because the jackets maintain divers in a more vertical position. Soft-touch or low-pressure inflator mechanisms, rather than oral inflators, are also recommended. Divers with paraplegia may want to attach one- or two-pound weights to their ankles to prevent their legs from floating.

Fins/Gloves

Although divers without use of their legs do not dive with fins, flexible vented fins are recommended for divers with weak or impaired lower extremities (Figure 29.4 a and b). Waterproof prostheses with fins attached provide lower extremity amputees with options other than hand propulsion. Powergloves or webbed neoprene hand fins increase stroke power for divers with lower extremity impairments who need compensatory arm power. With an efficient arm stroke, an individual with lower extremity disabilities may consume less oxygen than a diver without a disability.

Wetsuits

Wetsuits are helpful when temperature regulation is a safety concern. Getting into and out of suits may present challenges. Hanauer (1981) describes how a diver with paraplegia altered his wetsuit to meet his individual needs. Finding it extremely difficult to put on the pants portion of the suit over his atrophied legs, the diver had the pants cut along the outside seam and velcro strips sewn into the suit. A once difficult task was then reduced to overlapping velcro strips.

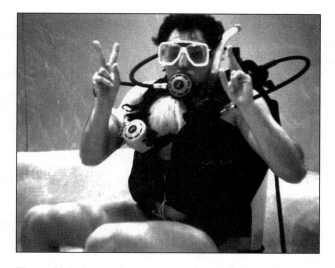

Figure 29.3. Low-volume masks and secondary regulators are standard scuba equipment. (Photo by Carmen Quintana)

Dive Propulsion Vehicles (DPVs)

Dive propulsion vehicles (DPVs) provide an alternative to arm propulsion for divers with lower extremity impairments. As all good instructors will indicate, diver's use of a DPV is not a substitute for basic swimming skills, but it is a means of increasing the diver's mobility in the water.

EQUIPMENT SUPPLIERS

For the most part, any scuba supply company is appropriate for divers with disabilities. A few of the larger on-line companies are listed below for the convenience of the reader. Specific needs can be addressed by contacting individuals at one of the local or national organizations for divers with disabilities.

Divers Discount
Website: http://diversdiscount.com/

Divers Supply
(800) 999-DIVE
Website: http://www.divers-supply.com/

Scuba Byte
Website: http://www.scubabyte.com/

Scuba Express
Website: http://www.scubaexpress.com/

Scuba Source
Website: http://www.scubasource.com/

ADDITIONAL RESOURCES AND WEBSITES

At this time, the number of websites related to diving for individuals with disabilities is growing including training programs and accessible dive resorts. Various sites are available throughout the world. By accessing the following sites, readers will have links to most other sites. Most participants will find the following sites satisfactory for gathering information.

American Association of Challenged Divers
John Ellerbrock
P.O. Box 8862
Sparren Way
San Diego, CA 92129
(619) 538-3483
Email: pinnacle@cts.com

Dis-A-Dive
C/o Bart Schassoort
3530 Warrensville Center Road, Suite 200
Shaker Heights, OH 44122
(216) 752-3483

Divers Unlimbited
724 Loranne Ave. #1100
Pomona CA, 91767
(909) 623-2412 (voice/fax))
Email: Info@DiversUnlimbited.org
Website: http://www.diversunlimbited.org/

Diving Medicine Online
Diving With Disabilities
Website: http://www.gulftel.com/~scubadoc/
This site provides information about medical issues facing divers with disabilities at
http://www.gulftel.com/~scubadoc/divdis.htm.

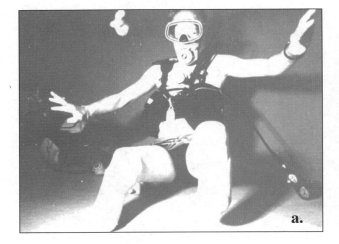

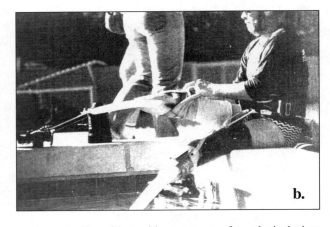

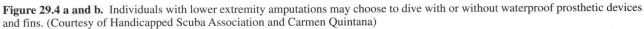

Figure 29.4 a and b. Individuals with lower extremity amputations may choose to dive with or without waterproof prosthetic devices and fins. (Courtesy of Handicapped Scuba Association and Carmen Quintana)

Eels on Wheels Adaptive Scuba Club
4020 Travis Country Circle
Austin, TX 78735
(512) 892-0863
Email: tskelley@sig.net
Website: www.eels.org/

Handicapped Scuba Association International (HSAI)
1104 El Prado
San Clemente, CA 92672
(949) 498-6128 (voice/fax)
Website: http://www.hsascuba.com
    HSAI has several excellent videos available.

International Association for Handicapped Divers (IAHD)
Vargmötesvagen 4, SE- 186 30
Vallentuna, SWEDEN
Email: info@iahd.org
Website: http://www.iahd.org/

Moray Wheels
P.O. Box 1660 GMF
Boston, MA 02205
Email: Info@MorayWheels.org
Website: http://www.moraywheels.org/

National Association of Underwater Instructors (NAUI)
9942 Currie Davis Drive, Suite H
Tampa, FL 33619-2667
(800) 553-6284
(813) 628-6284.
Email: nauihq@nauiww.org
Website: http://www.naui.org/index-top.html

National Instructors Association for Divers with Disabilities (NIADD)
P.O. Box 112223
Campbell, CA 95011-2223
(408) 379-6536 or
(408) 244-4433
(408) 244- 8652 fax
Email: degnan@degnandivers.com

Open Waters Program
Alpha One
127 Main Street
South Portland, ME 04106
(207) 767-2189 (voice or TTY)
(800) 640-7200 (voice or TTY)
(207) 799-8346 (fax)
Email: info@alpha-one.org or Owscuba@aol.com
Website: http://www.alpha-one.org/

Professional Association of Diving Instructors (PADI)
30151 Tomas Street
Rancho Santa Margarita, CA 92688-2125
(800) 729-7234
(949) 858-7234
(949) 858-7264 (fax)
Website: http://www.padi.com/

Underwater Safari's
2950 N. Lincoln Ave.
Chicago, IL 60657
(773) 348-3999
Email: info@uwsafaris.com
Website: http://www.uwsafaris.com

Scuba Diving For Everyone:
A Guide to Making Scuba Diving Training Accessible to People with Disabilities

   This 150-page guide is fully illustrated with photographs of real-life divers with disabilities in scuba diving situations. The guide is designed to help scuba instructors, certifying agencies, diving facilities and other interested parties promote scuba diving to people with disabilities. Available from Open Waters Program (see address above) for $40 + $5 s&h.

BIBLIOGRAPHY

Allen, A. (1991). Disabled athletes dive into scuba. *Rehab Management* 4(2):20.

Brabant, J. (1983). Scuba diving for the disabled. *Sports 'n Spokes* 9(4):9-1.

Degnan, F. (1998). *A Guide for Teaching Scuba to Divers with Special Needs*. Flagstaff, AZ: Best Publishing Co.

Elliott, G. (1996). Underwater Equity. *Sports 'n Spokes* 22(7):45-48.

Gulick, A. (1999). Go With the Tide. *Sports 'n Spokes* 25(2):37-41.

Gulick, A. (1998). Project Tide. *Alert Diver*. July/August. Pp. 39-44.

Hanauer, E. (1981). Sea legs. *Sports 'n Spokes* 8(6):27-30.

Larose, D. (1997). Reaching New Depths. *Disability Today* 6(2):42-44.

Myers, J. (1999). Gravity Be Damned. *Active Living* 8(5):11-13.

Petrofsky, J.S. (1994). Diving with a spinal cord injury. *Palaestra* 10(4):36-39,40.

Chapter 30

Shooting

SPORT GOVERNING BODIES:
National: USA Shooting
International: International Sport Shooting Federation (ISSF)

Official Sport Of: ____DAAA   ____USABA   ____USCPAA
                          ____DS/USA   ____USADSF   _x_WS/USA
                          ____SOI

DISABLED SPORTS ORGANIZATION:
National: NRA Disabled Shooting Services
International: International Shooting Committee for the Disabled (ISCD)

PRIMARY DISABILITY: Individuals with Physical Disabilities

SPORT OVERVIEW

Shooting is an official Olympic and Paralympic sport where athletes fire small arms (rifles/pistols) at a stationary target at distances of 10, 25, or 50 meters (Figure 30.1 a and b). The goal of shooting is to place a series of shots inside the center ring of the bulls eye. Athletes with disabilities shoot from standing, kneeling, sitting and/or prone positions.

USA Shooting is the national governing body for the sport in the United States, and as such, selects and trains United States shooting teams that compete in the Olympic Games, and various World Shooting Championships. Competition includes rifle events (air rifle, small-bore, and center fire), shotgun (trap and skeet), and .22-caliber rifles (moving game target).

Shooting competitions sponsored by disability sport organizations have been traditionally restricted to air guns. Interest in shotgun trapshoot competitions increased during the late 1980's through the efforts of the Paralyzed Veterans Association (PVA). Starting with the 1992 Paralympic Games in Barcelona, competition has been held in all the Olympic-style .22 caliber rifle and pistol events. Competitions for individuals with disabilities are governed under the International Shooting Committee for the Disabled while using International Sport Shooting Federation (ISSF) rules. Rules are modified to allow for differences existing between shooting for the able-bodied and shooting for persons with a disability. A functional classification system is used in Paralympic competitions. This system enables athletes from different disability classes with the same abilities to compete together, either individually or in teams. Competition in the 12 shooting events are open to both ambulatory and wheelchair athletes. Six of these events are open to both women and men, three are open to women only, and three are open to men only.

SPORT ORIGIN

It comes as no surprise to learn that the sport of target shooting has its origins in the military as soldiers practiced for war. As the practices became more competitive and enjoyable, target shooting quickly became a sporting event. Various sport-governing bodies were established during the 20th century to oversee the development of the sport.

The International Shooting Union (ISSF)

The Union Internationale de Tiro (UIT) now the International Sport Shooting Federation (ISSF), was founded in 1907 and is recognized today as the world governing body for shooting. The USA joined the ISSF in 1908. The organization is now based in Munich, Germany, and has roughly 130 member federations. This organization sanctions, and establishes guidelines and rules for international competitions.

USA Shooting

USA Shooting, established in 1994, is the national governing body for the Olympic shooting sports and those governed by the International Sport Shooting Federation (ISSF). The National Rifle Association (NRA) had previously accomplished this role. The organization is responsible for training and selecting the shooting teams to represent the United States at World Cups, World Shooting Championships, the Pan American Games, and the Olympic Games. In addition, USA Shooting manages development programs and sanctions events at the local, state, regional, and national levels, including the national shooting championships.

National Rifle Association

The National Rifle Association was founded in 1871 due a lack of marksmanship demonstrated by United States soldiers with the mission to "promote and encour-

age rifle shooting on a scientific basis". Today, this controversial organizations boasts membership of almost 3 million.

The NRA sponsors and promotes several excellent shooting clinics and workshops nationwide to assist individuals of all ages in developing appreciation for air guns and the proper skills to use them. Today, youth programs are still a cornerstone of the NRA, with more than one million youth participating in NRA shooting sports events and affiliated programs with groups such as 4-H, the Boy Scouts of America, the American Legion, U.S. Jaycees and others. Various programs can be found on the NRA website as well as other resource information.

National Rifle Association Disabled Shooting Services

Shooting competition for athletes with physical disabilities began in England in 1977 and was introduced to the Paralympic Games competition schedule at Arnhem, the Netherlands, in 1980. The NRA Disabled Shooting Services now coordinates shooting competition for ambulatory and wheelchair user participants. Over the years, the National Rifle Association has been instrumental in assisting individuals with disabilities to participate in target shooting competitions. The NRA Disabled Shooting Services was formed to improve shooting sports opportunities for active Americans with physical disabilities, and to foster research and development into the therapeutic benefits of marksmanship practice for many disabled citizens. The NRA Disabled Shooting Services provides assistance to individuals with disabilities to foster their participation in shooting sports.

Visually Impaired Shooters

Paralympic competition is open to athletes with visual impairments. ISSF and ISCD rules are used with

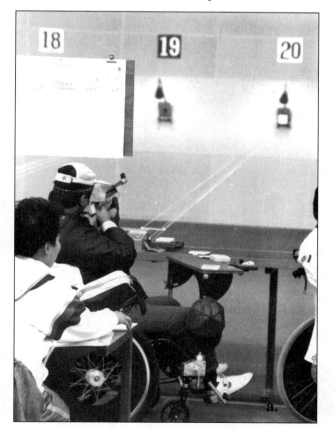

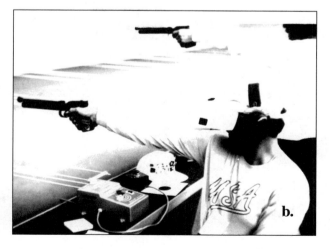

Figure 30.1 a and b. In both rifle and pistol air gun competition, the target is 10 meters from the shooting line. (Courtesy of Specialized Sports Unlimited)

specific modifications specifically related to the sighting system. An air rifle, equipped with a special scope, is used. This scope contains, or is connected to, an electronic circuit that transforms light into sound. A tone of higher or lower pitch is produced related to the intensity of the light on the target. The scope picks up the reflection of the light from the target allowing the shooter is able to "hear" the aiming on the target in the ear/headphone that is used. Each blind competitor is allowed to use a coach for safety purposes, to change targets, or to give results of shooting. Coaching is not permitted.

Trapshooting

Trapshooting has been a very popular sport throughout the United States for many years and is governed by the Amateur Trapshooting Association of America (ATA). Trapshooting requires the ability to hold an 8-pound shotgun with minimal movement to swing to the flying clay target. Individuals with a variety of disability conditions will find it possible to enjoy this sport. Trapshooting is an ideal sport for wheelchair shooters as the sport does not require physical exertion or extreme body movement. The ability to swing one arm to point the gun is the only requirement needed to shoot. Individuals with arm impairments will find the use of a brace or gun support helpful.

PVA National Trapshoot Circuit

The first recognized trapshoot shotgun invitational for individuals with disabilities was sponsored by the California Paralyzed Veterans Association in 1987. Many major trapshooting competitions now routinely include wheelchair shooters (Figure 30.2). The ATA has a special shoot just for Chair-Shooters at the Grand American World Championships, an event that draws tens of thousands of competitors. The PVA has sponsored its own national wheelchair trapshooting tournament since 1988. Trapshooting is one of the few sports where there are no rule distinctions between the wheelchair and standing competitor. The Amateur Trapshooting Association's (ATA's) Book of Rules ensures that wheelchair shooters are treated exactly the same as other shooters. This is a two-day competition with the first day open to PVA members and others with disabilities and the second open to those from the first day as well as able-bodied shooters, who also compete from a wheelchair.

Accessibility is generally not an issue with trapshooting. In most cases, each trap has concrete runways and access to all the traps are usually paved. Most gun clubs sponsoring large registered shoots are well paved and accommodate wheelchair shooters. The chair can be easily positioned to adjust for specific shooting stations

Cowboy Action Shooting

In 1998, a group in Charlestown, WV started a Cowboy Action Shooting group for individuals with disabilities. This sport involves contestants competing with firearms typical of those used in the old west; single-action rvolvers and lever-action rifles. Competition is conducted according to Old West Style and is governed by The Single Action Shooting Society (SASS).

EQUIPMENT

Special equipment used by shooters with disabilities is generally limited to shooting tables, shooting stands, slings, tripods and other support mechanisms (Figure 30.3 a and b). The use of these devices in international competitions is based on the classification of the shooter and event entered. See the IPC Shooting Rules Website at: <http://www.paralympic.org/ipc/handbook/section4/chapter12/content.htm#4.

There are many distributors of appropriate firearms throughout communities. Those needing additional information should check with local gun shops, clubs, sports dealers, and gun magazines.

EQUIPMENT SUPPLIERS

Many distributors of air guns are in existence and are easily accessed. Information on dozens of airgun distributors can be found on the following website:
<http://www.airguns.net/air_deal.html>

ADDITIONAL RESOURCES AND WEBSITES

Associations

Amateur Trapshooting Association of America
601 W. National Road
Vandalia, Ohio 45377

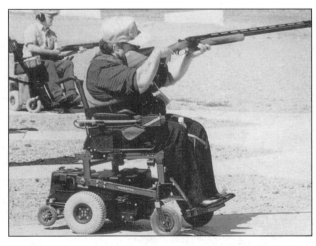

Figure 30.2. The Paralyzed Veterans of America offers several trap shooting competitions each year. (Courtesy of *Sports 'n Spokes* 1999, 25/3:32)

(937) 898-4638
(937) 898-5472 (fax)
Email: Shootata@bright.net
Website: http://www.shootata.com/

International Shooting Committee for the Disabled
(ISCD)
Email: wvl@bigfoot.com
Website: http://members.tripod.com/ShootISCD/

International Shooting Sport Federation (ISSF)
Bavariaring 21
D-80336 München, Germany
49-89-5443550
49-89-54435544 (fax)
Email: issfmunich@compuserve.com
Website: http://www.issf-shooting.org

National Wheelchair Shooting Federation
C/o David Baskin
NRA Disabled Shooting Services
11250 Waples Mill Road
Fairfax, VA 22030
703-267-1495
703-267-3941 (fax)
Website: http://www.nra.org/

Paralyzed Veterans of America (PVA) National Trapshoot
Circuit
Paralyzed Veterans of America
80l 18th Street, NW
Washington, DC 20006 USA

(202) 872-1300
(800) 424-8200
Email: info@pva.org
Website:
    http://www.pva.org/sports/trapshoot/trapoverview.htm

Single Action Shooting Society (TASS)
23255 La Palma Avenue
Yorba Linda, California 92887
(714) 694-1800;
(714) 694-1815 (fax)
Email: sasseot@aol.com
Website: http://www.sassnet.com

USA Shooting
One Olympic Plaza
Colorado Springs, CO 80909-5762
(719) 578-4670
Email: Admin.Info@usashooting.org
Website: http://www.usashooting.com

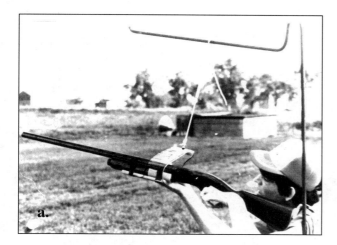

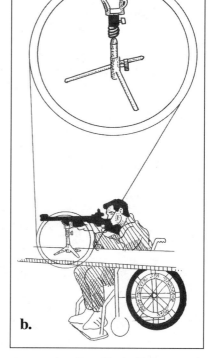

Figure 30.3 a and b. (a) A simple adaptation provides support for a shotgun in trap shooting. **(b)** A rifle support is allowed in USCPAA competition. (Courtesy of Human Kinetics Publishers)

Chapter 31

Showdown

SPORT OVERVIEW

Showdown is a table game that some refer to as a cross between table tennis and air hockey (Figure 31.1). It is actually a unique game with its own specific characteristics. Originally developed for people with visual impairments, Showdown is often played by people with sight.

A Showdown table is 12 feet long and 4 feet wide and stands 35 inches above the floor. The table is divided by a 15 inch wide screen called the "centerboard screen", which allows the ball to pass underneath, but effectively blocks the view of the opponent's goal by players who may be sighted to any degree. Sunken goals are at either end of the table.

The object of the game is to bat a ball filled with BBs (to provide auditory cues) off the side wall, along the table, under the centerboard screen, and into the opponent's goal. The first player to score 11 points through a combination of making goals and a variety of other means wins the game. If the game is tied at 16, the next goal wins.

Scoring

Points are awarded in one of six ways.

1. Player scores a goal-2 points. Either player may score points regardless of who is serving.

2. Player hits the ball into the centerboard screen, preventing it from passing through to the other side-1 point for the opponent.
3. Player hits ball over the centerboard screen-1 point for the opponent.
4. Player intentionally traps or stops the ball and does not immediately resume play-1 point for the opponent.
5. Player touches the ball with any part of his or her body other than the bat and the batting hand, up to and including the wrist-1 point for the opponent.
6. Player hits the ball off the table-1 point for the opponent.

A complete set of suggested rules can be found at the following Showdown website:

<www.casema.net/~jojejo/showdown.htm>

SPORT ORIGIN

Also known as Batbol in many countries, Showdown was adapted from an Australian game called Swish and first promoted by the Canadians in the 1960's. The invention of the game is credited to Joe Lewis with assistance from Patrick York, blind Canadians who were looking to develop recreational activities that could be played independently by people with and without visual impairments. The game has been played recreationally at every Paralympic Games since the 1980 games in Holland.

Showdown is being played in countries throughout Europe, Africa, Asia and North and South America. After the success of Showdown as a demonstration recreational sport at the 1996 Atlanta Paralympics, the IBSA Showdown Sub-committee is encouraging regional and national Showdown Tournaments in an effort to have international championships which may lead to sanctioning by the Paralympics.

EQUIPMENT

Goalball can be played in a small room. Equipment consists of a specially designed table, two paddles, specially designed ball into which metal BB's have been inserted, and perhaps a glove for the batting hand. Sound produced by the bee bees rolling around inside the ball helps indicate the location of the ball during the play.

Bats:

Specially designed bats are generally made of wood with a 5" x 1.2 inch handle and 10" x 3.5" blade (Figure 31.2).

Balls:

Balls are to be made audible by inserting small pieces of metal into them (e.g.: stainless steel metal bearings, BB's etc.) (Figure 31.2). Balls are six cm in diameter are usually made of a hard plastic material.

Hand Protection:

Gloves providing hand and finger protection are optional.

Blindfolds:

Players must wear blindfolds which completely obscures the player's vision.

Table:

The dimensions for a Showdown table are listed in the sport oversview section.

Plans for constructing your own Showdown table can be found at this IBSA Website:
<www.ibsa.es/sports/planos.html>

ADDITIONAL RESOURCES AND WEBSITES

Due to its mostly recreational nature, few Showdown websites have been developed. The IBSA web site is the most comprehensive and provides links to other pages. Some of the sites that provide the most information are as follows.

British Columbia Blind Sports and Recreation Association
317-1367 West Broadway
Vancouver, British Columbia
Canada V6H 4A9
(604) 325-8638
(604) 325-1638 (fax)

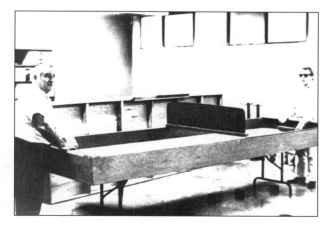

Figure 31.1. Showdown, a competitive sport for the blind, combines the skills of table tennis and air hockey. (Courtesy of the Canadian Blind Sports Association)

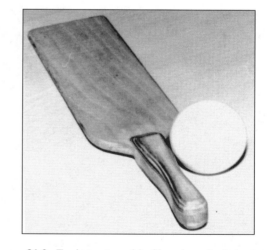

Figure 31.2. Equipment used in Showdown includes a paddle or "bat," and a plastic ball with pellets inserted for auditory cues. (Photo by Michael J. Paciorek)

IBSA Showdown Sub-committee
(604) 325-8638
(604) 325-1638 (fax)
Email: bcbs@express.ca
    Will provide information regarding playing, coaching, officiating, equipment specifications, or rules .

IBSA Showdown Site:
Website: http://www.ibsa.es/sports/showdown.html

IBSA Showdown Table Construction site:
Website: http://www.ibsa.es/sports/planos.html

Chapter 32

Skiing

SPORT OVERVIEW

Skiing is an excellent example of the growth of competitive and recreational sport for individuals with disabilities. Skiing dates back 5,000 years to Sweden and Finland as people used frames covered with leather to glide over snow. Modern skiing was begun in Norway in the 19th century where it quickly spread to Europe at about the same time the sport was developing in the United States, primarily in Minnesota and Canada. The International Ski Federation was founded in 1924 in Sweden and provided the impetus for competitive skiing. The popularity of skiing grew rapidly as resorts became more accessible with new resorts and ski lifts. Today skiing opportunities and competition have expanded to ski jumping, aerial competitions, and snowboarding. Events that combine shooting with Nordic skiing (biathlon) have been popular in many military organizations for years and has recently been added to competitions for individuals with disabilities.

Disabled European veterans were the first to discover the benefits of skiing as they looked for rehab and recreation opportunities after returning from World War II. In more recent years, adaptive ski programs have flourished in many countries. In the United States disabled skiing was lead by the development of the National Handicapped Sports and Recreation Association, now known as Disabled Sports USA. Disabled Sports USA has been a pioneer in disability skiing for over 30 years. Disability skiing is now fully integrated into the United States Skiing and Snowboarding Association. A combination of Alpine, Nordic, Snowboarding and snowshoeing events are offered by many disability sport organizations. Many resorts throughout the United States and Canada now offer lessons and programs specifically designed for individuals with disabilities.

This chapter will describe the two major types of skiing, Alpine and Nordic and will discuss the various techniques used by different disability groups to participate. Additional information will be provided on the related winter activities of snowboarding, biathlon, and snowshoeing. Disability ski programs have grown greatly over the past few years due to the development of adaptive equipment.

SKIING AND OTHER WINTER EVENTS

Many disability sports organizations offer competitive skiing opportunities at local, regional, national and international levels. Skiing is offered at the Special

Olympics World Games, World Games for the Deaf, and the Paralympic Games. Skiing events for athletes with disabilities are held in both Alpine (Figure 32.1) and Nordic (Figure 32.2) and include ambulatory and sitting competitions.

Alpine

Alpine (or "on the mountain") competition includes the following events:

Slalom:

A race in which each competitor skis as fast as possible down a zig zag course around tightly placed markers.

Giant Slalom:

A race that is similar to slalom but on a longer course and the markers are further apart. Thus turns are less frequent but at higher speeds.

Super Giant Slalom:

Similar to the giant slalom but on a much longer course with fewer turns which results in very fast racing.

Downhill:

The fastest of all the ski races. The skier negotiates a course with even fewer turns than the Super Giant Slalom.

Nordic

Nordic skiing, the oldest form of skiing, originated in northern Europe. It is called Nordic Skiing because the sport developed in the Nordic countries and is pursued over flat areas or a combination of flat and hilly terrain. Nordic skis are long and narrow and are fastened to a cross country ski boot at the toe. The skier is also equipped with poles to help with balance and forward motion. Nordic skiing competition consists of biathlon and cross-country. In biathlon, the skier combines the strenuous nature of cross-country skiing with the precision of shooting. Nordic skiing is much like jogging, alternating left and right while gliding over the terrain. In fact, many hand cyclists and wheelchair racers use a cross-country sit-ski during the winter to stay in shape year-round. Wax is applied on the bottom of each ski to grip on the snow as the alternating motion takes place. Nordic skiing takes place on surfaces where tracks have been made by previous skiers or courses prepared by race organizers. Disability sport organizations compete in Nordic skiing in varying distances based on abilities and classification. Nordic sit-skiing has gained greater popularity since the development of bi-skis. First introduced in Norway many years ago, Nordic sit-skiing enjoys its greatest popularity in Europe. It appeared in the United States in the 1980s (Kauffman, 1990). Technique and equipment are distinctly different from Alpine ski equipment.

Snowboarding

In just a few years the popularity of snowboarding has increased greatly. Technology has advanced as

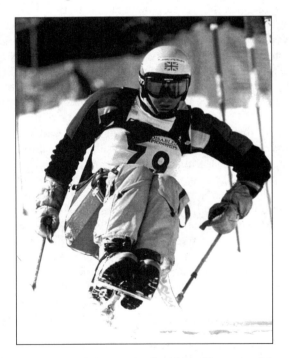

Figure 32.1. Alpine events for sit-skiers. (Courtesy of *Sports 'n Spokes* 5/90:49, 64 and Brooks Dodge)

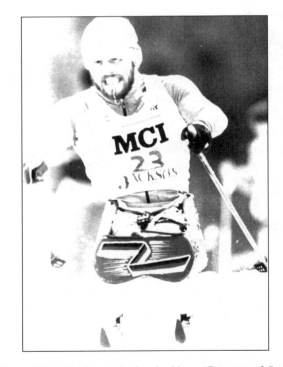

Figure 32.2. Nordic events for sit-skiers. (Courtesy of *Sports 'n Spokes* 5/90:49, 64 and Brooks Dodge)

quickly as the sport with special boots that lock into bindings. Anyone who can stand with reasonable balance can enjoy snowboarding. Already, two of the disability sport organizations, the U.S. Deaf Sports Federation and Special Olympics (nationally popular sport) offer competitive snowboard opportunities. Adaptations can include moving the binding placements on the board or using outriggers to help with balance.

Snowshoeing

Snowshoeing for recreation or competition is an excellent cardiovascular activity. It is an excellent activity for older individuals as an alternative to skiing. Ski poles can even be used for those people who desire additional support. Competitive snowshoe competition is held by some Special Olympic chapters. In fact, Special Olympics Michigan boasts over 1,700 snowshoe competitors throughout the state (Figure 32.3).

SKIING TECHNIQUES

There are primarily four skiing methods or techniques from which an individual with a disability may choose.

Buddy System (Visual Guide)

The Buddy System involves the use of a second skier or guide (usually able bodied) to assist a skier with a disability in negotiating a ski slope or trail (Figure 32.4. Used initially with skiers who were blind or visually impaired, the concept has been employed in programs for other disabilities as well. Skiers with visual impairments learn to ski auditorially with a sighted guide who uses communication and touch to replace the function of vision. Visually impaired skiers can become very proficient in skiing moderate to difficult terrain, including moguls. This technique usually requires no additional pieces of ski equipment although some skiers may choose to use outriggers for stability.

The Buddy System involves a 50-50 relationship between the guide and the skier, with the guide assuming a great deal of responsibility for the safety of the skier with a disability. Effective communication plays a key role in the guide's task of safely navigating a skier who in many cases may have poor balance, rigid and uncoordinated movements, and a poor sense of speed.

Three-Tracking

One of the largest categories in disability skiing are those who "three-track", or use one ski and two outriggers. This method is used by those who cannot effectively use one of their legs or feet for skiing. Outriggers are an adapted version of a Lofstrand or forearm crutch and a shortened ski or mini-ski attached to the bottom of the crutch. Commonly known as either "flipskis" or outriggers, they provide additional balance and steering maneuverability that a standard ski pole does not.

Similar to crutches, most outriggers are height-adjustable. The ski portion is attached with a hinge that only allows approximately 30 degrees of movement. When activated by a cord attached to the handgrip, it "flips up" the ski, locking it in an upright position enabling it to be used as a walking crutch (Kegel, 1985, p. 47) (Figure 32.5 a and b).

Three-trackers are usually single-leg amputees or individuals with some type of hemiplegic impairment (such as post-polio), that results in leg weakness and the inability to support the weight of the ski boot and/or ski. For the latter group, an adaptive support can be attached to the ski on which the weaker leg can rest to prevent it from

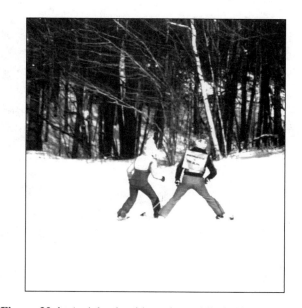

Figure 32.4. A sighted guide assists a blind skier down the slopes. (Courtesy of Specialized Sports Unlimited)

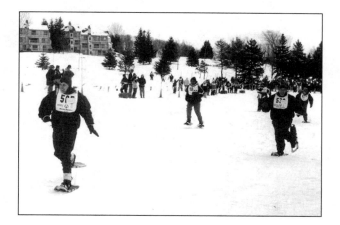

Figure 32.3. Special Olympic Snow Shoe competition (Photo by Michael J. Paciorek)

dragging and becoming injured (Figure 32.6. When skill increases, the three-tracker may choose to replace the outriggers with standard ski poles if a greater sense of balance and stability have been achieved.

Four-Tracking

Four-track skiing is virtually the same as three-track except the skier uses the second ski (Figure 32.7). The purpose and use of the outriggers remains the same. This technique is used by people with poor balance such as skiers with mental retardation, cerebral palsy, muscular dystrophy, multiple sclerosis and others.

Sit-Skiing

The sit-skiing method is used primarily by individuals with paraplegia, quadriplegia and people with disabilities who cannot use their legs for support or do not wish to four-track or three-track. Sit-skiing involves the use of a mono-ski, bi-ski, or sled-type devices. Sit-skis come in both Alpine and Nordic models. Both Mono- and Bi-skis

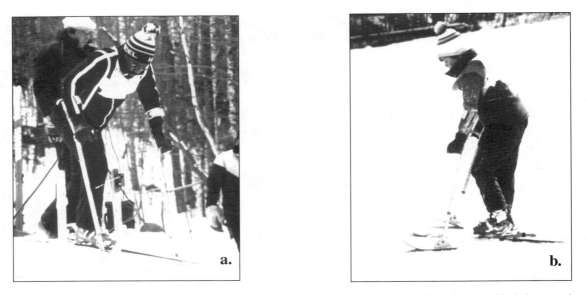

Figure 32.5 a and b. Outriggers, in the up position at the start of the race, are easily repositioned to provide balance and steering while skiing. (Courtesy of Specialized Sports Unlimited)

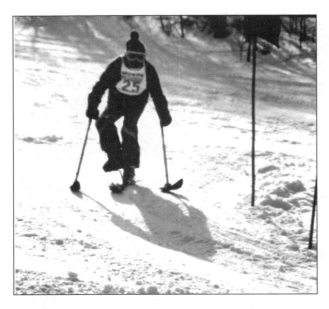

Figure 32.6. Skier's non-support leg is maintained in position by a metal support attached to the other ski boot. (Courtesy of Specialized Sports Unlimited)

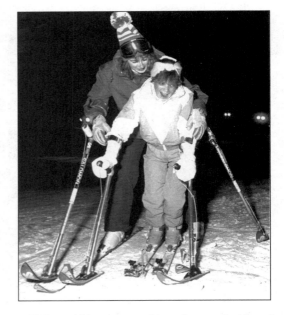

Figure 32.7. A ski instructor guides a four-track skier who is also using a ski bra. (Courtesy of Disabled Sports USA)

are chairlift accessible by releasing a lock that extends the ski allowing the chair to slide under the bucket of the ski (Figure 32.8 a and b).

Sleds

The sled is a type of sit-ski with a slippery plastic bottom. It is not as maneuverable as the mono or bi-skis, but can be the best choice for people with highly involved disabilities (Figure 32.9).

Mono-Ski

The mono-ski is essentially a custom-molded bucket with only one ski underneath. The advantages of a mono-ski versus other sit-down methods are more speed and maneuverability (Figure 32.10). The mono-ski is the most difficult sit-down equipment to use because it re-

quires more muscle strength to handle. It is designed primarily for individuals with double amputations and low level spinal cord injuries. The technique used by mono-skiers is not that different than that used by non-disabled skiers. To push across a level or uphill terrain, outriggers are used to push forward the same way a non-disabled skier would use ski poles. Unlike a non-disabled skier, however, who lifts the skis alternately to push up a steep terrain, absent extremely strong upper body muscles, the mono-skier, in many cases, becomes dependent on ski

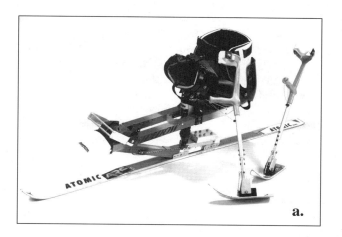
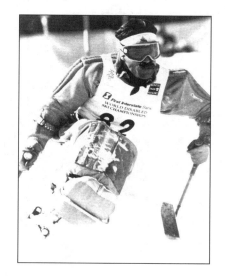

Figure 32.8 a and b. Sit skis are designed specially for easy loading and unloading on most chair lifts. (Courtesy of *Sports 'n Spokes* 5/91:58 and Robert Turtil)

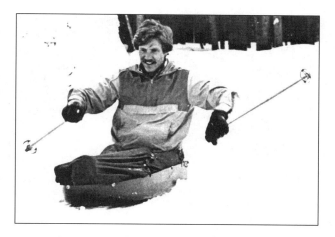

Figure 32.9. The original sit ski or pulk was introduced to the United States in the late 1970s. (Courtesy of *Sports 'n Spokes* 11/79:6)

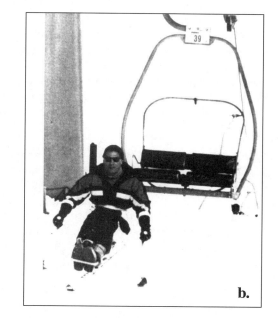

Figure 32.10. The transition from pulk skiing to mono-skiing has revolutionized sit-skiing. (Courtesy of *Sports 'n Spokes* 5/90:62 and Brooks Dodge)

buddies and instructors to push up a steep terrain (Petrofsky, 1997).

Bi-Ski

The bi-ski is similar to a mono-ski having a custom-molded bucket with two asymmetrically cut skis underneath. Outriggers are used for pushing and to increase stability. Bi-skis are used for better balance and support when the skier's disability is too great, such as with an individual who has quadriplegia or severe spasticity due to cerebral palsy.

When first learning to sit-ski, most instructors use a technique called tethering. Two tethers are attached to the sit-ski to allow the instructors to control balance and turn the ski while the beginning skier moves toward independence. Tethering is not only limited to sit-skiers. The use of tethers is a common technique when teaching ambulatory children to ski. A variety of other safety equipment is avaiable for the competitive sit-skier (Figure 32.11).

The Role of the Disabled Sports USA

Disabled Sports USA is a cross-disability programming organizing dedicated to providing individuals with disabilities of all ages opportunities to participate in vigorous sports for psychological and physical rehabilitation. Challenging outdoor activities develop self-confidence, increase sociability, foster organizational skills and responsibility, and improve mobility (Figure 32.12). The Disabled Sports USA motto is: "If I can do this, I can do anything".

Disabled Sports USA was founded in 1967 as the National Handicapped Sports & Recreation Association by disabled Vietnam veterans in California. Some of these original members became certified professional ski instructors and are among the nation's experts in adaptive skiing. Although Disabled Sports USA offers a year-round program of activities, they are best known for their winter sports offerings. Many of the Disabled Sports USA chapters and affiliates offer skiing and other programming for individuals with disabilities. Since space limitations preclude listing all chapters individually, the website where each local Chapter may be found is listed in the resource section of this chapter.

United States Skiing and Snowboarding Association

The United States Skiing and Snowboarding Association (USSA) is the national governing body for Olympic skiing and snowboarding. USSA is the designated representative for skiing and snowboarding in the USA by the International Ski Federation, and USSA is recognized by the U.S. Olympic Committee as the representative for Olympic skiing and snowboarding. Athletes with disabilities are fully integrated within the USSA structure and as such, the USSA coordinates the selection of the US Disabled Ski Team. USSA coordinates a nationwide program in six distinctly different disciplines-alpine skiing, cross country, disabled alpine and cross country, freestyle, ski jumping and nordic combined and snowboard.

Deaf Skiing

Founded in 1968, The U. S. Deaf Ski & Snowboard Association, USDSSA, is a non-profit recreational and competitive organization of Deaf skiers and snowboarders. USDSSA is affiliated with USA Deaf Sports Federation (USADSF) and is recognized by U. S. Ski & Snowboard Association, USSA. Services provided by the USDSSA include a biennial Deaf Ski and Snowboard Week Convention, which includes the U.S. Deaf Ski &

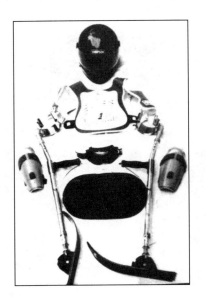

Figure 32.11. Sit skiers who decide to race should consider the use of safety equipment. (Courtesy of *Sports 'n Spokes* 11/88:30)

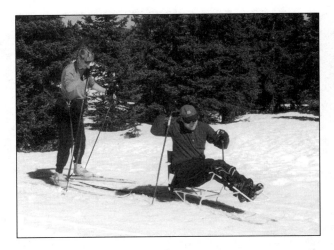

Figure 32.12. Nordic or cross-country skiing is a perfect family activity. (Courtesy of Cory Nagel)

Snowboard Championships and the North American Deaf Ski & Snowboard Championships. USDSSA is responsible for selecting members of the U.S. Deaf Ski and Snowboard Teams, which compete at the North American Deaf Ski & Snowboard Championships every 2 years as well as at the Winter Deaf World Games every 4-years.

The USDSSA maintains a calendar of upcoming Deaf ski and snowboard activities, a list of resorts which offer free or discount lift tickets to Deaf skiers and snowboarders, and plans recreational trips to popular winter sports resorts. Further information on the programs offered by the USDSSA can be found on their website (see Additional Resources).

Blind Skiing

Alpine and Nordic skiing are official sports of the United States Association for Blind Athletes (USABA). As mentioned earlier, blind skiers may choose to use a sighted guide depending on the amount of residual vision. B-1 skiers are required to wear black shaded goggles and to use guides while guides are recommended for B-2 and B-3 skiers. These skiers wear jackets that display the words Blind Skier as a means of identification by non-disabled skiers. The guide wears a jacket that displays the words Blind Skier Instructor to alert other skiers not to go between them. The skier controls his/her descent by traversing the face of the hill. The guide facilitates this activity by calling out turns to be made. USABA sponsors Alpine competitions in regional, national and international levels in slalom, giant slalom, super giant slalom, and downhill.

In Nordic competition the skier keeps their skis in the tracks made by previous skiers or race organizers. This facilitates the sport for blind skiers and decreases their reliance on sighted guides. Guides are needed however, in navigating turns, by calling directions to the skier. USABA Nordic events include men's 15k and 30k, and women's 5k, 10k and 4x10 relay races.

A variety of other organizations exist to promote skiing for individuals who are blind or visually impaired such as the American Blind Skiers Federation (ABSF). Founded in 1971, the purpose of ABSF is to provide an educational skiing program that is open to any blind or visually impaired person in the hope of providing both and physical and psychological therapeutic value to that person.

Paralympic Skiing

Both Alpine and Nordic (cross-country and biathlon) skiing are offered as official Paralympic events for all athletes with physical disabilities and those who are blind or visually impaired. Alpine events include slalom, giant slalom, super giant slalom and downhill. Men and women Nordic competitors vie in classical or free techniques and there are individual and team events ranging between 2.5 km to 20 km in distance (Figure 32.13 a-c). For this competition, the competitors are divided into three categories: sitting, visually impaired and standing. This is the only sport in the Paralympic Winter Games program to include athletes with an intellectual disability.

Biathlon

Biathlon is a combined event of cross-country skiing and shooting. This event consists of skiing three 2.5 km legs (7.5 km total), with two targets at five shots each between each leg. Air guns are mounted on stands and are used by each competitor to shoot the targets, which are 10 meters away. Each miss of the target is penalized by an increase in the competitor's overall time. A sound-system is used to aid visually impaired competitors. The strength of the signal helps to indicate when to fire. Both men and women compete in this event.

A complete set of technical rules may be found at the International Paralympic Committee website (see Additional Resources).

Special Olympics

Special Olympics offers both Alpine and Nordic skiing as part of their official program. Alpine skiing made its first appearance at the 1977 World Special Olympic Winter Games. Today, events are held in downhill, slalom and giant slalom at three different ability levels, advanced, intermediate or novice. Courses are set for appropriate ability levels. Unified competition is also held in these three events as athletes with mental retardation are paired with peer athletes who are not mentally retarded. In this category, the times of the athlete and the partner are combined to create the Unified team score.

Nordic events offered by Special Olympics range from a 500 meter race to a 10 kilometer race (Figure 32.14). Team competition is held in a 3 x 1 km or a 4 x 1 km races. Similar to Alpine skiing, Unified competition is held in Nordic skiing where the individual times of the racers are combined to form a team score.

Developmental Alpine events are also held for those athletes with lower ability or just beginning, such as the 10 Meter Walk, Glide and Super Glide and a 10-meter ski race is offered as a developmental Nordic event.

National Sports Center for the Disabled and The National Ability Center

Many programs exist across the country providing instruction in skiing for individuals with disabilities. Two of the largest and most successful in the world are the National Sports Center for the Disabled (NSCD) in Winter Park, Colorado founded in 1970, and the National Ability Center, in Park City Utah. The National Sports Center for the Disabled (NSCD), is an innovative non-profit organization that provides recreation for children and adults with disabilities. In addition to recreational downhill and

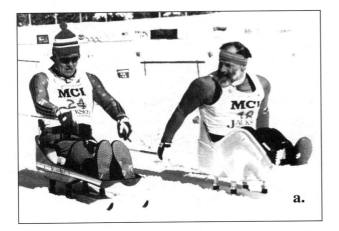

a.

Figure 32.13 a-c. Nordic sit skis have several different designs and models. (Courtesy of Holl Meditronics, Inc., and *Sports 'n Spokes* 5/90:48, Brooks Dodge and Cory Nagel)

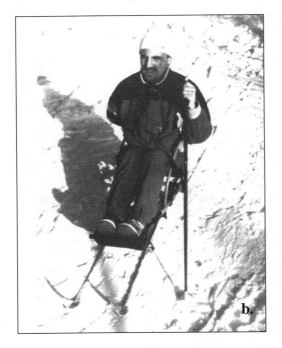

b.

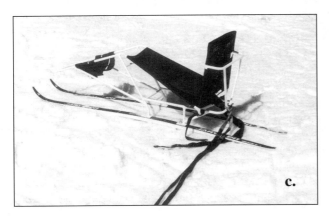

c.

cross-country skiing, snowboarding and snowshoeing lessons, NSCD provides year-round competition training to ski racers with disabilities.

The NSCD is recognized as a leader in therapeutic recreation. Ski school instructors and outdoor recreation specialists from around the country and the world visit the NSCD throughout the year for clinics or travel to Winter Park for the NSCD's annual adaptive sports symposium to learn how to develop or improve their own programs. In addition, the NSCD competition program hosts learn-to-race camps for teens and young adults at ski resorts nationally.

The National Ability Center has been a leader in teaching individuals with disabilities to ski since 1985 (Gillwald, 2000). The Center offers an extensive program in skiing and snowboarding in addition to a version of bobsledding (ice rocket) for individuals with disabilities.

EQUIPMENT

New Ski Designs

In addition to the types of sit-skis described above, conventional skis have also undergone changes recently that have benefited skiers with disabilities. The new design skis feature a curved ski, very wide at the tips and narrow at the center, compared to a conventional ski that is fairly flat throughout its length, although a little wider at the tips and tail. With curved skis, by merely leaning on one ski or the other, the ski bends to expose the outer curved edge to the snow causing the skier to turn. By the ski initiating the turn, less leg and hip strength is required by the skier, and smooth turns can be initiated with little effort. This new technology has allowed skiers with weak muscles to raise the level of their skiing and enabled people who would not be able to ski standing to at least ski beginning terrain's (Petrofsky, 1997).

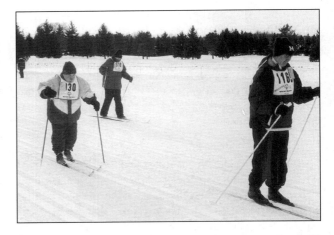

Figure 32.14. Special Olympic Nordic events range from 500 meters to 10 kilometers. (Photo by Michael J. Paciorek)

Specialized Support Device

A specially designed device (Figure 32.15) provides balanced support for Nordic skiing, snow shoe activities, or even walking on snowy surfaces.

Ski-Bra

A ski-bra is a unique device that consists of two metal parts that attach to the front tips of skis. When the parts are attached, the ski-bra prevents the skier from crossing tips, a common problem for all skiers. The ski-bra is a standard piece of equipment used by ski schools for beginning skiers.

The hook on one side attaches through the eyelet of the other and helps to maintain the skis in a consistent position while allowing flexibility in movement for snowplow and parallel skiing. Although used primarily with ski poles, they are commonly used by four-track skiers

Equipment for Amputee Skiers

Several devices are available for individuals with upper extremity amputations. The Ski-Hand (Figure 32.16) provides a force fit over the ski pole. New ski poles from TRS (Figure 32.17) allow a person with an upper extremity amputation to ski easily. The Ski-2 Td. can be used passively (without a cable) or with a cable for quick, precision pole plants. It is especially useful for nordic skiing where upper body strength is required for propulsion and in alpine mogul skiing and for helping to maintain balance and body posture. The Ski-2 Td. has a quick detach pole system (pole not provided) and a rubber shock absorber mounted in-line to accommodate for pole flexion during a fall. The device does not have a pole "break-away" system but the pole will tear free if snagged from behind. The pole is easily removed for chair lift safety. The pole is held in a retracted position by an adjustable tension elastic bungii until extended by a cable pull. Rubber shock absorbers for both beginner/novice and intermediate/experienced skiers are provided.

EQUIPMENT SUPPLIERS

The number of adaptive equipment suppliers precludes listing all of them. The National Sports Center for the Disabled offers a web page with suppliers with whom they have had success and a partial list follows.

National Sports Center for the Disabled: Equipment Web Page
Website: http://www.nscd.org/adequip/index.html

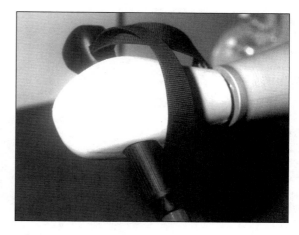

Figure 32.16. The Ski Hand is available in three sizes and can be used with all Hosmer wrists. (Courtesy of Hosmer Dorrance Corp.)

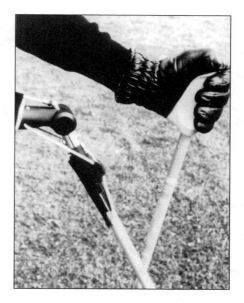

Figure 32.17. The All-Terrain Ski Terminal Device (AT-SKI-TD) can be used for both Nordic and Alpine Skiing. (Courtesy of TRS)

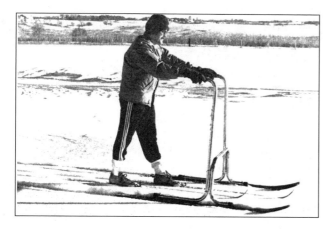

Figure 32.15. A specially designed device by Stuart G. Oxford, M.D., provides balanced support for cross-country skiing, snow shoe activities, or even walking on snowy surfaces. (Courtesy of *Disabled Outdoors*)

Mono-Skis and Bi-Ski Suppliers

Beneficial Designs, Inc.
5858 Empire Grade
Santa Cruz, CA 95060-9603
(831) 429.8447
(831) 423.8450 (fax)
Email: mail@beneficialdesigns.com
Website: http://www.beneficialdesigns.com/

Enabling Technology
2225 S. Platte River Dr.
Denver, CO 80223
(303) 922-0605

Freedom Factory
Rt. 5, Box 50734
Winnsboro, TX 75494
(903) 629-3945
(903) 629-3946 (fax)

Grove Innovations
120 W Church Box 185
Centre Hall PA 16828
(814) 364-2677
(814) 364-2760 (fax)
Email: willinnovate@hotmail.com
Website: http://www.sitski.com/grove.html

Mogul Master
AT's Freedom Factory
Rt. 5 Box 50734
Winnsboro, TX 75494
(903) 629-3945

Mountain Man
FFS Dual Ski
720 Front Street
Bozeman, MT 59715
(406) 587-0310

New Hall's Wheels
P.O. Box 380784
Cambridge, MA 02238
(617) 628-7955
(800) 628-7956
Website: http://www.newhalls.com/

Radventures, Inc.
20755 SW 238th Place
Sherwood, OR 97140
(503) 628-2895
(503) 628-0517 (fax)

Email: radyetti@aol.com
Website: http://www.radventures-yetti.com

Shadow Rehabilitation Equip. Assn.
8030 S. Willow St. Unit 4
Manchester, NH 03103
(603) 645-5200

Skistar Technologies
PO Box 7466
Tahoe City, Ca. 96145
(916) 581-2441
Website: http://www.northtahoe.com/skistar/index.htm

Spokes 'n Motion
2225 S Platte River Drive West
Denver, CO 80223
(303) 922-0605
(303) 922-7943 (fax)
Email: info@spokenmotion.com
Website: http://www.spokesnmotion.com/

Strange Research and Development
Box 2247
Banff, Alberta
Canada T0L 0C0
(403) 762-5003
(403) 762-5860 (fax)
Email: strange@telusplanet.net
Website: http://www.sitski.com/strangerd

Nordic Sit-ski

New Hall's Wheels
(see above)

Outriggers

Spokes N Motion
(see above)

Ski Doctor: Shockshaft
609 Munroe St
Sacramento, CA 95825
(916) 488-5398

LaCome, Inc
PO Box 1026
Questa, NM 87556
(505) 586-0356

Tip Retention, Ski Bras

Ski Eze
4401 Devonshire
Lansing, MI 48910
(517) 882-4608

ADDITIONAL RESOURCES AND WEBSITES

At this time, the number of websites related to skiing for individuals with disabilities are numerous. A limited number of major sites and resources is provided below. By accessing the following sites, readers will have links to most other skiing-related sites and local programs.

American Blind Skiing Foundation (ABSF)
227 East North Avenue
Elmhurst IL 60126
Email: ABSF@bigfoot.com
Website: http://www.absf.org/

Canadian Association for Disabled Skiing
P.O. Box 307
Kimberly, B.C. V1A 2Y9
(250) 427-7712
(250) 427-7715 (fax)
Email: info@disabledskiing.ca
Website: http://www.disabledskiing.ca/

Disabled Sports USA
The following website has a complete list of DSUSA chapters
Website: http://www.dsusa.org/chapter-state.htm

International Paralympic Committee
Website: http://www.paralympic.org
For a complete set of rules.

Extreme Adaptive Sports
This monoski and adaptive sport resource provides links and reviews of ski manufacturers
Website: http://www.sitski.com/

International Ski Federation (FIS)
Blochstrasse 2
3653 Oberhofen/Thunersee, Switzerland
Email: webmaster@fisski.ch
Website: http://www.fis-ski.com/home/default.sps

National Ability Center
P.O. Box 682799
Park City, UT 84068
(435) 649-3991
Website: http://www.nationalabilitycenter.org/

National Sports Center for the Disabled
P.O. Box 1290
Winter Park, CO 80482
(970) 726-1540
(970) 726-4112

Email: info@nscd.org
Website: http://www.nscd.org/

Ski Central
An internet site to skiing for the disabled. Includes equipment and instructional programs.
Website: http://skicentral.com/adaptive.html

Special Olympics Director of Alpine and Nordic Skiing
1325 G Street, NW, Suite 500
Washington, DC 20005-3104
(202) 628-3630
(202) 824-0200 (fax)
Email: SOImail@aol.com
Website: http://www.specialolympics.org
The Special Olympics Sports Skills Program Guides are available for purchase through Special Olympics. These guides provides a developmental approach to teaching Alpine and Nordic skiing for all individuals.

The U.S. Deaf Ski & Snowboarding Association (US-DSSA)
C/o U.S. Deaf Sports Federation
Website: http://www.usdssa.org/

U.S. Ski and Snowboard Association
Box 100
1500 Kearns Blvd.
Park City, UT 84060
(435) 649-9090
(435) 649-3613 (fax)
Email: special2@ussa.org
Website: http://www.usskiteam.com

United States Ski and Snowboard Association: Disabled Home Page
Linda Johnson
Prog. Mgr./Team Mgr.
(435) 647-2055
Email: ljohnson@ussa.org
Website: http://www.usskiteam.com/disabled/disabled.htm

BIBLIOGRAPHY

Axelson, P. (2000). It's All Downhill. *Sports 'n Spokes* 26(7).49-55.

Kegel, B. (1985). Sport and recreation for those with lower limb amputations or impairments. *Journal of Rehabilitation Research and Development*, Clinical supplement #1, Washington, D.C.:Veterans Administration.

Petrofsky, J.S. (1997). Skiing with a disability. *Palaestra* 13(1)28-31.

Rawland, A. (1997). Going Cross Country: Scrap the Sofa and Settle into a Sit Ski. *Active Living* 6(5)25-27.

Rawland, A. (1997). Just Say Snow. *Sports 'n Spokes* 23(1)12-17.

Sports Skill Program Guide: Alpine Skiing Washington, D.C.: Special Olympics.

Sports Skill Program Guide: Nordic Skiing Washington, D.C.: Special Olympics.

Will, S. (1998). Monoskiing 101. *New Mobility* 9(62)19-20.

Chapter 33

Skydiving

SPORT GOVERNING BODIES:
National: United States Parachute Association (USPA)
International: Fédération Aéronautique Internationale (FAI)

DISABLED SPORTS ORGANIZATION:
National:
International:

RECREATIONAL ACTIVITY ONLY

PRIMARY DISABILITY: Amputee, Spinal Cord Injuries, Blind, Deaf

---

SPORT OVERVIEW

Blue Skies! The motto of the serious skydiver indicates the perfect weather for skydiving. Skydiving is a high-risk recreational activity available to individuals with a variety of disabilities. It should not be attempted by anyone without training and supervision by experts. This chapter will discuss several modifications used by individuals with lower and upper extremity impairments.

Ever since Jim McGowan became the first publicly documented paraplegic to skydive (Glasser, 1982; Jenkins, 1991), it seems that no recreational activity is off-limits to individuals with disabilities. Tandem jumping is by far the most popular technique used by skydivers with disabilities, although documentation exists of skydivers performing water landings and blanket catches. Water landings have been used by jumpers with spinal cord injuries who are not able to adequately absorb the shock of landing. Logistical problems make this technique not very practical for most people. Blanket catches seem to be even more impractical although records exist of its use in the early 1980's. This technique involves the use of approximately 30 people and a 15- to 20- foot blanket or canvas. With the advanced design of today's chutes, skydivers have much more control than in years past. Anecdotal records exist of a blind jumper who packs his own chute. After jumping, his wife uses a radio to guide him in!

SPORT HISTORY

Airborne (parachute) operations during World War II were very successful and received much exposure by the media due to its glamorous nature. It is not surprising that the popularity of the sport as a recreational activity exploded after the war.

At the international level, The Fédération Aéronautique Internationale (FAI), the world's air sports federation, was founded in 1905. It is a non-governmental and non-profit making international organization with the basic aim of furthering aeronautical and astronautical activities worldwide including skydiving through it's technical advisory committee, the FAI Parachuting Commission. It brings together people who participate in air sports from around the world.

Skydiving is governed in America by The United States Parachute Association (USPA), a 34,000 member not-for-profit organization dedicated to promoting the safe enjoyment of skydiving. USPA works with skydiving centers and clubs, member skydivers, and the Federal Aviation Administration (FAA) to promote the sport in a safe environment and publishes The Parachutist, a monthly magazine with news, events, and current trends in skydiving. The USPA was formed in 1946 as the National Parachute Jumpers & Riggers Association headquartered in Mineola, New York. The name was changed in 1957 to the Parachute Club of America and in 1967 received it's current name with it's headquarters in Alexandria, Virginia. The USPA hosts a variety of competitions sanctioned by the FAI including: Freefall Style and Accuracy Landing; Formation Skydiving; Para-Ski; Freeflying; Freestyle, Skydiving and Skysurfing; and Canopy Formation. Although it appears that there are very few skydiving clubs or programs specifically for people with disabilities, almost all clubs welcome individuals with disabilities into their programs. It is best to call ahead when considering a club.

Pieces of Eight Amputee Skydiving Team

For more than twenty years, an amputee skydiving team called Pieces of Eight, has been providing individuals with amputations an opportunity to skydive in Perris Valley, CA. Founded in 1972 by a French nationalist, Larry Yohn, who traveled to the United States because French laws prohibited amputees to skydive, the group has members with between 80-3,000 jumps to their credit. See Additional Resources for contact information.

Tandem Jumping

A Tandem Skydive is where a person is attached to an instructor (tandem master) by a harness. In essence, the tandem master is making the jump while the student goes along for the ride. Although used with beginning skydivers, it is also a very effective method for individuals with disabilities (Figure 33.1 a and b). This method provides the thrill of freefall with the comfort of an experienced instructor. Tandem jumping is made possible by the use of an enlarged canopy (parachute built for two). Tandem jumping by individuals with disabilities, including quadriplegia is now a common occurance.

EQUIPMENT

Similar to scuba diving, equipment used by skydiver's with disabilities is no different than any able-bodied skydiver. Round parachutes are seldom seen these days and have been replaced by modern, rectangular "ram-air" canopies that have better directional control and offer softer landings (Poynter & Turoff, 1998). Reserve parachutes are typically worn on the back above the main parachute, as opposed to the older front mount assembly, and parachute fabrics today are more durable with many made of zero-porosity nylon fabric.

A variety of technical skydiving equipment is available through most skydiving clubs and suppliers. Beginning skydivers may want to consider the use of an Automatic Activation Device (AAD). An AAD is a self-contained device that calculates rate of descent and altitude and deploys either the main or reserve canopy at a preset altitude. AADs are backup devices required for student gear, and optional but recommended for experienced jumpers.

Jumpsuits, helmets and goggles should all be worn by all skydivers. Jumpsuits have different functions depending on the skydiving discipline involved. Fabrics and size help control descent speeds and give the skydiver more control with certain parts of their bodies. Tight, slippery materials allows a faster fall rate, while large cotton-like jumpsuits allow for a slower fall rate. There are several options for jumpsuits to suit different needs.

Detachable Pylon

Kegel (1985) describes the use of a prosthetic socket with a removable pylon for lower extremity amputees who choose to jump without their regular prostheses. Although the residual limb is adequately padded for protection on landing, the jumper is faced with a mobil-

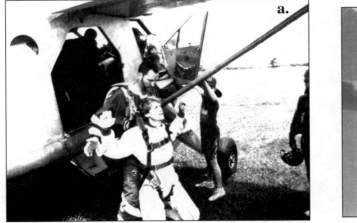
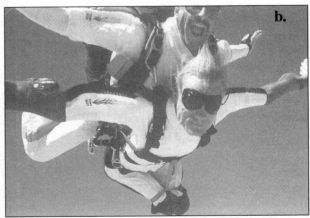

Figure 33.1 a and b. Tandem jumping has become a very popular method of instruction for disabled and nondisabled students. (Courtesy of *Sports 'n Spokes* 11/87:64, 2 and 1997 3/5:34)

ity problem once on the ground. The socket prostheses with removable pylon provide independence upon landing.

Extended Freefall

During extended freefalls, mid- to high-level paraplegics have great difficulty maintaining the stability necessary to execute the jump. An assistive device called the Wenger Cocoon can help (McGowan, 1983). The device resemble s a heavy nylon straitjacket that wraps around the body from just beneath the arms to the knees. The instructor uses the handles on each side to maneuver and hold the body in a stable position.

EQUIPMENT SUPPLIERS

The number of skydiving equipment suppliers precludes the listing of all. A few of the larger online suppliers are listed below.

Skydivers Depot
9981 SW 130th Street
Miami, Florida 33176
(888) 667-3285
(305) 251-8303 (fax)
Email: skydive@who.net for
Website: http://www.skydiversdepot.com/products.htm

Square One Parachutes, Inc.
(800) 877-7191 (Order Line)
(909) 657-8260
(909) 657-8179 (fax)
Email: sales@square1.com
Website: http://www.square1.com/

Enclave.com
Website: http://www.enclave.com/
Complete resources organizations/equipment etc.

ADDITIONAL RESOURCES AND WEBSITES

At this time, no websites related to skydiving for individuals with disabilities exist although there are numerous sites for any advocate of the sport. A limited number of major sites and resources is provided below. By accessing the following sites, readers will have links to most other skydiving-related sites and local programs.

Fédération Aéronautique Internationale (FAI)
Avenue Mon Repos 24
CH-1005 Lausanne, Switzerland

+41 21 345 1070
+41 21 345 1077 (fax)
Website:
http://www.fai.org/
Email: info@fai.org

Landings: Skydiving links
Website: http://www.landings.com/_landings/pages/
skydiving.html

Pieces of Eight Amputee Skydiving Team
Mike DiMenichi
13700 Alton #154
Irvine, CA 92718 or

Dan Dalton
P.O. Box 1618
New Brunswick, NJ 08903-1618.
Email: skydive@wishmail.net
Website: http://home.wish.net/~skydive/

Skydiving Magazine Online
Website: http://www.skydivingmagazine.com/

United States Parachute Association (USPA)
1440 Duke St.
Alexandria, VA 22314
703-836-3495
703-836-2843 (fax)
Email: USPA@USPA.org
Website: http://www.USPA.org/

BIBLIOGRAPHY

Glasser, P. (1982), Spring). Skydiving: Paraplegic jumpers hit on target-for first. *Accent on Living*, 36-41.

Jenkins, T. (1991, September). A spirit undaunted: Skydiving has helped this paraplegic man realize his dream. Independent Living.

Kegel, B. (1985). Sport and recreation for those with lower limb amputations or impairments. *Journal of Rehabilitation Research and Development*, Clinical Supplement No. 1. Washington, D.C.: Veterans Administration.

McGowan, J. (1983) Chuting for the stars. *Sports 'n Spokes* 9(2):8-12.

Mitcehll, A. 91998). Pieces of Eight fly again. *InMotion* 8(4):34-36.

Poynter, D. & Turoff, M. (1998). The Skydiver's Handbook: USPA: Alexandria, VA.

Chapter 34

Soccer

SPORT GOVERNING BODIES:
National: United States Soccer Federation (USSF)
International: Federation Internationale de Football Association (FIFA)

Official Sport Of: _____DAAA   _____USABA   _x__USCPAA
                         _____DS/USA   _x__USADSF   _____WS/USA
                         _x__SOI

DISABLED SPORTS ORGANIZATION:
National: United States Cerebral Palsy Athletic Association (USCPAA)
                     United States of America Deaf Soccer Association (USADSA)
                     American Amputee Soccer Association (AASA)
International: International Amputee Football Federation (IAFF)

PRIMARY DISABILITY: Mentally Impaired, Deaf, Amputees and other Physical Disabilities

SPORT OVERVIEW

Although professional soccer in the United States has not yet achieved great popularity, soccer continues to be an excellent and very popular sport among young people. Minimal equipment needs, combined with undisputed physical and social benefits have made soccer an appealing sport for interscholastic athletics and youth leagues, especially compared with other sports requiring high capital outlays. The increase in indoor soccer facilities has allowed soccer to become a year-round sport in northern climates.

Modifications to the game by disabled sport organizations are limited to the size of the field and goal, and the number of players. One modification is usually the result of another. When the standard team size of 11 is reduced, it increases the number of competitive teams in a given geographic area. This is necessary simply because the number of individuals with similar disabilities within a given location is usually limited. Field size may be reduced accordingly so players are not forced to cover a standard-sized field with fewer than 11 players.

Changes in goal size relates to disabilities. The United States Cerebral Palsy Athletic Association (USCPAA) uses a smaller goal since goalies with cerebral palsy are often faced with various types of locomotor problems, making guarding a standard-size goal extremely difficult (Figure 34.1).

SPORT ORIGIN

Soccer in various forms dates back to ancient China when Chinese soldiers would play the game as part of their training using the head of an enemy soldier as a ball. Greece, England, Germany, and many other countries also lay claim to its origin. Standardized soccer rules were developed in the mid-1800s. Soccer is the most played and watched sport in the world.

Headquartered in Chicago, the United States Soccer Federation, or U.S. Soccer, is the National Governing Body for the sport of soccer in the United States. Known originally as the U.S. Football Association, U.S. Soccer's name was changed to the United States Soccer Football Association in 1945 and then to its present name in 1974. U.S. Soccer, is a non-profit organization serving approximately 3 million youth players 19 years of age and under;

300,000 senior players over the age of 19; and the professional division.

Soccer is an excellent team sport for people with disabilities. Currently, Special Olympics, the United States Cerebral Palsy Athletic Association and the USA Deaf Sports Federation offer soccer as part of their official programming. Amputees play soccer through the American Amputee Soccer Association or the United States Amputee Soccer Program. All of the disabled sports organizations that offer soccer have affiliations with U.S. Soccer.

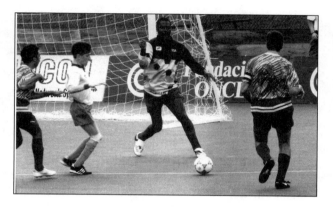

Figure 34.1. The smaller goal used in USCPAA soccer competition measures 5 meters wide by 2 meters high. (Courtesy of Oscar Izquierdo)

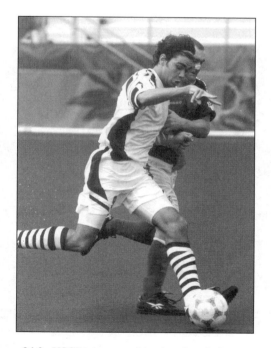

Figure 34.2. USCPAA competition involves 7 players on each side. (Courtesy of Specialized Sports Unlimited)

USCPAA

The United States Cerebral Palsy Athletic Association offers two versions of the games, ambulatory soccer and wheelchair soccer for athletes with cerebral palsy, traumatic brain injuries or stroke survivors. Throughout the year USCPAA also hosts training camps for members of the squad. On a national and international level, the United States Men's Paralympic Soccer Team also competes in non-Paralympic events such as the World Championships, and the Pan American Games.

Ambulatory Soccer

USCPAA has implemented all the above mentioned modifications into its competitive soccer program for athletes who are ambulatory. Teams consist of seven players on a reduced playing field, with goals smaller than the official United States Soccer Federation size (Figure 34.2). USCPAA competitions follow USSF rules with only slight modifications incluidng field size (Figure 34.3). Games consist of two 25-minute halves. The offside rule does not apply and players may conduct throw-ins with one arm if needed. Ambulatory soccer is limited to athletes in class 5, 6, 7, or 8. One class 5 or 6 athlete must be on the field at all times or the team shall play with one less player. Players are not allowed to use crutches. More specific rules may be found in the USCPAA rule book or by accessing the International Paralympic Committee webpage.

Wheelchair Soccer

Formerly known as Wheelchair Team Handball, Wheelchair Soccer represents one of four team sports offered by USCPAA (Figure 34.4). Wheelchair soccer is one of the most exciting sports available to athletes with disabilities requiring skills of catching, throwing and maneuvering of the wheelchair. Nine players per team

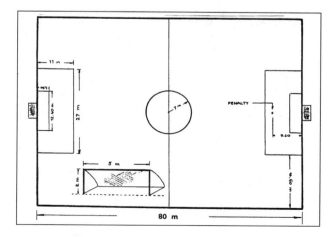

Figure 34.3. USCPAA soccer field dimensions. (Courtesy of CP-ISRA)

(seven court players, two goalies) play on a court the size of a basketball court for two 30-minute halves. The game is similar to Team Handball as players attempt to throw the ball into the goal.

SPECIAL OLYMPICS

Special Olympics offers a variety of soccer official events in which athletes can participate, ranging from full team competition to individual skills competition. Special Olympics soccer is offered in all 50 states and in 130 nations around the world and is played by over 150,000 Special Olympic athletes. Rules for the team competition are based upon Federation Internationale de Football Association (FIFA) rules for Football (soccer).

Events include:

1. Eleven (11)-A-Side Team Competition
   Rules for the team competition are based upon the FIFA Rules for Football (soccer) with certain modifications developed by Special Olympics.

2. Five (5)-A-Side Team Competition
   Rules are the same as for the regulation game but with fewer players to allow for more teams, or for players of lesser ability. The maximum field size allowed is 50m x 35m although a smaller size (40m x 30m is recommended for players of lesser skill. The goal size is 4m x 2m.

3. Indoor Soccer (Futsal)
   Although not an official offering through Special Olympics, indoor soccer is strongly encouraged in areas that have appropriate facilities.

4. Unified Sports® Team Competition (11-a-side and 5-a-side)
   Unified Sports® allows for inclusion of athletes with and without mental retardation. During competition, the line up shall include six athletes and five partners (three athletes and two partners for five-a-side).

5. Individual Skills Contest
   The individual skills competition is recommended for athletes with lower ability levels or for athletes who use assistive devices for walking (Figure 34.5). It is not recommended for athletes who can play the game. This contest provides practice in dribbling, shooting; and run & kick. The Unified Sports® Individual skills competition consists of one athlete and one unified partner. Specific instructions can be found in the Official Special Olympics Summer Sports Rules.

Special Olympics Soccer Sports Skills Guide

A copy of the *Soccer Sports Skills Program Guide* is available for purchase through Special Olympics. This guide provides a developmental approach to teaching and coaching soccer. It is an excellent resource for physical education classes.

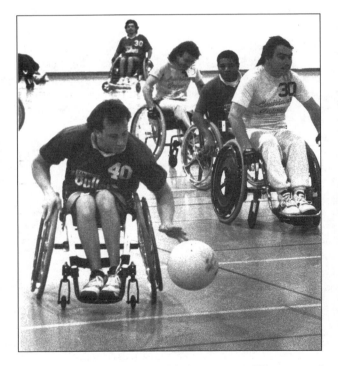

Figure 34.4. Indoor wheelchair soccer. (Courtesy of USCPAA)

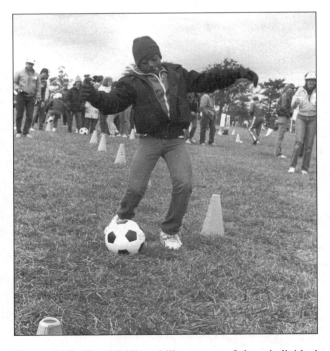

Figure 34.5. The dribbling skills are one of three individual skills tested in Special Olympics soccer competition. (Courtesy of Special Olympics Michigan)

BLIND

Although no official leagues for the blind are recognized at this time in the United States, soccer can be played by the visually impaired with a few modifications in addition to the ones already mentioned. Soccer for individuals who are blind were held in Spain in 1986 and tournaments have spread throughout Europe and parts of South America. The International Blind Sports Association (IBSA) have developed official rules for soccer using a sound ball. Complete rules may be found on the IBSA website. Matches are played by two teams, each consisting of a maximum of 4 totally blind (B1) players and 1 goalkeeper who may be Sighted or Visually Impaired (B2 or B3). Sighted guides positioned in various sectors assist in positioning.

Some other suggested adaptations that may be used in less formal situations are to increase the size of the ball and use brightly colored or beeper or bell balls, use flags or cones to mark sidelines, use sighted guides, use an audible goal locator, and wrap goal posts with brightly colored tape. Handi Life company is a supplier of bell balls that can be used for blind soccer (see Equipment Suppliers).

DEAF

Deaf soccer is governed by the United States of America Deaf Soccer Association. FIFA rules are used with adjustments made regarding visual signals for the stop of play.

POWER SOCCER

Power soccer was founded in 1982 as Motor Soccer at Queen Alexandria Hospital in Victoria, British Columbia and was accepted as on official sport of the Canadian Wheelchair Sports Association at the British Columbia Games for the Physically Disabled in July 1983 (Davis, 1998). It is fast-growing, competitive, and the first team sport created by and for power chair users. The objective of the game is to push the game ball over the opponent's goal line using a power wheelchair (Figure 34.6). Power soccer is similar in concept to the sport of quad rugby. It is usually played in two 25 or 30-minute halves. It is an ideal game for physical education classes and can provide meaningful competition for individuals with more severe disabilities.

The game is played throughout Canada, and is popular on the United States west coast. The Bay Area Outreach and Recreation Program (BORP), a Berkeley-based wheelchair sports non-profit organization appears to offer the most extensive Power Soccer program. They have offered Power Soccer since 1986 and are an excellent resource for individuals interested in developing power soccer programs. Plans are to take the sport to national and international levels.

Power Soccer Rules

The game is usually played on a basketball court with a 25' x 12' goal zone at each end. Court size and surface can be changed to meet the needs of the program. To score, players push a ball using bumpers attached to their wheelchairs, around opposing players to the goal line (Figure 34.7). Teams consist of four players including the goalie and all players must use power wheelchairs. Due to a lack of standardized rules and variations with footguards and wheelchair bumpers, the size of the ball has not been consistent. The size of the ball can vary from 12" up to a 37.5" The Gymnic ball is the most popular ball to use and it is available from most equipment suppliers. The ideal ball size is considered to be 16-18".

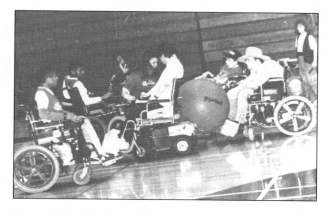

Figure 34.6. Similar in concept to quad rugby, the object of power soccer is to get the ball over the opponent's goal line.

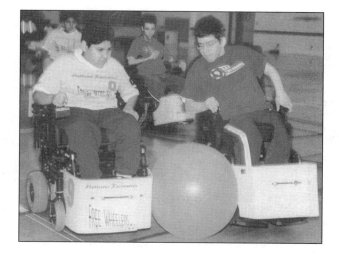

Figure 34.7. The wheelchair bumper helps propel the game ball in power soccer while protecting the players feet and the lower legs. A player can direct the ball without getting it caught under the foot pedals or the wheelchair.

AMPUTEE SOCCER

Soccer opportunities for persons with amputations have increased greatly during the past 5 years. Amputee Soccer in this country traces its origins to the northwest where official amputee soccer programs were developed in the mid-1980's in Seattle and west coast area. Although quick to grow in traditional soccer countries and especially in the Soviet Union, in the United States amputee soccer remained primarily a high level competitive sport, with teams participating in a number of international events. But the game remained relatively unknown outside the Seattle area. During the mid 1990's the sport experienced some growth on the east coast and further growth is anticipated with the formation of the American Amputee Soccer Association and the more recent formation of the international governing body for amputee soccer, the International Amputee Football Federation (IAFF). Prior to the time these organizations were established, rules for amputee soccer were not well defined. In the United States, two organizations exist that promote amputee soccer.

United States Amputee Soccer Association

The United States Amputee Soccer is administered through Disabled Sports USA—Northwest from their Seattle office. Amputee soccer networks and programs can be found in Seattle, WA, Portland, OR, Southern California, and Philadelphia, PA.

American Amputee Soccer Association

The American Amputee Soccer Association was formed to develop recreational and competitive amputee soccer programs for adult, new and youth amputees, and to develop athletes to represent the United States in elite International and Paralympic amputee soccer competition.

Amputee soccer is a co-ed sport that follows the same basic rules as the two-legged version, with some unique modifications:

Strikers and sweepers may have two hands but only one foot. Goalies may have two legs, but only one hand. Players with missing legs must use metal crutches but are not allowed to use crutches to strike or advance the ball. The use of a crutch in this manner is considered the same as a hand ball. Players with two legs do not use crutches, but must wear a red sock around one leg and are not allowed to use that leg for striking, trapping or trapping the ball, or for any use which might give them an advantage. The use of this leg results in a hand ball. Although incidental contact is allowed, residual limbs may not be used to advance the ball. Players with longer residual limbs would have a distinct advantage over those with shorter residuals. Goalies with two legs must play one-handed. Throw-ins are taken as indirect kicks and the offside rule does not apply.

Amputee soccer is played with 7 players per team including the goalie with unlimited substitution permitted. Play consists of 2 periods of 25 minutes each on a field measuring between 55m-70m in length and 30m-60m in width. Goals measure 2.2m high x 5m wide.

A form of amputee soccer can also be played indoors in an arena or high school gym. In these cases, the use of walls and bank shots are allowed.

Although prosthesis are not permitted in amputee soccer competition, for those hand amputees who complete in traditional soccer, the Super Sport prosthesis (Figure 34.8) is an ideal solution for a missing hand. Super Sports are designed to enable two-handed performance in all types of recreational and athletic activities, especially soccer. The prosthesis comes in a variety of sizes and is available through TRS, Inc.

A complete copy of all amputee soccer rules can be found on the AASA website.

International Amputee Football Federation

The International Amputee Football Federation (IAFF) was established in December 1998, in Moscow, Russia and is affiliated with the International Sports Organization for the Disabled (ISOD). The IAFF is recognized by FIFA. The goal of the IAFF is to make amputee soccer a world wide sport, included as a gold medal sport in the Paralympic Games. The American Amputee Soccer Association is the United States representative to the IAFF.

TOPSoccer

Affiliated with the United States Youth Soccer Association (the largest member of the United States Soccer Federation), TOPSoccer is a feeder program to recruit, assess, and train players with disabilities age 8-18, to par-

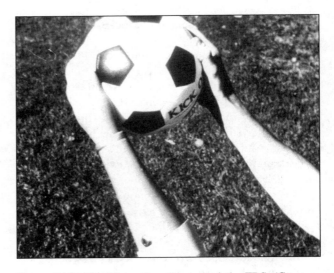

Figure 34.8. The "Super Sport" prosthesis by TRS. (Courtesy of TRS)

ticipate in soccer competitions offered by existing disabled sports organizations, and to help include higher ability players onto regular youth soccer teams. For more information, contact the United States Youth Soccer Association.

EQUIPMENT SUPPLIERS

Sound Balls

Handi Life
Blakke Moellevej
18B 4050
Skibby, Denmark
47 52 60 22
47 52 60 97 (fax)
Email: hls@handilifesport.com
Website: http://www.handilifesport.com/

Super Sport Prosthesis

T.R.S., Inc.
2450 Central Avenue, Unit D
Boulder, CO 80301-2844
(800) 279-1865
(303) 444-5372 (fax)
Website: http://www.oandp.com/trs

Power-Soccer Ball (26")
Hollister Recreation Division
300 West Street
Hollister, CA 95023
(831) 636-4390
Website: http://www.hollisterrecreation.org

ADDITIONAL RESOURCES AND WEBSITES

American Amputee Soccer Association
Website: http://www.ampsoccer.org
    This site provides a wide range of information on amputee soccer with links to other soccer organizations including the IAFF.

Bay Area Outreach and Recreation Program (BORP)
830 Bancroft Way
Berkeley, CA, 94710
(510) 849-4663
(510) 849-4616 (fax).
Website: http://www.borp.org
    Provides a full range of range of programming for individuals with disabilities. Has an extensive program for Power Soccer.

Federation Internationale de Football Association (FIFA)
Case Postale 85 (Hitzigweg 11)

8030 Zurich, Switzerland
(41-1) 384-9595
(41-1) 384-9696 (fax)
Website: http://www.fifa.com

International Amputee Football Federation
Website: http://www.ampsoccer.org/iaff/index.htm
    Full set of rules and field dimensions are available on this web site.

International Paralympic Committee 7-A-Side Soccer Rules
Website:
http://www.paralympic.org/ipc/handbook/section4/chapter13/content.html

International Blind Sports Association
Website: http://www.ibsa.es/ibsa/ibsa.html

Soccer Net
Website: http://www.soccernet.com
    The ultimate soccer website.

United States of America Deaf Soccer Association
Farley Warshaw (temporary)
(301) 662-9340
(301) 662-1371 (FAX)
Email: farwar@aol.com

United States Amputee Soccer Association
% Disabled Sports USA – Northwest
117 E. Louisa St., #202
Seattle, WA 98102
(260) 467-5157
Email: USAsteam@aol.com

United States Soccer Federation
U.S. Soccer House
1801-1811 South Prairie Avenue
Chicago, IL 60616
(312) 808-1300
(312) 808-9566 (fax)
Email: socfed@aol.com
Website: http://www.us-soccer.com
    The National Governing Body of Soccer in the United States

US Youth Soccer Association
899 Presidential Drive, Suite 117
Richardson, TX 75081
(800) 4-Soccer
Website: http://www.youthsoccer.org

This site provides information on all aspects of youth soccer. This is a great website for the young soccer enthusiast. Contact USYSA for information on TopSoccer.

BIBLIOGRAPHY

Davis, B. (1998, September). We've Got the Power. *Sports 'N Spokes*.

Official Special Olympics Summer Sports Rules (1996-1999). Special Olympics International: Washington, D.C.

Chapter 35

Softball

SPORT GOVERNING BODIES:
National: Amateur Softball Association
International: International Softball Federation

Official Sport Of: _____ **DAAA**   _____ **USABA**   _____ **USCPAA**
                               _____ **DS/USA**   _x_ **USADSF**   _____ **WS/USA**
                               _x_ **SOI**

DISABLED SPORTS ORGANIZATION:
National: National Wheelchair Softball Association, National Softball Association of the
                   Deaf
International:

PRIMARY DISABILITY: Individuals with physical disabilities and mental retardation

SPORT OVERVIEW

Softball is known as "America's game". Played in almost every city in America, softball is a popular summer recreational and competitive sport. Three disability sport organizations, the Dwarf Athletic Association of America, Special Olympics, and the USA Deaf Sports Federation, offer it as a competitive activity. The National Wheelchair Softball Association (NWSA) oversees a highly competitive program involving players with physical disabilities.

Rules governing each organization's version of softball mirror standard softball rules with minor changes that will be discussed in this chapter. A version of sport for individuals with visual impairment called Beep Baseball was discussed in Chapter 4 of this book.

DEAF SOFTBALL/BASEBALL

The USA Deaf Sports Federation has sponsored competitive softball since 1976 through the National Softball Association of the Deaf (NSAD), a non-profit recreational and competitive organization serving Deaf and Hard-of-Hearing regional softball organizations and players. The National Softball Association of the Deaf is

divided into eight (8) regional member organizations throughout the United States.

In addition to its extensive softabll program, the USDSF is also promoting baseball for its members with the hosting of the first World Deaf Baseball Tournament in 2000.

SPECIAL OLYMPICS SOFTBALL

Softball competition for athletes with mental impairments involves slow-pitch team competition with 10 players per side and Unified Sports competition where athletes with and without mental retardation are paired on teams. Athletes with lower ability compete in various developmental events such as, tee-ball competition, and individual skills contests that focus on teaching the fundamentals of the game. Athletes are grouped in competition divisions according to their ability level, age and gender. International Softball Federation (ISF) rules are used in all Special Olympics competition.

A unique program recently started by Special Olympics is called the Special Olympics Officials Program for Athletes®, where interested athletes train to become American Softball Association certified officials.

The athletes pass the same requirements as all other officials and are certified to referee softball competition.

WHEELCHAIR SOFTBALL

Wheelchair Softball began over 25 years ago in the Midwest by a few individuals with spinal cord injuries and lower extremity impairments that still wanted to play even though they lacked the full use of their legs. The game was played on a hard surface that allowed for easy maneuvering of the wheelchair. A 16-inch softball was introduced to the game, allowing wheelchair players to catch the softball without using a glove, since players need both hands to maneuver the wheelchair.

The National Wheelchair Softball Association (NWSA) was founded in 1976 and serves as the independent governing body for the dozens of wheelchair softball teams throughout the United States. The NWSA is not affiliated with Wheelchair Sports USA. Rather, it provides sport-specific programming primarily to individuals with spinal cord injuries. Individuals with other physical disabilities such as amputations, cerebral palsy, and several les autres conditions also compete in the NWSA on a regular basis. The game is played under the official rules as approved by the Amateur Softball Association of America with 14 exceptions that are geared toward the wheelchair user (Figure 35.1 a and b). Teams throughout America compete on a regular basis and the NWSA hosts several tournaments throughout the summer. A national wheelchair softball tournament is hosted annually by the National Wheelchair Softball Association.

Predictably, rules for wheelchair softball are slightly different from standard softball rules; however, those changes are only incorporated to accommodate wheelchairs. Some rule modifications are:

1. Players must participate in a wheelchair and all chairs must have foot platforms.
2. The playing field must have a smooth, hard surface such as blacktop or similar material.
3. The pitching stripe is 28 feet from home and bases are 50 feet apart.
4. Each base consists of a 4-foot-diameter circle centered on a 1-foot square flat base, all of which is located in fair territory (Figure 35.2).
5. If fielders leave their chairs to gain fielding advantage, all base runners will be awarded two bases.
6. If the ball leaves the playing area because of a throwing error, all runners receive an additional base.
7. All teams are required to have a person with quadriplegia in active play. On defense, this person must play one of the positions in the field; on offense they must take their turn batting. A team that fails to include a person with quadriplegia plays with only nine players and receives an automatic out every 10th batter.
8. Teams are balanced by the following point system:

WSUSA Classes 1A, 1B, 1C = 1 point
WSUSA Class 1 = 1 point
WSUSA Class 2 = 2 points
WSUSA Class 3 = 3 points

At no time in a game shall a team member points total more than 22.

Further information can be received from the National Wheelchair Softball Association.

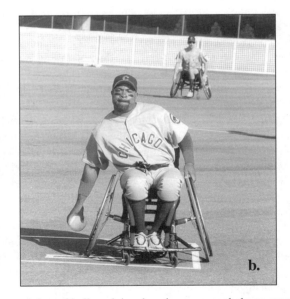

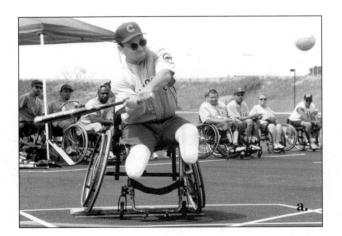

Figure 35.1 a and b. Wheelchair softball uses a 16-inch Chicago-style softball and is played on an asphalt or paved surface. (Courtesy of Rehabilitation Institute of Chicago's Wirtz Sports Program)

LITTLE LEAGUE CHALLENGER DIVISION

Many communities throughout the United States now offer baseball opportunities to children with disabilities through a unique program affiliated with Little League Baseball. Children with physical or mental disabilities ages 6-18 are eligible to play Little League Baseball in the Challenger Division. Players participate in tee-ball, coach pitch, or player pitch. For further information on organizing or joining a team, contact the Little League Headquarters in Williamsport, PA.

OVER-THE-LINE SOFTBALL

An adapted version of wheelchair softball called wheelchair over-the-line (OTL) was first introduced as a way to play softball without the standard 20 players (Figure 35.3). One ball, one bat, and two teams of three players apiece are the only requirements for OTL. Shepard (1989) and Bianchi (1993) outline the following OTL rules.

Over-The-Line Rules

Players: Three per team

Divisions: For World-Class the three players must include one woman and one person with quadriplegia. For Unlimited Class the three players must include one nondisabled player.

Equipment: Gloves are used only by women and individuals with quadriplegia. Taping of hands and use of golf gloves for batting allowed. Softball and Little League bats are used except for individuals with quadriplegia who may use plastic bats and balls.

Games: Games consist of three innings. If the score is tied after four innings, the team with the most hits wins. If hits are tied, the game continues until the tie in hits or runs is broken.

Hits: Defined as any ball hit in fair territory not caught on the fly or after one bounce, or any ball dropped by a fielder. For individuals with quadriplegia, a hit is any ball hit past the 10- or 15-foot line (depending on division) and not caught on the fly or after one bounce. A home run is any ball hit past the farthest wheelchair outfielder in fair territory on the fly without being touched.

Outs: Two foul balls, one strike for player other than the individual with quadriplegia who gets two strikes.

Scoring: Three hits in an inning scores one run. Each additional hit in the same inning scores one more run. A home run clears the bases.

At-bat Positions: Bat from home. Team pitches from anywhere in front of THE LINE or its extension but not in the field of play.

Fielding Positions: Fielders may play anywhere past the line (A) or its extension, except when a player with quadriplegia is at bat. In this situation, one fielder may play in front of the 10-foot line. In the Unlimited Class, the batter must hit the ball over the 15-foot line; thus one fielder may be behind the 15-foot line.

EQUIPMENT

Very little modified or adaptive equipment is needed to play softball beyond the standard equipment. For wheelchair users a good sports chair is advantageous in addition to the 16-inch softball used in regulation play. For individuals with upper extremity amputations, certain pieces of adaptive equipment are available.

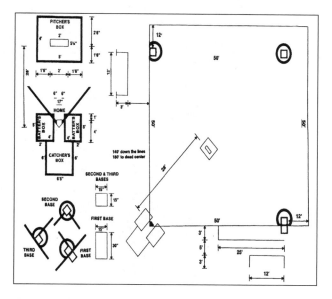

Figure 35.2. Field dimensions for wheelchair softball. (Courtesy of Courage Center)

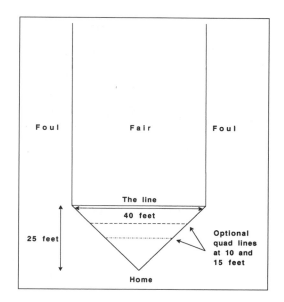

Figure 35.3. Field dimensions for wheelchair "over-the-line" softball.

Hi-Fly Fielder

Playing softball is easier for people with upper extremity amputations with pieces of adaptive equipment (Radocy, 1992). A versatile baseball catching device is available for one-handed players. The Hi-Fly Fielder (or Hi-Fly Jr. for children) (Figure 35.4) is patterned after lacrosse equipment and features a bilateral pocket allowing the player to catch a ball using either a forehand or backhand technique eliminating the need for forearm rotation. The Hi-Fly Fielder attaches directly into any standard prosthesis and does not require a cable for operation. Other adapted catching devices for people with amputations include one that fits into a standard glove (Figure 35.5) and another one that is a specially made terminal device (Figure 35.6).

Power Swing Ring

The Power Swing ring is a special accessory for batting that screws directly into the bottom of any wooden or plastic bat (Figure 35.7 a and b). The player, using a regular prosthesis, simply grasps or engages the ring. Swivel action of the ring simulates the wrist break or rollover not available in a standard prosthesis. The power Swing ring allows a one-handed person to swing hard and smoothly with the control and power of two arms. The device accommodates any style prehensor or hook finger or thumb, and allows for "wrist break" (roll-over) not available in prosthetic wrist systems.

Grand Slam Tds.

The Grand Slam Tds. is a prosthetic device from TRS for batting with no cable needed. This device is designed to fit aluminum bats with one inch diameter handles (straight or tapered). It features a high strength flexible coupling and long cylindrical channel allows for natural grip and powerful unrestricted swing and follow-through and fits all standard body-powered, mechanical prosthetic wrists.

EQUIPMENT SUPPLIERS

Hi Fly Fielder, Power Swing Ring, Grand Slam Tds
T.R.S., Inc.
2450 Central Avenue, Unit D
Boulder, CO 80301-2844

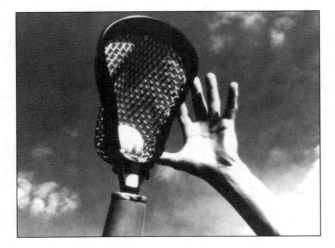

Figure 35.4. The "Hi Fly Fielder" attaches directly to any standard prosthesis. (Courtesy of TRS)

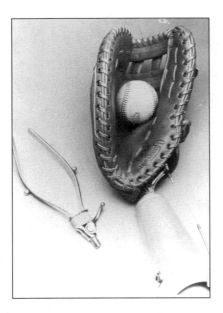

Figure 35.5. This adapted prosthetic device can be inserted into any standard softball glove. (Courtesy of TRS)

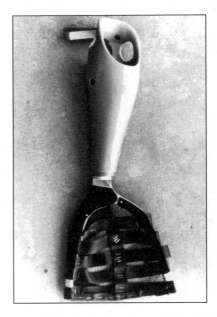

Figure 35.6. An all-inclusive prosthetic arm and glove is another option for the amputee softball player. (Courtesy of TRS)

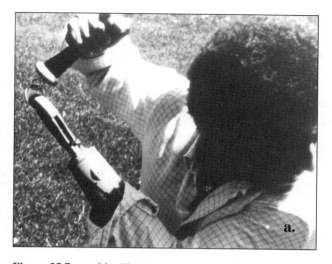

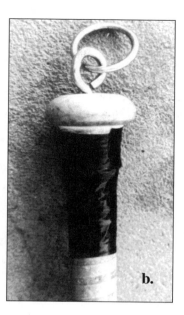

Figure 35.7 a and b. The Power Swing Ring is a simple adaptation that allows for a smooth two-handed swing despite a prosthetic hand. (Courtesy of TRS)

(800) 279-1865
(303) 444-4720
(303) 444-5372 (FAX)
Website: http://www.oandp.com/trs

ADDITIONAL RESOURCES AND WEBSITES

At this time, the number of websites related to softball for individuals with disabilities is limited to various local wheelchair softball teams. By accessing the following sites, readers will have links to most other softball-related sites.

Amateur Softball Association (USA Softball)
2801 N.E. 50th Street
Oklahoma City, OK 73111-7203
Email: info@softball.org
Website: http:www.usasoftball.com/
                  (national team information only)
Website: http://www.softball.org/

International Softball Federation
1900 S. Park Road
Plant City, FL 33566-8113 USA
(813) 707 7204
(813) 707 7209 (fax)
Email: isfsoftball@ci.plant-city.fl.us
Website:
   http://www.worldsport.com/worldsport/sports/softball/home.html

Little League Baseball
Website: http://www.littleleague.org/
Challenger Division
Website: http://www.littleleague.org/divisions/chall.htm
   Contact the regional Little League center servicing your state

National Softball Association of the Deaf (NSAD)
USA Deaf Sports Federation
3607 Washington Blvd., Suite 4
Ogden, UT 84403-1737
(801) 393-7916 Office (tty: use your state relay service)
(801) 393-2263 (fax)
Email: Officers@NSAD
Website: http://www.nsad.org/

National Wheelchair Softball Association
1616 Todd Court
Hastings, MN 55033
Website: http://www.wheelchairsoftball.com/

Special Olympics Sports Skills Program

Special Olympics
1325 G Street, NW, Suite 500
Washington, DC 20005-3104
(202) 628-3630
(202) 824-0200 (fax)
Email: SOImail@aol.com
Website: http://www.specialolympics.org
   The Special Olympics Sports Skills Program Guide is available for purchase through Special Olympics. This guide provides a developmental approach to teaching and coaching softball for all individuals.

BIBLIOGRAPHY

Bianchi, A. (1993). Over-the-Line: 15 years & still growing. *Sports 'n Spokes* 19(1):75.

Radocy, B. (1992). Adapted equipment for people with upper extremity amputations: HiFly Fielder & Power Swing Ring. *Palaestra* 8(4):52.

Shepderd, M.E. (1989). 11th annual over-the-line tournament. *Sports 'n Spokes* 15(4):15.

Sports Skill Program Guide: Softball. Washington, D.C.: Special Olympics

Chapter 36

Swimming

SPORT GOVERNING BODIES:
National: USA Swimming (USAS)
International: Federation Internationale de Natation Amateur (FINA)

Official Sport Of:

x DAAA	x USABA	x USCPAA
x DS/USA	x USADSF	x WS/USA
x SOI		

DISABLED SPORTS ORGANIZATION:
National: USA Swimming (Adapted Section)/US Wheelchair Swimming
International:

PRIMARY DISABILITY: All

SPORT OVERVIEW

The therapeutic nature of swimming makes it one of the most popular and beneficial forms of physical activity for individuals with disabilities. Movement problems that exist on land are very often negated once in the water. The value of aquatic activities is so important that P.L. (94-142-The Individuals with Disabilities Education Act) specifically identifies water skill development as a part of all physical education curricula. Although all of the major disability sport organizations (DSO's) offer swimming events as part of their competitive programming, swimming ranks third (behind track and field) in the number of competitors. However, its greatest value is as a recreational and therapeutic activity. Adults who are interested in swimming should contact the United Masters Swimming (see Additional Resources) for local chapters. Competitively, many athletes with disabilities swim the same events, strokes and distances as their nondisabled counterparts; however, strokes and distances can be adjusted to accommodate various disabilities.

USA Deaf Sports Federation and Special Olympics are the only organizations to offer competition in diving in addition to swimming. Both offer one-meter springboard diving.

Within the competitive swimming ranks in the United States, USA Swimming is the National Governing Body. USA Swimming was established in 1978 replacing the Competitive Swimming Committee of the Amateur Athletic Union (AAU). USA Swimming is responsible for the conduct and administration of swimming in the United States including formulating rules, implementing policies and procedures, conducting national championships, disseminating safety and sports medicine information and selecting athletes to represent the United States in international competition. The Adapted Swimming Section of USA Swimming oversees aspects related to swimming for individuals with disabilities. The USA Swimming Official Rulebook includes a section on officiating meets for athletes with disabilities.

On the international level the Federation Internationale de Natation Amateur (FINA) has much the same responsibility but is the ultimate authority in competitive swimming world-wide.

SPORT ORIGIN

An excellent but brief description of the origin of swimming can be found on the USOC website <http://www.usoc.org>. Competitive swimming probably began in England in the early to mid 1800s as pools were being constructed throughout the city of London, but early depictions of swimming goes back to the days of ancient Rome and Greece. The breaststroke was the stroke of choice for Londoners. Freestyle events were held at the first modern Olympic Games and other strokes were established through the years as coaches and individuals looked for ways to increase speed.

Adapted swimming began in the 1930s as Dr. Charles Lowman, a physician, systematized hydrotherapy for people with disabilities. Swimming for individuals with disabilities has been a part of disability sports since its beginning. Swimming has been a part of just about all of the DSO's inaugural games including the 1924 World Games for the Deaf in Paris, and the 1960 Paralympic Games in Rome. An indication of the strides made, and growth of expectations in disability sports is reflected in the first Special Olympic Games in 1968. At these games, organizers were so worried about the capabilities of athletes, they made the longest event 25 yards, even allowing athletes to stop and touch the bottom during the race if they became tired! Today, Special Olympians compete in races up to 1,500 meters with official FINA rules applying.

Swimming is an important component of all the disability sport organization programming. Swimming programs for athletes with disabilites are designed to accommodate swimmers of all ages and skill levels, from recreational participants to elite international competitors. Participants learn to swim at programs offered by their schools and communities, as well as at learn-to-swim camps held in conjunction with the annual specific disability sport national games and regional events. Top-level swimmers may qualify to compete at the USA Swimming Disability Championships, Paralympic Games, or IPC World Swimming Championships.

Sport Classification

As will be evident in many of the sports described in this book, each of the disability sport organizations have their own specific classification systems. These classification systems help to ensure that competition is equitable and that individuals who win, do so because of training and talent and not because their disability happens to be less severe then their opponents.

For international competitions the system changes. Since the late 1980's international swimming for athletes with disabilities has used a functional classification system. This approach was first implemented at the 1992 Barcelona Paralympic Summer Games, and combines over 2 dozen different classes of the disability sports organizations (excepting the blind) into a 10-class system for freestyle, backstroke, butterfly and individual medley, and a 9 class system is used for breaststroke competition. Although a need to combine the many classes exists, the current system may not be the most equitable. Many athletes, especially those with cerebral palsy, are being left behind, not because of their ability or training, but because their disability is more severe than others. Athletes who are blind use their tradition 3 classification system based on visual acuity, since organizers have realized how unfair it would be for these athletes to compete head to head with athletes with other physical disabilities.

USA Swimming Adapted Swimming utilizes a 15 class system for athletes with physical disabilities (class S1-S-10), athletes who are blind (class S11-S13), athletes who have cognitive impairments (class S14), and athletes who are deaf or hard of hearing (class S15). The International Paralympic Committee website <http://www.paralympic.org> offers a complete description of the international swimming classification guidelines while the USA Swimming website describes their classification in detail

The remaining portion of this section will discuss pool accessibility, flotation devices, and several suggestions and considerations specific to certain disabilities.

POOL ACCESSIBILITY

For swimmers with mobility problems, whether ambulatory or nonambulatory, the ability to access the swimming pool is a major concern (Figures 36.1 and 36.2). Unless a pool is specifically designed as a therapeutic pool, there is a good chance that it will not be easily accessible to individuals with lower extremity disabilities.

The easiest and most inexpensive way around an inaccessible pool is to train the aquatic staff in the proper methods of manual lifts and transfers. Manual lifts can be done with a two-person lift, a four-person lift, or with a large towel or blanket. Floor mats for padding the pool's side and gutter help to prevent bruising of the feet, legs, and buttocks. Various commercial lifts and portable stairs used to safely assist the swimmer from the pool deck and/or wheelchair in to the water, are also available from most pool suppliers and medical supply companies (Figure 36.3).

The Polymedic Pool Wheelchair from Achievable Concepts is used to assist people with limited mobility to get into swimming pools. It is a lightweight, durable, and rustproof pool wheelchair. The wheelchair is suitable for swimming pools with ramps into the water, and it can be fully immersed. As the wheelchair enters the pool, the frame of the wheelchair fills with water to prevent it from floating. The water drains out of the frame as the wheelchair leaves the water.

The implementation of the American's with Disabilities Act (ADA) has boosted the number of companies producing both pool lifts and portable stair devices (Figure 36.4). A list of some popular manufacturers is provided at the end of this chapter. Many public and private pools are upgrading their aquatic facilities to meet the increasing demands for accessible pools.

CONSIDERATIONS FOR SWIMMERS WITH AMPUTATIONS

Swimming is regarded as a preferred fitness activity for individuals with amputations for both its physical conditioning and for the absence of trauma to the residual limb area. This is an important consideration, especially for swimmers who have experienced a recent loss of an extremity.

Prostheses

Prostheses devices may provide balance in the water through even weight distribution. Examples of lower limb prostheses include the Otto Bock Hollow Ultra Light (hollow chambered leg for BK or AK amputations), Aqualite (peg leg used for BK or AK amputations), and ActivAnkle (swim ankle for fins).

Swim Fins

Various styles fo swim fins exist for amputee swimmers. The Viau-Whiteside Swimming Attachment (Fig-

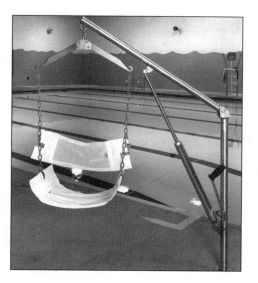

Figure 36.1. Econo-Life is designed for budget-conscious facilities that may have only occasional need for access. (Courtesy of Spectrum Pool Products)

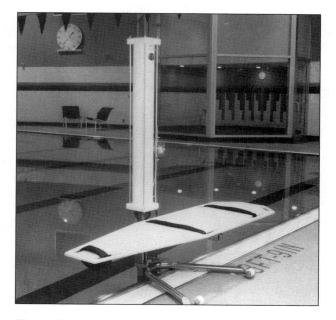

Figure 36.2. Certain models of lifts also allow for an optional rescue board attachment. (Courtesy of Spectrum Pool Products)

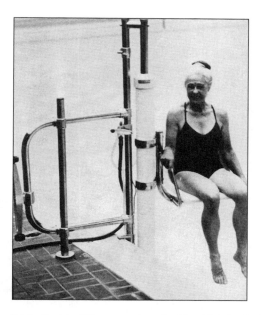

Figure 36.3. Certain lifts are equipped with a high-back rigid seat. (Courtesy of Access to Recreation)

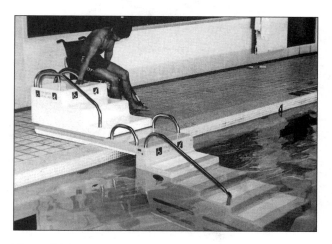

Figure 36.4. Portable stairs provide easy access from a wheelchair to the water. (Courtesy of Triad Technologies, Inc.)

ure (36.5) and the P.O.S.O.S./Tablada swimming hand prosthesis (Figures 36.6 a and b) represent some of the earlier attempts at designing swim fins for amputeen swimmers.

One of the best devices available for the person with an upper limb amputation is the Freestyle TSD (therapeutic swim device) by Therapeutic Recreation Systems (TRS) (Figure 36.7 a and b). The Freestyle Swimming Terminal device is a recreational accessory designed to be used with a custom swimming prosthesis for those interested in high performance or competitive swimming capability. The design which mimics a folding wing reduces resistance during stroke recovery but flares open to provide maximum resistance during the power stroke. The device can be rotated to optimize various swimming strokes and styles. The wings can be fixed in a flared position for treading water and water aerobic exercise. The

Freestyle comes in an adult size but can be easily modified down to conform to smaller hand displacements using standard shop equipment such as band or jig saws and belt sanders. Threaded stainless stud fits all standard body powered, mechanical prosthetic wrists. It is a passive device (no cables) that can best be utilized with a custom-shortened prosthesis which is designed to place the Freestyle device as proximally as limb length allows. The Freestyle is also acceptable for competition in high school athletics. TRS offers a Swim Fin Kit as an alternative to the Freestyle (Figure 36.8 a and b). The kit uses the same flexing fin system, but is designed to eliminate the prosthesis. Advantages over the freestyle are cost, weight, and convenience of use.

Although it should be noted that swimmers with amputations may not use any prosthetic or swim fin device during competitive events, the use of such items may be very appropriate for recreational use depending on individual preferences.

CONSIDERATIONS FOR BLIND SWIMMERS

Generally, blind or visually impaired swimmers have little need for adaptations in the pool. Some may use beeper devices at each end of the pool to provide auditory directional clues to assist them in swimming straight lines. Some coaches will use a "tap stick" to tell swimmers when to begin their flip turns, or that the edge of the pool is within reach (Figure 36.9). In backstroke competitions, backstroke flags are lowered to 3.5 feet above the water's surface.

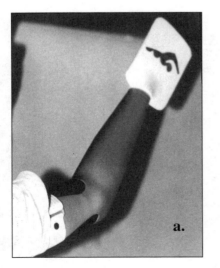

Figure 36.5. The Viau-Whiteside Swimming Attachment. (Courtesy of TRS)

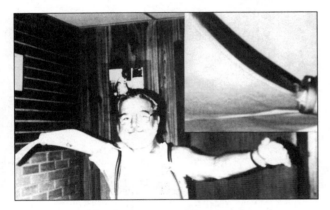

a.

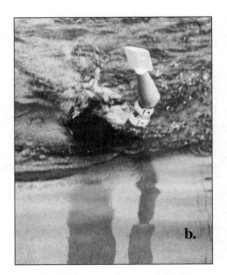

b.

Figure 36.6 a and b. The P.O.S.O.S./Tablada Swimming Hand Prosthesis. (Courtesy of TRS)

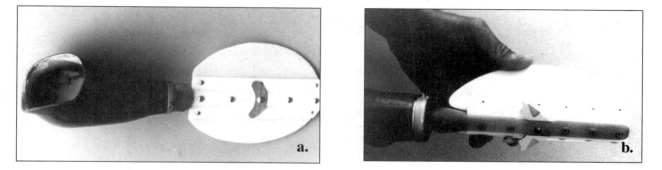

Figure 36.7 a and b. The Freestyle T.S.D. (Therapeutic Swim Device) is designed to reduce resistance during the recovery portion of the stroke. (Courtesy of TRS)

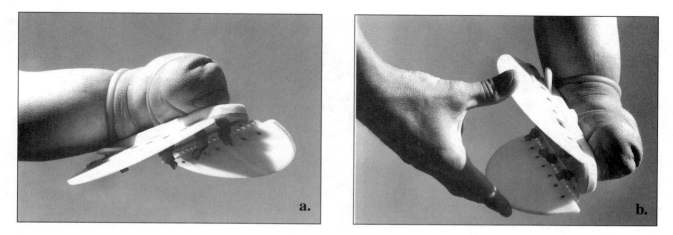

Figure 36.8 a and b. The Swim Fin Kit eliminates the need of the prosthesis thus reducing cost and weight and increasing convenience. (Courtesy of TRS)

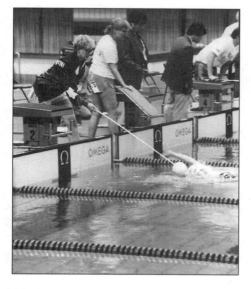

Figure 36.9. The use of "tap sticks" tells blind and visually impaired swimmers when to begin their flip turns. (Courtesy of Specialized Sports Unlimited)

FLOTATION DEVICES

The use of flotation devices in competitive swimming for individuals with disabilities is limited to two of the eight classes in cerebral palsy sports, and 2 developmental events in Special Olympics for athletes with lower ability levels. However, since most swim programs for individuals with disabilities are not run for competitive swimmers, the use of flotation devices is common and highly recommended (Figure 36.10 a and b). The individual's swimming ability (determined by physical strength, flexibility, and buoyancy), swimming style or technique, experience in the water, and any related disability (i.e., seizures) should be considered when selecting a flotation device.

Tire tubs, Styrofoam bubbles, inflatable collars, water ski waist belts, old gym mats (floating on the surface), personal flotation devices (PFD's), life vests, and life-jackets have all been used in swimming programs for individuals with disabilities. A number of multipurpose swim rings and head floats allow instructors to work with the swimmer's arms and legs. Other floats compensate for lateral rotation due to uneven muscle development. Danmar Products is a major supplier and distributor of flotation devices for individuals with disabilities. By accessing their website (see Equipment Suppliers at the end of the chapter), the reader the will be able to locate local suppliers of Danmar products.

A swimmer's need or dependence on a float may change as confidence, strength, and skill are acquired in a particular stroke. The bulky PFD is often replaced by streamlined waist belts or waist bubbles, which in time may be replaced by water wings. Progression to independent swimming will be as individual as the initial selection of a float.

Although water-therapy or aqua-fitness are not covered here, it should be noted that several companies do manufacture exercise and therapy-related flotation devices (Figures 36.11 and 36.12). Some of these are listed under Equipment Suppliers.

Modifications to Rules

Although rule modifications are minimal in swimming, some modifications or adaptations to FINA rules may be allowed based on the disability of the athlete. For instance:

- Starting position (in or out of the water) is optional
- During starts, the use of strobe light in conjunction with an auditory signal may be appropriate for individuals who are deaf, while the use of a whistle for individuals with cerebral palsy is preferred over the use of a gun. The use of a gun may stimulate an unwanted reflex effect in an athlete with cerebral palsy
- During relays, a light touch on the shoulder of a

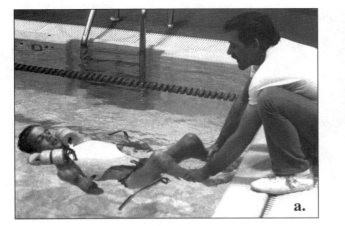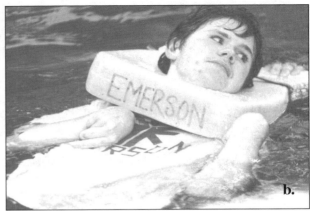

Figure 36.10 a and b. Various commercially available flotation devices provide reassurance and safety to many swimmers. (Courtesy of Human Kinetics)

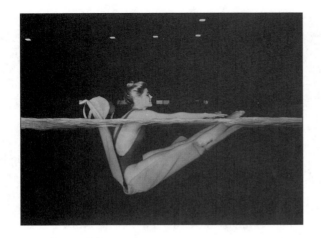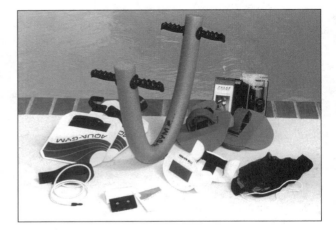

Figure 36.11. The Bodyciser is a unique aquatic fitness device and low-impact method of exercise. (Courtesy of Bodyciser International Corp.)

Figure 36.12. The Aqua-Gym complete water system allows the user to simulate cycling, running, kicking, strength training and calisthenics while the participant is immersed in water. (Courtesy of Aqua-Gym Inc.)

- blind athlete signals them when to begin their leg of the race, while other disabilities may use an optional deck or water start
- Since strict stroke mechanics may be impossible for some athletes due to their disability, stroke judgement should be concerned with the action of the non-impaired limbs

EQUIPMENT SUPPLIERS

The number of reputable aquatic equipment suppliers is tremendous. The following is a sample of some of these companies and is not meant to be inclusive.

Flotation Devices

Danmar Products, Inc.
221 Jackson Industrial Drive
Ann Arbor MI 48103
(800) 783-1998
(734) 761-1990
(734) 761-8977 (fax)
Email: danmarpro@aol.com
Website: http://www.danmarproducts.com/
Danmar is one of the largest suppliers of head floats, stabilizers, headfloat/stabilizer, swim rings, hydrotherapy equipment in the world.

Floating Swimwear Inc.
1725 East Wassall
Wichita, KS 67216-2143
(800) 341-8110
(316) 524-0444
(316) 524-0411 (fax)
Email: info@floatingswimwear.com
Website: http://www.floatingswimwear.com/

Rothhammer International Inc.
P.O. Box 3840
San Luis Obispo, CA 93403
(800) 235-2156
(800) 541-5339 (fax)
Email: info@sprintaquatics.com
Website: http://www.sprintaquatics.com/

Polymedic Pool Wheelchair

Achievable Concepts
P.O. Box 361
Moonee Ponds 3039
Victoria , Australia
(61) 3 9752 5958
(61) 3 9754 4798 (fax)
Email   sales@achievableconcepts.com.au
Website: http://www.achievableconcepts.com.au

Pool Lifts (above and in-ground pools)

Arjo, inc.
50 N. gary Ave.
Roselle, IL 60172
(800) 323-1245
(888) 594-2756 (fax)
Website: http://www.arjo.com

Aquatic Access Inc.
417 Dorsey Way
Louisville, KY 40223 USA
(800) 325-5438
(502) 425-5817
(502) 425-9607 (fax)
Email: info@aquatic-access.com
Website: http://www.aquaticaccess.com/

Barrier Free Lifts, Inc
9230 Prince William Street
Manassas VA 2011
(800) 582-8732
(703) 361-6531
(703) 361-7861
Email: bflinc@erols.com
Website: http://www.bfl-inc.com/

Disability Mall
Disability mall is an online resource that features many companies that provide pool lifts as well as other products for individuals with disabilities
Website: http://www.disabilitymall.com

Mengo Industires Inc.
4611 Green Bay Rd.
Kenosha, WI 53144
(800) 279-4611
(262) 652-3070
(262) 652-9910 (fax)
Email: dotline@mengo-ind.com
Website: http://www.mengo-ind.com

PAL-Portable Aquatic Lift
RehaMed International, LLC.
14260 SW 136th Street #9
Miami, FL 33186
(800) 577-4424
(305) 969-LIFT
(305) 969-2155 (fax)
Email: info@poollifts.com
Website: http://www.rehamedlifts.com

Spectrum Pool Products
7100 Spectrum Lane

Missoula, MT 59808
Email: info@SpectrumProducts.com
Website: http://www.spectrumproducts.com/
(800) 776-5309
(800) 728-7143 (fax)

SureHands International
982 Route 1
Pine Island, NY 10969
(800) 724-5305
(914) 258-6634 (fax)
Email: surehand@warwick.net
Website: http://www.surehands.com/

Stairs

Quaker Plastic Corp.
"The Swim Step System"
103 South Manor St.
Mountville, PA 17554
(717) 285-4571
(717) 285-7740 (fax)
Email: Info@QuakerPlastic.com
Website: http://www.quakerplastic.com/

Rehab System LLC
610 N. University
Fargo, ND 58102
(800) 726-8620
(701) 297-9702 (fax)
Email: AquaTrek2000@aol.com
Website: http://www.rehabsystems.net

Swim Fin Device

Therapeutic Recreation Systems (TRS), Inc.
2450 Central Avenue, Unit D
Boulder, CO 80301-2844
(800) 279-1865
(303) 444-4720
(303) 444-5372 (fax)
Website: www.oandp.com/trs

ADDITIONAL RESOURCES AND WEBSITES

Swimmers will find many websites and support organizations related to their sports. Most participants will find the following sites satisfactory for gathering information.

Federation Internationale de Natation Amateur (FINA)
Ave. de Beaumont 9
1012 Lausanne, Switzerland
Website: http://www.fina.org

Harvard Swimming and Diving
Website: http://www.hcs.harvard.edu/~swim/
Although not disability related, this website contains over 1500 links related to the broad field of aquatics.

US Aquatic Association of the Deaf (USAAD)
Carrie Miller, Director
6808 40th Ave NE
Seattle, WA 98115
(206) 616-6143 TTY
Email: cmiller@ocean.washington.edu
Website: http://members.tripod.com/USAAD/
Email: USAAD@hotmail.com

US Wheelchair Swimming
Liz DeFrancesco
5730 Chambertin Drive
San Jose, CA 95118
(408) 267-0200
(408) 2672834 (fax)

USA Swimming
One Olympic Plaza
Colorado Springs, CO 80909
(719) 578-4578
Email: ussinfo@usa-swimming.org
Website: http://www.usa-swimming.org/
This website provides a tremendous amount of links for every state. Just about any needed information can be found here. Go to programs for information on the adapted swimming section.

United States Masters Swimming
P.O. Box 185
Londonderry NH 03053-0185
phone (603) 537-0203
fax (603) 537-0204
Email: usms@usms.org.
Website: http://www.usms.org/

BIBLIOGRAPHY

Amputee Coalition of America (1997). Prosthetic components enhance swimming. *In-Motion* 7(3)42.

Broadrick, T. (1997, August). In the swim. *Exceptional Parent*. P64-65, 69.

Greene, E. (1998). The fin. *In-Motion* 8(3) 21-22, 24.

Mace, R. (1993). Make pools accessible. *Athletic Business* 17(8)34, 36.

Myers, J. (1999). A new twist in therapetuic swimming. *Active Living 8*(3)27-28.

Popke, M. (1994, May) Water's edge. *Athletic Business.* P. 39-43.

Suomi, J. & Suomi, R. (2000). Cretating an inclusive early childhood swim program-Special needs aquatic program (SNAP). *Palaestra 16*(2)20-29.

Chapter 37

Table Tennis

SPORT GOVERNING BODIES:
National: USA Table Tennis (USATT)
International: International Table Tennis Federation (ITTF)

Official Sport Of: __x__ **DAAA**   ____ **USABA**   __x__ **USCPAA**
                           __x__ **DS/USA**   __x__ **USADSF**   __x__ **WS/USA**
                           __x__ **SOI**

DISABLED SPORTS ORGANIZATION:
National: American WheelchairTable Tennis Association (AWTTA)
                     USATT Disabled Players Committee
International: International Table Tennis Committee for theDisabled

PRIMARY DISABILITY: All

SPORT OVERVIEW

Table tennis is probably more popular and recognized as a recreational activity than as a competitive sport. As with many of the activities described within this text, modifications to allow participation by individuals with disabilities are limited and simple to implement.

Table tennis probably began as an after dinner activity in England in the later 1800's. It has been known by many names over the years especially the very common term "Ping-Pong". The sport became a competitive event sometime in the early 1900's as it grew in popularity. Within the United States the USA Table Tennis (USATT), founded in 1933, is the National Governing Body (NGB) for table tennis, with the goal to promote table tennis, recreationally and professionally. It has been an Olympic sport since 1988 and is an official sport of the first Paralympic Games in 1960, World Games for the Deaf and Special Olympics.

All sanctioned competitions conducted under the auspices of the disability sport organizations follow USA Table Tennis (USATT) and International Table Tennis Federation (ITTF) rules with a few modifications for wheelchair players. All matches are played best of three

games to 21. Both organizations have committees established for inclusion of athletes with disabilities. Rule modifications for individuals with disabilities have been included in both National Governing Bodies Official Rule Books indicating the continued inclusion of athletes with disabilities into able bodied NGBs. These rules are available on the USATT and International Paralympic Committee websites. The USATT Disabled Players Committee works for the promotion of table tennis among individuals with disabilities. Two styles of table tennis are played by individuals with disabilities, standing and wheelchair. Each of the 6 disability sports organizations (DSO's) listed previously offers competitive table tennis on the local, regional, and national levels. Disabled Sports USA, Special Olympics, and USCPAA offer both wheelchair and standing divisions. USA Deaf Sports Federation and the Dwarf Athletic Association of America conduct only ambulatory competition, while Wheelchair Sports USA offers only wheelchair competition through the American Wheelchair Table Tennis Association (Figure 37.1). Each DSO uses a different sport classification to group players into competitive categories and divisions. Within the United States each DSO competes separately. International competition for individuals with disabilities divides participants into wheelchair and standing categories, and then separates them into more specific competition classes based on functional ability. The current international classification system consists of 5 wheelchair classes (1-5) and 5 standing classes (6-10). A complete guide to the classification system is provided on the International Paralympic Committee website.

STYLES OF PLAY

Standing Table Tennis

According to ITTF Rules, no exceptions to existing table tennis rules are made for individuals with disabilities who play standing up. Individuals may choose to play with or without assistive devices such as crutches (Figure 37.2), and without or without prosthetic devices.

Wheelchair Table Tennis

Only a few exceptions to existing rules are needed for athletes who use wheelchairs. The height of the table remains at 2'6" but players may add cushions to their wheelchair to adjust their sitting height. Some of the more common exceptions are as follows:

- a let is called if while serving, the ball leaves the table by either of the *receiver's sidelines* (on one or more bounces), or on bouncing on the receiver's side returns in the direction of the net, or comes to rest on the receiver's side of the playing surface (unless server returns ball);
- during play, a player may touch the playing surface with the free hand, only to restore balance *after striking the ball* (provided the playing surface is not moved);
- during doubles play, a player's wheelchair can not protrude an imaginary extension of the center line of the table. If it does the umpire awards the point to the opposing pair;

- tables must be accessible for wheelchair players;
- no strapping of players is allowed (upper torso) except for medical reasons, although below knees strapping is allowed;
- strapping of the paddle to the hand is permitted in all classes.

Special Olympics

Table tennis has been offered in Special Olympics programming since 1987. Currently, table tennis is considered to be a nationally popular or demonstration sport and not one of the official Special Olympic sports. A variety of competitions may be offered including singles, doubles, mixed doubles, unified sports doubles, unified sports mixed doubles, wheelchair competition, and the Individual Skills Contest. Unified sports competition pairs athletes with and without mental retardation while the individual skills competition consists of events for lower skilled athletes. These contests include the Target Serve where the athlete serves 5 balls into the service area, getting one point for each successful performance; the Racket Bounce, where the athlete attempts to bounce a table tennis ball on their racket as many times as possible during two 30 second rounds; and the Return Shot where the athlete attempts to return a ball, served to him by a feeder, into the opposite service box.

EQUIPMENT

Only three pieces of equipment are used in the game, a table, a ball, and a paddle with rubber backing. Very few adaptations or modifications are available, so the basic concept of table tennis stays intact. The only exception allowed in sanctioned play is to the paddle, which will be discussed below.

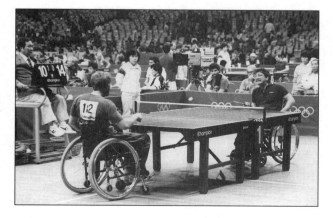

Figure 37.1. Wheelchair Sports USA offers both singles and doubles competition in table tennis. (Courtesy of Specialized Sports Unlimited)

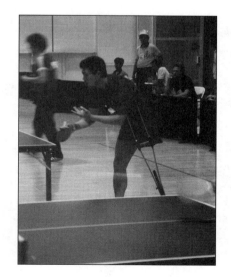

Figure 37.2. Athletes have the option of using crutches during competition.

Tables

There are several ways to modify the table to provide greater recreational opportunities. Adams and McCubbin (1991, pp.181-187) describe an adapted version of the game called "surface table tennis", which uses a standard table with wooden rails attached to the sides and an elevated net (Figure 37.3).

The object of surface table tennis is to keep the ball on the surface of the table under the net. Points are awarded to the opposing player if the ball is hit *over or into* the net. The side rails are used to keep the ball in play as much as possible. Scoring is similar to a standard game.

Versatility is important when different disability groups participate in the same sport. Height-adjustable tables can be constructed that can be raised from 24 to 30 inches. Ideal for children and wheelchair users, the table can also be constructed with side guards that can help the beginning or recreational player keep the ball in play (Figure 37.4). Table height can also be adjusted in other ways. Six-inch floor risers have been seen in Dwarf Athletic Association of America (DAAA) competition when short-statured players needed additional height allowances to play at official tables.

Paddles

For players with grasp difficulties severe enough to prevent them from effectively holding paddles, there are several alternatives. Strap-on paddles can be created by adding velcro strips to standard table tennis paddles (Figure 37.5). This represents the simplest and most inexpensive option.

The concept of a strap-on paddle advanced with the development of the table tennis cuff or activity glove (Figure 37.6). Use of the cuff provides a more natural and secure placement of the paddle in the player's palm and allows participation by individuals with virtually no hand or wrist function. The Action Life Glove (Figure 37.7)

available through Access to Recreation is an example of a glove that allows the person to grasp various objects such as table tennis paddles.

Arm Support

Muscle weakness and increased vulnerability to fatigue in certain disabilities, most notably muscular dystrophy, prevent some people from raising their paddle arms for prolonged periods. A ball-bearing feeder arm support, as described by Adams and McCubbin (1991, p. 183), can eliminate this problem and still provide a full range of movement (Figure 37.8). The device supports the weight of the arm by using gravity to substitute for loss of power.

EQUIPMENT SUPPLIERS

Equipment needed to play table tennis is available at any local sporting goods store and listing of suppliers is unnecessary. However, for the enthusiast who wishes to support USATT sponsors, a listing of USATT approved distributors can be found at the following website: http://www.usatt.org/equipment/dealers.shtml

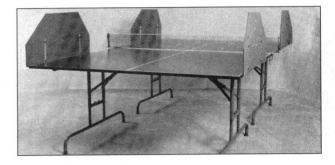

Figure 37.4. Height-adjustable table with removable side guards can be used for beginning and recreational players. (Courtesy of Access to Recreation, Inc.)

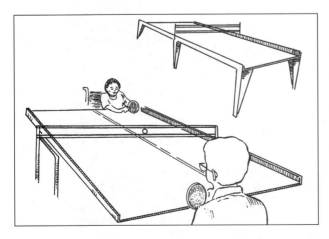

Figure 37.3. Surface table tennis uses a different net and adapted rules.

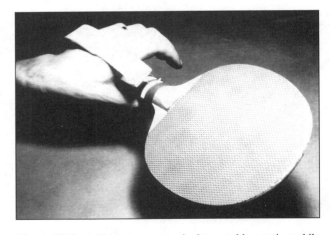

Figure 37.5. A Velcro strap attached to a table tennis paddle provides an easy solution to grasp problems. (Courtesy of Maddak, Inc.)

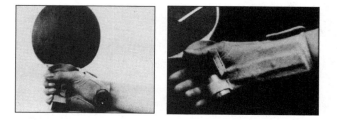

Figure 37.6. Table tennis cuffs enable individuals with little or no hand or wrist function to participate. (Courtesy of Access to Recreation, Inc.)

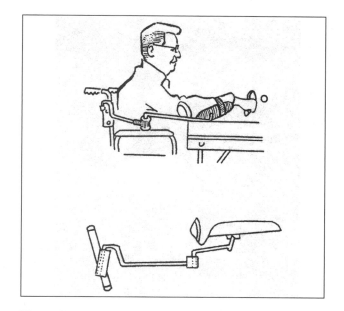

Figure 37.7. The Action Life Glove by Patton is another alternative to the table tennis cuff. (Courtesy of Patton Enterprises)

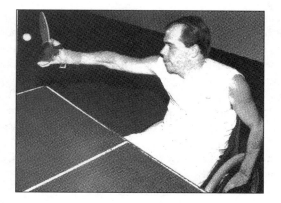

Figure 37.8. The arm support moves freely through the use of a ball-bearing mechanism.

A listing of official USA Table Tennis Approved Equipment available from the above dealers can be accessed at the following website:
http://www.usatt.org/equipment/index.shtml

Access to Recreation, Inc (Action Life Glove)
8 Sandra Court
Newbury Park CA 91320
(800) 634-4351
(805) 498-7535
(805) 498-8186 (fax)
Email: dkrebs@gte.net
Website: http://www.accesstr.com

ADDITIONAL RESOURCES AND WEBSITES

Individuals interested in table tennis will find many websites related to their sport. Because this sport is accessible for those with and without disabilities, most participants will find the following sites and organizations satisfactory for gathering information.

American Wheelchair Table Tennis Association (AWTTA)
Attn: Jennifer Johnson
23 Parker Street
Port Chester, NY 10573
(914) 937-3932

International Table Tennis Federation (ITTF)
53, London Road
St. Leonards-on-Sea, East Sussex
TN37 6AY, Great Britain
Email: http://www@ittf.com
Website: http://www.ittf.com

International Table Tennis Committee for the Disabled
Website: http://www.tabletennis.org/ittc/
This website provides extensive information on players rankings, profiles, rules, competition updates, and links

USA Table Tennis (USATT)
USATT Disabled Athletes & Tournaments Committee
One Olympic Plaza
Colorado Springs, CO 80909-5769
(719) 578-4583
(719) 632-6071 (fax)
Email: usatt@iex.net
Website: http://www.usatt.org/

BIBLIOGRAPHY

Adams, R.C. & McCubbin, J.A. (1991). *Games, Sports & Exercises for the Physically Handicapped.* (4th Ed.). Philadephia: Lea & Febiger.

Chapter 38

Team Handball

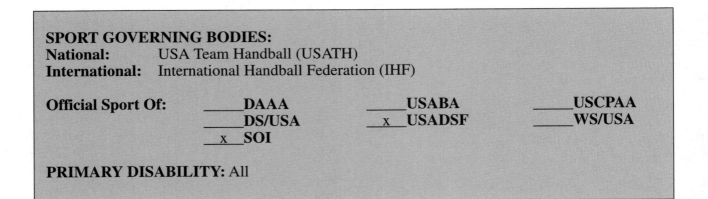

SPORT GOVERNING BODIES:
National: USA Team Handball (USATH)
International: International Handball Federation (IHF)

Official Sport Of: ____DAAA   ____USABA   ____USCPAA
                          ____DS/USA   _x__USADSF   ____WS/USA
                          _x__SOI

PRIMARY DISABILITY: All

SPORT OVERVIEW

Team handball combines the basic skills of catching, passing, dribbling, running, and throwing into a fast-moving, semi non-contact sport. On a court slightly larger than a basketball court, team handball is played with seven players, six court players and a goalie, who play both offense and defense. The object of the game is to move the ball up the court into the opponent's end and attempt to score by throwing the ball past the goalie into the goal. Athletes also have to react quickly as they are only allowed to take three (3) steps while in possession of the ball or hold the ball for three (3) seconds—without moving. A player may run three steps, dribble any number of times, pick the ball up, and run three more steps. Once they have stopped their dribble, players are not allowed to dribble again. Team handball promotes excellent physical conditioning and a good working knowledge of team play. Good strategy, planning and training are essential to successful competition in team handball.

Currently, only two disabled sport organizations offer team handball. Team handball is one of the seven *nationally popular* sports in Special Olympics, while the USA Deaf Sports Federation offers the sport through the U.S. Deaf Team Handball Association with no modifications to the official game.

The United States Cerebral Palsy Association (USCPAA) offered the sport of Wheelchair Team Handball until the name of the game was changed recently to Wheelchair Soccer (see the Soccer Chapter).

SPORT ORIGIN

Team handball was developed in Europe in the 1920's and was reintroduced as an Olympic sport 1972 after an absence of 34 years. Team handball can claim worldwide participation by 136 countries and 12 million International Handball Federation affiliated players. Only 5 years ago the numbers of countries playing totaled about 36 with approximately 3 million affiliated players. It is surprising that even though team handball is fast-paced, exciting to watch, and even more exciting to play, it has not become more popular in the United States. Known throughout the world as "handball", the name Team Handball is used in the United States due to the other game of handball. For years the game has enjoyed great appeal in the United States military, and many of the U.S. world class athletes in this sport have been from the military. Through the educational and promotional efforts of USA Team Handball, many universities throughout the country now include team handball instruction for physical education majors. The game remains a popular activity in physical education classes.

USA Team Handball founded in 1959, serves as the sport's National Governing Body; developing team handball through schools, recreation leagues and colleges; providing multiple levels of competition for all ages, skill levels, and interests as well as developing the Men's and Women's teams for the Pan American Games and the Olympic Games. USA Team Handball is a member of the United States Olympic Committee (USOC), Pan American Team Handball Federation (PATHF), and the International Handball Federation (IHF).

EQUIPMENT AND SET-UP

Team handball is an ideal sport for physical education classes since the only equipment needed is a ball and a goal.

The Playing Court:

The playing court is slightly larger than a basketball court and measures 20 meters (65' 7") by 40 meters (131' 3") (Figure 38.1). The length may be shortened when space is limited.

Goal and Goal Area:

The goal is two meters (6.6') high by three meters (9.8') wide. The net is 1 meter (3.3') deep at the base of the goal. The goal area line, or 6-meter line (19' 8"), is the most important line. No one except the goalie is allowed to stand in the goal area. The goal opening is 2 meters by 3 meters. When shooting for a goal, players may jump into the area if the ball is released before landing in the area.

The Ball:

Team handball is played with a 32-panel leather ball and is slightly larger than a 16" softball. For women, the ball is 54 to 56 centimeters and 325 to 400 grams. For men, it is 58 to 60 centimeters and 425 to 475 grams. A youth training ball is available through USA Team Handball for use with beginners or in physical education classes although any standard foam ball that is easily grasped would be appropriate.

Number of Players:

There are seven players on each team (six court players and one goalie). A maximum of 12 players may dress and participate in a game for each team. Substitutes may enter the game at any time through own substitution area as long as the player they are replacing has left the court.

Game Duration:

Generally, for players 18 years and over, the game consists of 2, 30-minute halves with a 10-minute half-time. Youth games may consist of 2, 15-minute or 20-minute halves.

A complete set of rules, resource materials, films, and video-tapes are available from the USA Team Handball national office or online through the International Handball Federation website.

SPECIAL OLYMPICS TEAM HANDBALL

Team handball is offered through Special Olympics as one of their nationally popular sports. The game was first played internationally at the 1991 International Summer Special Olympic Games in Minneapolis, with 15 teams competing.

Special Olympics offers a variety of team handball official events in which athletes can participate, ranging from full team competition to individual skills competition. Rules for the team competition are based upon the International Handball Federation (IHF) Rules for Team Handball. Rules for other events were developed in close cooperation with USA Team Handball. Events include:

1. Team Competition

Rules for the team competition are based upon the International Handball Federation (IHF) Rules for Team Handball.

2. Five (5)-A-Side Competition

Rules are the same as for the regulation game but with fewer players to allow for more teams, or for players of lesser ability. A foam ball is recommended.

3. Unified Sports® Team Competition

Unified Sports® allows for inclusion of athletes with and without mental retardation. At least four of the players on the court must be athletes with mental retardation. Three shall be unified partners without mental retardation.

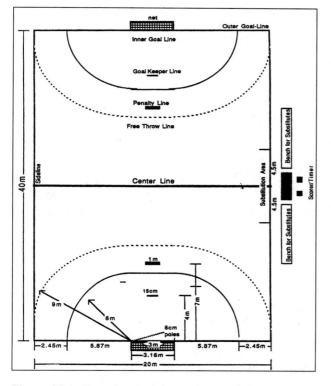

Figure 38.1. Team handball court dimension. (Courtesy of SOI)

4. Unified Sports® Individual Skills Competition

Individual skills competition consists of one athlete and one unified partner.

5. Individual Skills Contest

The individual skills competition is recommended for athletes with lower ability levels. It is not recommended for athletes who can play the game. This contest provides practice in passing, dribbling, and shooting. Specific instructions can be found in the Official Special Olympics Summer Sports Rules.

Special Olympics Team Handball Sports Skills Guide

A copy of the *Team Handball Sports Skills Program Guide* is available for purchase through Special Olympics. This guide provides a developmental approach to teaching and coaching team handball. It is an excellent resource for physical education classes.

EQUIPMENT SUPPLIERS

Equipment used in team handball is similar for those with or without disabilities. Information on hundreds of athletic equipment suppliers can be found on the Athletic Business Buyers Guide at <www.athleticbusiness.com>. Within the last few years more of the larger physical education equipment distributors have started to carry a full line of team handballs and goals. In addition to carrying official team handball equipment, Sportime also carries the youth training ball of USA Team Handball. Refer to Appendix A for more equipment manufacturers.

Team Handball Balls

Baden Sports Inc.
34114 21st Ave. S.
Federal Way, WA 98003
(253) 925-0500
(253) 925-0570 (fax)
(800) 544-2998

D. Hauptman Co. Inc. (also goals)
4856 W. Jefferson Blvd.
Los Angeles, CA 90016
(216) 734-2597 (in California)
(800) 542-4625 (al others)

Scoring Sports Corp. (also nets/goals)
505 Broadway
P.O. Box 1396
Tacoma, WA 98401
(253) 272-9764
(253) 627-7274
(800) 743-4117
Email: dtisoccer@dtisoccer.com

Sportime (also nets/goals)
One Sportime Way
Atlanta, GA 30340
(770) 449-5700
(770) 263-0897 (fax)
(800) 523-8176
Email: jgooden@sportime.com
Website: http://www.sportime.com

Tachikara USA Inc.
8000 W. 110th St., Suite 150
Overland Park, KS 66210
(913) 498-1881
(913) 498-1882 (fax)
Email: office@tachikara.com
Website: http://www.tachikara.com

Goal Nets & Frames

All Goals Inc.
P.O. Box 2201
Inver Grove Heights, MN 55076
(651) 306-1500
(651) 455-4024 (fax)
Email: allgoals@usinternet.com

Jason Mills Inc.
220 Kinderkamack Road
Westwood, NJ 07675-3601
(201) 358-6500
(201) 358-8915 (fax)
Email: inquiry@jasonmills.com

U.S. Team Handball Supply Co.
400 Hillside Ave.
Hillside, NJ 07205
(201) 973-6000

ADDITIONAL RESOURCES AND WEBSITES

Team handball players will find many websites related to their sport. Because this sport is accessible for those with and without disabilities, most participants will find the following sites satisfactory for gathering information.

International Handball Federation
Case Postale 312 (Lange Gasse 10)
4020 Basel, Switzerland (4052)
(41-61) 272-1300
 (41-61) 272-1344 (fax)
Email: IHF@magnet.ch
Website: http://www.ihf.ch/or
            http://www.worldsport.com/sports/handball/home.html

The IHF operates their website through worldsport.com, a website with links to dozens of sports.

A complete set of team handball rules can be found at this site.

Select Team Handball
Website: http://www.mts.net/~bcrocket/selects.html

This site provides hundreds of links to team handball sites throughout the world.

Special Olympics Director of Team Handball
1325 G Street, N.W., Suite 500
Washington, DC 20005
(202) 628-3630
(202) 824-0200 (fax)
E-Mail: SOImail@aol.com
Website: http://www.specialolympics.org

United States Deaf Team Handball Association
Gene Duve

(510) 862-2907
Email: geneduve@aol.com

USA Team Handball
1903 Powers Ferry Rd., Suite 230
Atlanta, Ga. 30339
(770) 956-7660
(770) 956-7976 (fax)
(888) Play-THB
Email: info@usateamhandball.org
Website: http://www.usateamhandball.org

This is the site for the national governing body of team handball in the United States.

BIBLIOGRAPHY

Official Special Olympics Summer Sports Rules (1996-1999). Special Olympics International: Washington, D.C.

Chapter 39

Tennis

<table>
<tr><td colspan="3">SPORT GOVERNING BODIES:
National: United States Tennis Association (USTA)
International: International Tennis Federation (ITF)</td></tr>
</table>

SPORT GOVERNING BODIES:
National: United States Tennis Association (USTA)
International: International Tennis Federation (ITF)

Official Sport Of:

_____DAAA	_____USABA	_____USCPAA
_____DS/USA	_x__USADSF	_x__WS/USA
_x__SOI		

DISABLED SPORTS ORGANIZATION:
National: National Foundation of Wheelchair Tennis (NFWT)
International: International Wheelchair Tennis Association (IWTA)

PRIMARY DISABILITY: All

SPORT OVERVIEW

Widely enjoyed as a favorite leisure activity for all individuals, regardless of ability, tennis is a sport that athletes with disabilities can enjoy and benefit from even when not competing in an official competition. Tennis gives athletes the opportunity to learn and perform a variety of skills that can be played throughout life. Tennis is played in two versions by people with disabilities, ambulatory tennis and wheelchair tennis.

The world's first national governing body for tennis was formed in New York in 1881 as the United States National Lawn Tennis Association. The new organization was created to standardize tennis rules and regulations and to encourage and develop the sport. The name was eventually shortened to the current United States Tennis Association (USTA) in 1975. Although traditional tennis had its origins over 100 years ago, the development of tennis for individuals with disabilities did not occur until much later. Wheelchair tennis within the United States and internationally is now fully integrated with traditional tennis governing bodies.

A limited need for adaptations, high availability of facilities, low-cost equipment, availability of college wheelchair tennis programs, and good national leadership has made tennis a very appealing sport for individuals with physical disabilities throughout the world.

Nationally, The United States Tennis Association, through its publications, activities, and the sponsoring of wheelchair tennis tournaments, has succeeded in providing opportunities in tennis to people with a wide variety of disabilities. By working with existing disability sport organizations, the USTA wants to serve all individuals expressing an interest in the sport. The USTA publication *Tennis Programs for the Disabled* is a tremendous guide for individuals who wish to organize programs. Included are how-to sections on teaching tennis to people with disabilities, guidelines on starting programs, and a state-by–state directory of existing programs.

WHEELCHAIR TENNIS

Wheelchair tennis began in 1976 with the founding of the National Foundation of Wheelchair Tennis (NFWT) occurring in 1980. Led by Brad Parks, the NFWT did for wheelchair tennis and tennis for people with disabilities what Wimbledon and the U.S. Open have done for traditional tennis. Currently, the functions of the NFWT have been assumed by the United States Tennis Association within the Adult Tennis Department as USA Wheelchair Tennis.

Wheelchair tennis is one of the fastest growing and most challenging of all wheelchair tennis sports. To meet this demand, USA Tennis offers programs geared towards the wheelchair player. In wheelchair tennis, the player must master the game and the wheelchair. Learning mobility on the court is exciting and challenging, and helps build strength and cardiovascular ability. Wheelchair tennis provides persons with disabilities the opportunity to share in activities with their peers and family, whether able-bodied or disabled. Playing wheelchair tennis adds to socialization and the normalization of life after sustaining a disabling injury. Proficient wheelchair users can play and actively compete against stand-up players.

In response to enormous global growth, the International Wheelchair Tennis Federation (IWTF) was founded in 1988 as the organizing body at the international level. As of 1998, the IWTF became fully integrated with its able-body counterpart, the International Tennis Federation, making it the first disabled sport to achieve such a union on an international level. In order to maintain links to national wheelchair tennis associations, the IWTF became the International Wheelchair Tennis Association (IWTA). The IWTA acts as the advisory body to the ITF Wheelchair Tennis Committee and represents the views of all those involved in the game.

Wheelchair tennis was first played as an exhibition sport in the 1988 Paralympic Games in Seoul and has grown rapidly with 16 nations competing at the 1992 Barcelona Paralympic Games and 24 nations competing in the sport at the 1996 Atlanta Paralympic Games. In addition to the Paralympic Games, wheelchair tennis athletes may compete in many other events and tournaments around the world. At the end of each calendar year, the International Wheelchair Tennis Federation (IWTF) considers NEC Wheelchair Tennis Rankings, National Rankings, and other relevant information to determine recipients of World Champion Awards.

The choice of a suitable tennis wheelchair is critical to involvement in competitive tennis. Mobility is enhanced by the use of chairs designed specifically for tennis. These chairs have one front caster with cambered wheels allowing more maneuverability (see Equipment Suppliers).

General Wheelchair Tennis Rules

A complete set of wheelchair tennis rules can be found on the website of the USTA. The game of wheelchair tennis follows the same rules as able-bodied tennis as endorsed by the International Tennis Federation with few exceptions:

- The server shall be in a stationary position prior to commencing the serve, but shall then be allowed one push before striking the ball as long as the wheel does not come in contact with the baseline.

- The served ball may, after hitting the ground in the service court, hit the ground once again within the bounds of the court or it may hit the ground outside the court boundaries before the receiver returns it.
- If conventional methods for the service are physically impossible for a quadriplegic player, then another individual may drop the ball for such a player.
- The wheelchair tennis player is allowed two bounces of the ball (Figure 39.1 a and b). The player must return the ball before it hits the ground a third time. The second bounce can be either in or out of the court boundaries.
- The wheelchair is part of the body and all applicable ITF Rules which apply to a player's body shall apply to the wheelchair.

Wheelchair/Able-Bodied Singles or Doubles Tennis

- Where a wheelchair player is playing with or against an able-bodied person in singles or in doubles, the rules of wheelchair tennis shall apply for the wheel-

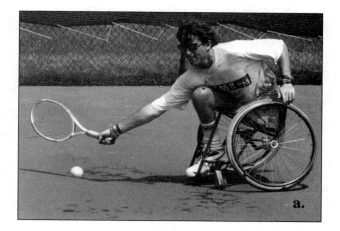

Figures 39.1 a and b. Wheelchair tennis incorporates a two-bounce rule, although it is rarely used by elite wheelchair tennis players. (Courtesy of Specialized Sports Unlimited)

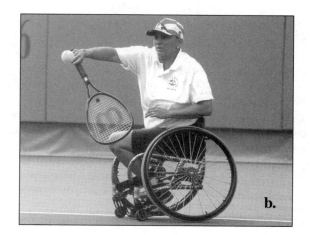

chair player while the rules of tennis for able-bodied tennis shall apply for the able-bodied player. In this instance, the wheelchair player is allowed two bounces while the able-bodied player is allowed only one bounce.

Wheelchair Tennis Eligibility

To be eligible to play sanctioned wheelchair tennis, a player must have a medically diagnosed permanent mobility-related physical disability. This disability must result in a substantial or total loss of function in one or more lower extremities. If, as a result of these functional limitations, the player is unable to play competitive able-bodied tennis and does not have the mobility to cover the court with adequate speed, then the player is eligible to play in sanctioned competitive wheelchair tennis events. A quadriplegic division is used for players who have permanent physical disability in at least three limbs.

AMBULATORY TENNIS

Tennis is played by two disability sport organizations, the United States Deaf Sports Federation and Special Olympics.

Deaf Tennis

Tennis is offered as an official sport throughout the United States Deaf Sports Federation. ITF and USTA rules are used with no modifications.

Special Olympics Tennis

Tennis is one of the newer official sports offered in Special Olympics. The game is expanding rapidly within Special Olympics since it was played as a demonstration sport at the 1983 World Summer Special Olympic Games.

Special Olympics athletes compete in all typical events, such as singles and doubles. Unified Sports® (with non-mentally retarded peers) singles and doubles events and individual skills contests are also offered. The individual skills contest provides athletes of lower ability to compete in events such as target serve, target bounce, return shot, racket bounce and return shot. The Official Special Olympics Sports Rules govern all Special Olympics tennis competitions. Specific rules for these modified contests may be found here.

A copy of the *Tennis Sports Skills Program Guide* is available for purchase through Special Olympics. This guide provides a developmental approach to teaching and coaching tennis. It is an excellent resource for physical education classes.

USTA Special Programs

USA Tennis Special Populations supports adaptive wheelchair and ambulatory tennis programs, providing grant money, equipment and resources for specifically-tailored programs that provide fun, fitness and a positive social experience for participants. Regional clinics and instructional programs are held throughout the country, often in conjunction with agencies devoted to serving special populations within the respective communities.

USA Tennis Special Populations programs recognizes four main categories of differently-abled players:

- Developmentally disabled (learning disabilities, autism, Down's Syndrome, mental retardation).
- Physically disabled (birth defects, multiple sclerosis, traumatic brain injury, muscular dystrophy, etc.).
- Consumers of mental health services.
- At risk/environmentally disabled (substance abusers, mentally and physically abused, homeless, HIV positive individuals, persons within the juvenile justice system, etc.).

EQUIPMENT

The only significant items of equipment, other than positioning straps and a good wheelchair tennis chair, are grip devices. Depending on the type and severity of the disability, a player may be able to swing a racquet but unable to maintain a proper grip throughout a game because of inconsistent hand strength. Several solutions are available.

Two of the simplest are the use of athletic tape or an ACE bandage wrapped around the hand for additional support (Figure 39.2). If more support is needed, commercial devices provide even greater stability. Nesbitt (1986) describes the use of the InHous orthopedic racquet holder, a plastic molded device that fits over the fist of the player and is padded for assistance in pushing (Figure 39.3).

Individuals with arthrogryposis, Guillan-Barre syndrome, and juvenile rheumatoid arthritis, as well as spinal cord-injured players, have successfully used the racquet holder. Any rehabilitation center's orthotics department may consider investigating local resources for a custom-made orthotic grip device. As with all adapted sports, adaptability is the key to successful participation (Figure 39.4).

EQUIPMENT SUPPLIERS

Most serious wheelchair tennis players will want to consider expensive but essential customized chairs. Several manufacturers should be contacted in order to compare information on warranties, guarantees, and cost. Many medical supply companies now routinely carry tennis wheelchairs such as Eagle, Quickie, and Top End. *Sports 'n Spokes* magazine conducts a yearly survey of a variety of sport and tennis wheelchair companies. This review is based on the response of the companies them-

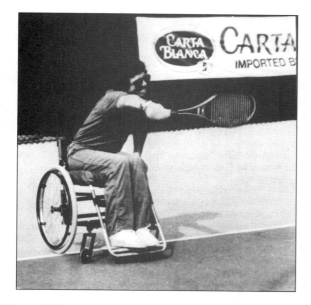

Figure 39.2. One of the several ways to secure one's grip on a tennis racquet is by using an Ace bandage. (Courtesy of *Sports 'n Spokes* 1/93:16; Curt Beamer)

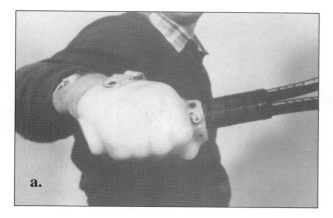

a.

Figure 39.3 a and b. The InHous orthopedic racquet holder has assisted many tennis players with varying disabilities in successfully playing the game. (Courtesy of InHous Orthopedics, Inc.)

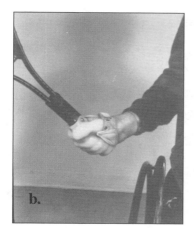

b.

selves, but it should provide an example of some of the manufacturers and types of wheelchair designs available. A list of some of the lightweight wheelchair suppliers can be found below but this list is not meant to be inclusive, only representative.

Allegro Home Health Care Supplies
(888) 462-5534
Website: http://www.goallegro.com
    Allegro is an online discount source for a variety of wheelchairs.

Care
1877 NE Seventh Avenue
Portland, OR 97212
(800) 443-7091
(503) 287-3957 (fax)
Email: ccs@caremedical.com
Website: http://www.caremedical.com/ccs

Eagle Sportchairs
2351 Parkwood Road
Snellville, GA 30039
(800) 932-9380

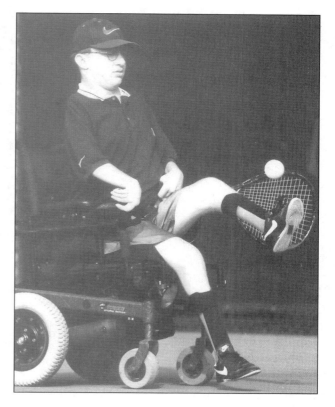

Figure 39.4. Adaptability is often key to successful participation in sports for individuals with disabilities. (Courtesy of *Sports 'n Spokes* 1997 23/1:14)

(770) 972-0763
(770) 985-4885 (fax)
Email: beweing@bellsouth.net
Website: http://www.harb.net/EagleSportchairs

Invacare Corporation (Action, Top End)
One Invacare Way
P.O. Box 4028
Elyria, OH 44036-2125
440-329-6000
Email: info@invacare.com
Website: http://www.invacare.com

New Hall's Wheels
P.O. Box 380784
Cambridge, MA 02238
(617) 628-7955
(617) 628-6546 (fax)
Email: newhalls@tiac.net
website: http://www.newhalls.com/

Spinlife.com
(800) 850-0335
Website: http://www.spinlife.com

Spokes N Motion
2225 S Platte River Drive W
Denver, CO 80223
(303) 922-0605
(303) 922-7943 (fax)
Email: info@spokenmotion.com
Website: http://www.spokesnmotion.com/

Sportaid
78 Bay Creek Rd.
Loganville, GA 30252
(800) 743-7203
(770) 554-594 (fax)
Website: http://www.sportaid.com

Sunrise Medical (Quickie)
7477 East Dry Creek Parkway
Longmont, CO 80503
(800) 333-4000
(800) 300-7502 (fax)
Website: http://www.sunrisemedical.com

TiSport
1426 East Third Avenue
Kennewick, WA 99337
(800) 545-2266
(509) 586-6117

Zebra Sport
16014 North 47th Place
Phoenix, AZ 85032
(602) 672-1901
Email: corbin8or@prodigy.net

ADDITIONAL RESOURCES AND WEBSITES

Tennis and wheelchair tennis players will find many websites related to their sport. Because this sport is accessible for those with and without disabilities, most participants will find the following sites satisfactory for gathering information.

Wheelchair Tennis Department
C/o International Tennis Federation
Bank Lane, Roehampton
London SW15 5XZ, United Kingdom
(011) 44-181-878-6464
(011) 44-181-392-4745 (fax)
Email: ITF@ITFTennis.com
Website: http://www.itftennis.com
Website:
    http://www.usta.com/usatennis/wheelchair/index.html

United States Tennis Association
70 West Red Oak Lane
White Plains, NY 10604-3602
(800) 990-8782
(914) 696-7008 (fax)
Website: http://www.usta.com

Special Olympics Director of Tennis
1325 G Street, NW, Suite 500
Washington, DC 20005
(202) 628-3630
(202) 824-0200 (fax)
Email: SOImail@aol.com
Website: http://www.specialolympics.org

BIBLIOGRAPHY

Nesbitt, J. (1986). *The International Directory of Recreation-Oriented Assistive Device Sources*. Marina Del Rey: Lifeboat Press.

Official Special Olympics Summer Sports Rules (1996-1999). Special Olympics International: Washington, D.C.

Chapter 40

Track & Field

SPORT GOVERNING BODIES:
National: USA Track & Field (USATF)
International: International Amateur Athletic Federation (IAAF)

Official Sport Of: __x__DAAA   __x__USABA   __x__USCPAA
                             __x__DS/USA   __x__USADSF   __x__WS/USA
                             __x__SOI

DISABLED SPORTS ORGANIZATION:
National:
International:

PRIMARY DISABILITY: All

SPORT OVERVIEW

Track & Field (Athletics) competition represent the single largest area of participation for athletes with disabilities, both in terms of number of events and overall number of participants. Athletes compete in either ambulatory or wheelchair categories for both track and field events. Track events range from the 10-meter assisted walk for Special Olympic athletes, 20-meter dashes for Class II athletes with cerebral palsy, to the marathon for wheelchair athletes and athletes who compete in Special Olympics. In between are a variety of events of varying distances including hurdles for Special Olympic athletes and race walking athletes who are dwarfs or Special Olympians. Due to the unique nature of long-distance running, this portion of athletic competition is covered separately in the chapter on Road Racing.

Conventional field events are held in all of the disability sport organization (DSO) competitions including the throwing events of shot-put, discus and javelin (discus and javelin are prohibited in Special Olympics competition) (Figure 40.1). The USA Deaf Sports Federation (USADSF), Disabled Sports USA (DSUSA), United States Association for Blind Athletes (USABA), and Special Olympics, Inc. (SOI) offer competition in the high

jump, while these four plus the United Cerebral Palsy Athletic Association (USCPAA) also offer long jump competition. A variety of uniquely modified field events are offered by some of the disability sport organizations that are described later in this chapter.

In 1960, the Division of Rehabilitation Education Services of the University of Illinois at Urbana-Champaign founded the first collegiate wheelchair track and field and road racing program in the world. Many of their athletes have gone on to win gold medals at national and international competitions. This program remains one of the elite programs of its type in the country. An annual track and field clinic and competition is offered for coaches and athletes.

USA Track and Field (USATF) is the National Governing Body of competitive track and field in the United States. USA Track & Field is responsible for the conduct and administration of track and field, including formulating rules, implementing policies and procedures, conducting national championships, disseminating safety and sports medicine information and selecting athletes to represent the United States in international competition. On the international level the International Amateur Athletic Federation (IAAF) has much the same responsibility, but is the ultimate authority in competitive athletics world-wide. All athletic competition (unless specifically modified by the individual DSO) are conducted under either USA Track & Field or International Amateur Athletic Federation (IAAF) rules.

SPORT ORIGIN

There is no more exciting sport in the Olympic and Paralympic Games than the competition in track and field. It is from this arena that the greatest Olympic athletes typically emerge. Races were a part of the ancient Olympic Games in 776 BC until the end of the games in 394 AD. The sport enjoyed its revival in the early 1800s in England and were an important part of the first modern Olympic Games.

Competition in track and field has been a part of all of the DSO's inaugural games including the 1924 World Games for the Deaf in Paris, and the 1960 Paralympic Games in Rome as well as the inaugural Special Olympic Games in 1968. Competitive track and field events for wheelchair users began in 1948 at the Stoke Mandeville Games in England and have been part of every Paralympic Games program. Wheelchair racing began in 1952 at Stoke Mandeville as a means of competition for the injured veterans of World War II. The 60-meter tarmac between the hospital and the helicopter pad became the standard distance for wheelchair competitions for many years.

Track competition received much publicity at the 1992 Barcelona and 1996 Atlanta Paralympics with the emergence of superstar Tony Volpentest. Volpentest, a double-leg-and-arm amputee set world records in the 100 meter and 200 meter dashes for his class (Figure 40.2 a and b). In Atlanta, he ran the 100 meter dash in a world record 11.36 seconds, approximately 1.5 seconds behind the world record set by Canada's Donovan Bailey at the 1996 Olympic Games.

An indication of the strides made, and growth of expectations in disability sports is reflected in the first Special Olympic Games in 1968. At these games, organizers

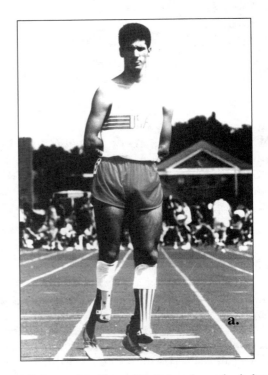

Figure 40.2 a and b. Specially designed prosthesis by Flex Foot have helped Tony Volpentest be the world's fastest amputee at the 1996 Paralympic Games. (Courtesy of Specialized Sports Unlimited)

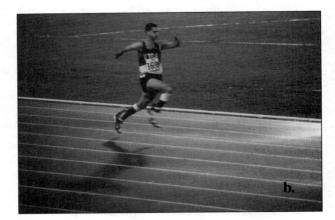

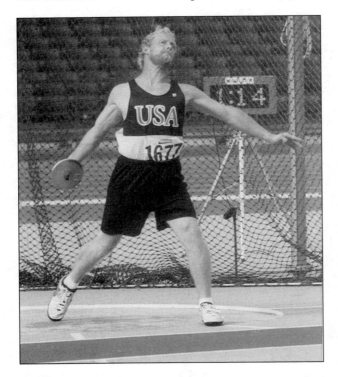

Figure 40.1. The discus throw is for athletes with Cerebral Palsy one of several traditional field events that are part of the Paralympic program. (Courtesy of Specialized Sports Unlimited)

were so worried about the capabilities of athletes, they made the longest event 100 yards. Today, Special Olympians complete the marathon in less then 3 hours!

Another indication of the strides being made in disability came when, in 1984, the International Olympic Committee approved the inclusion of the 1,500 meter wheelchair race for men, and 800 meter wheelchair race for women as demonstration events in Olympic competition. Although the Olympic and Paralympic Games may never be fully merged, this is an indication of the great respect athletes with disabilities have earned.

An excellent but brief description of the origin of athletics can be found on the USOC website <http://www.usoc.org>.

Sport Classification

As has been evident in many of the sports described in this book, each of the disability sport organizations have their own specific classification systems. These classification systems help to ensure that competition is equitable and that individuals who win, do so because of training and talent and not because their disability happens to be less severe then their opponents (Figure 40.3). Each organization also implements specific age categories to foster junior development.

For international competitions the classification system used changes. Since the late 1980's international athletic competition for athletes with disabilities has used a functional classification system. This approach was first

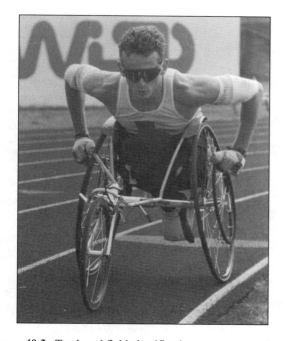

Figure 40.3. Track and field classifications are not completely integrated as is swimming. Athletes with cerebral palsy still have a separate system for track and field. (Courtesy of Specialized Sports Unlimited)

implemented at the 1992 Barcelona Paralympic Summer Games, and combines over 2 dozen different classes of the disability sports organizations (excepting athletes who are blind or who have cerebral palsy) into a system where athletes with spinal cord injuries, amputees, and les autres conditions competed against each other in wheelchair races, as did ambulatory amputee or les autres athletes. Athletes who are blind use their traditional 3 classification system based on visual acuity. Athletes who have cerebral palsy also use their own classification system although events at the Paralympic level are limited to less than one quarter of the official cerebral palsy track & field events.

Athletes who use wheelchairs have various levels of ability and disability. All athletes must go through a medical examination to test the function and strength of their muscles. Athletes are then classified according to abilities. There are 4 classes in track (T1, T2, T3, T4) and 8 classes in field (F1- F3 and F4 - F8). The lower classification numbers represent athletes with quadriplegia. The higher numbers consist of athletes with more muscular function and strength (paraplegics).

Quadriplegic Track (T1, T2)
Paraplegic Track (T3, T4)
Quadriplegic Field (F1-F3)
Paraplegic Field (F4-F8)

The International Paralympic Committee website <http://www.paralympic.org> offers a complete description of the international track & field classification guideline.

TRACK COMPETITION

Track competition is divided into two major categories, wheelchair track and ambulatory track. Specific rule modifications have been made based on the specific disability of the competitors. For instance, where a competitor has a hearing impairment, a flag or any other visual device may be used as well as a pistol. Some additional modifications are described below.

Wheelchair Track

Approximately 50% of athletes with physical disabilities participate in track events while using a wheelchair. A wide variety of wheelchair designs is needed to meet the various functional abilities and physical characteristics of the athletes involved. Better training and advancements in wheelchair design have contributed to improvements in finishing times.

Generally, the same rules used in able-bodied track events apply to wheelchair track. Drafting an opponent, similar to that used in cycling, is permitted in track and road racing. Racers use 3-wheel chairs with push rims attached to the rear wheels. A compensator device is used to set front wheels to the curvature of the track, removing the need for the athlete to steer around bends. This frees the athlete's hands for using the push rims. Most racers wear specially designed racers gloves (or tape) which requires the athlete to push the wheelchair rim as opposed to gripping the rim. During relays, each relay team is assigned to two lanes. Relay wheelchair athletes do not carry a baton, but rather touch their partner within the normal take-over zone.

Most athletes who are serious about their sport purchase racing chairs customized to their specifications. It is important for an athlete who competes using a wheelchair to stay abreast of current technology in the design and use of racing wheelchairs. With typical costs for a racing wheelchair ranging from $1,500-$2,500 per chair, it is important to make an informed and intelligent purchasing decision. Many manufacturers and suppliers of racing wheelchairs exist. *Sports 'n Spokes* magazine offers a yearly guide on the latest in racing designs by many manufacturers.

Wheelchair racing involves much more than the wheelchair itself. Other factors include the right tires, push rims, seating position, racing gloves, bad weather training methods, racing strategies, and equipment maintenance (Figure 40.4). A variety of workshops that focus on the specific of wheelchair racing are held at various locations around the country. One of the best resources for this information is the annual track & field clinic held at the University of Illinois-Champaign.

The category of wheelchair racing also includes those athletes who use power wheelchairs. Power wheelchair racing events are offered in Special Olympics competition for athletes with lower ability levels and in USCPAA competition for Class 1 athletes.

Crutch And Assistive Racing

Although several disability groups include athletes who ambulate with crutches or other assistive devices, only Special Olympics and the United States Cerebral Palsy Athletic Association offer a separate class of track events for crutch and assistive device users. In USCPAA competition, all athletes using crutches, canes, or walkers compete in one class despite the type or number of assistive devices used (Figure 40.5). Special Olympics offers a variety of events for their athletes with lower ability levels including assisted walking events of varying distances.

Running for Athletes Who Use Prostheses

Little modifications are needed for athletes who have amputations. Although athletes may choose to compete with or without their prosthesis during field events, athletes must wear a prosthesis during running events as no hopping is allowed.

Running For Athletes Who Are Blind

Simple adaptations are incorporated into USABA track events depending on the class within which the visually impaired athlete is participating. The international caller system is used for Class B-1 and B-2 athletes for the 100-meter dash. Runners compete individually against the clock as all lanes of the 100-meter straightaway are cleared. Runners follow auditory signals, usually numbers representing the lanes in which they are running. If a runner begins to swerve into another lane, the number being yelled is changed to indicate the runner is off course. It is important for the crowd to remain silent during all events where auditory cues are being used.

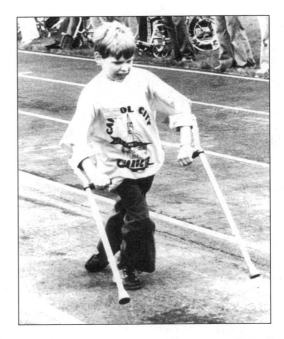

Figure 40.5. The predominant assistive device used by Class 5 CP athletes is the forearm crutch. (Courtesy of Specialized Sports Unlimited)

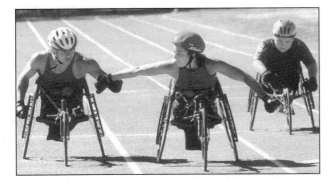

Figure 40.4. Wheelchair track racers must consider a variety of additional equipment including helmets, pushing gloves and push rim size. (Courtesy of Specialized Sports Unlimited)

Modifications are not permitted for B-3 (greater visual acuity) runners who follow IAAF rules in their entirety.

For longer distances the use of sighted guides depends entirely on the athlete's visual classification and the particular event. The method of guidance is the choice of the athlete. He/she may choose to use an elbow lead, or a tether with a sighted guide, or to run free. Sighted guides facilitate the activity by running alongside the visually impaired athlete, both runners holding on to a tether made of flexible non-elastic material not longer than 50 cm in length (Figure 40.6 a and b). Alternatively, stationary guides may be positioned around the track calling to the runner giving directional signals. Sighted guides are not allowed to run ahead of or to pull their blind partner. Each pair is given two lanes in which to run races 200-meters or longer. The tightness of the tether acts as a kinesthetic indicator assisting the blind runner in keeping proper position. In addition, the runner may receive verbal instruction from the guide. For races further than 400 meters two guides are allowed. Only one exchange of guides is permitted for each athlete. The exchange must take place without any hindrance to other athletes, and must take place on the straight, within 50m of the finish line. Other adapted devices have been used as well (Figure 40.7). For specific rules regarding the use of guide runners, refer to USABA track and field rules.

United States Of America Deaf Track And Field

Founded in 1986 as the Deaf Athletics Federation of the United States (DAFUS), until its recent name change in 1998, The United States of America Deaf Track and Field (USADTF), is an affiliate of the United States of America Deaf Sports Federation (USADSF) and USA Track & Field (USATF). The organization was founded to bring together the fragmented and disorganized groups of athletes representing state schools for the Deaf, Gallaudet University, the National Technical Institute for the Deaf, and other schools and colleges having Deaf athletes among their teams.

The group also helps to coordinate numerous activities including the development and refinement of basic skills of deaf track athletes, the training of deaf and hearing coaches by arranging for them to attend clinics sponsored by the United States Olympic Committee (USOC), the selection of national championship meet sites, and the selection of athletes and coaches to represent the United States in quadrennial World Games for the Deaf as well as national and international meets.

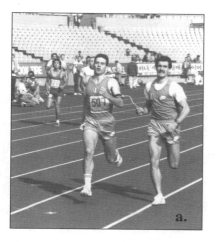

Figure 40.6 a and b. Blind runners in the B-1 class use tethers and sighted running guides to compete in track events ranging from the 200-meter dash to the 10,000-meter run where B-2 runners may use guide runners without tethers. (Courtesy of USABA)

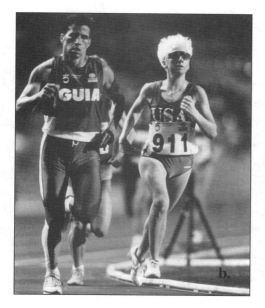

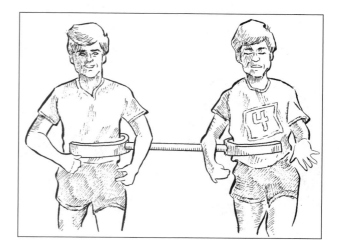

Figure 40.7. An adapted device allows a blind runner to train at moderate speeds with a sighted partner.

Special Olympics

High level Special Olympic athletes have achieved very competitive times in many running events. Special Olympics offers 69 official events in track and field including events for athletes with lower ability levels. Additionally, Unified events are held that pair athletes with and without mental retardation. The sum of the partners scores is used in determining the winner.

The classification system used for Special Olympics events is unique and different to other disability sport organizations. Evenness of each heat is an extremely important component of SOI events (Figure 40.8). Athletes are placed in heats according to age, gender, and performance level. Prior to competition, coaches submit scores or times on their athletes in their specific event(s). Athletes are then placed in heats with other athletes having similar performance scores. Implementation of even heats continues to be a challenge due to inaccurate submission of scores. This policy has the potential of not rewarding athletes who train hard for their events. Theoretically, one athlete with lesser ability who trains very hard to reach their maximum potential may be placed in a heat with an athlete with higher functional ability who did not train as hard. In this case the less trained athlete may come out ahead due to the fact they have a less severe disability.

Special Olympic athletes compete in many traditional field events in addition to developmental contests for athletes of lower skill level (Figure 40.9 a-c).

In part it may have been this policy that has brought about the creation of the International Sports Federation for Persons with an Intellectual Disability (INAS-FID). This organization is the newest international disability

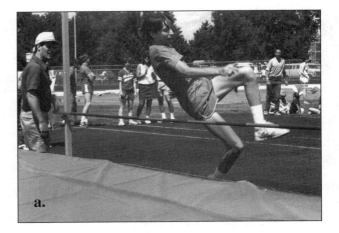

Figure 40.9 a, b, c. (a) Special Olympics athlete clears the bar in high jump at local summer games competition. **(b)** The standing long jump is a developmental field event offered by Special Olympics. **(c)** The shot put is one of the many field events offered by Special Olympics. (Courtesy of Special Olympics Michigan)

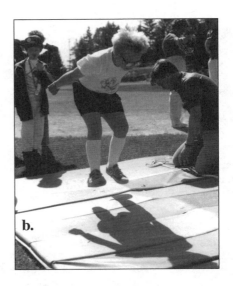

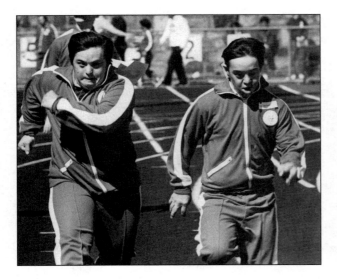

Figure 40.8. Due to a classification system based on ability, Special Olympic track races are usually very competitive. (Courtesy of Special Olympics Michigan)

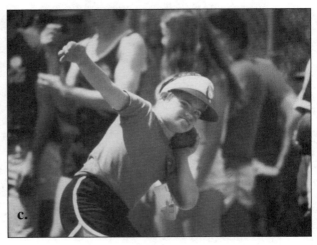

sports federation participating in the Paralympic Games. The difference between INAS-FID and Special Olympics are the strict qualifying standards established by INAS-FID.

FIELD COMPETITION

A variety of field competitions are offered by each of the disability sports organizations although most of the events follow traditional able-body field events and rules usually follow IAAF guidelines. Field competition is divided into wheelchair and standing categories and further divided by disability classifications. Athletes with amputations may compete with or without their prosthesis Figure 40.10 a and b). Athletes who compete from a wheelchair may use specialized throwing chairs (see Specialized Equipment).

Paralympic Field Events

Eight field events (including the pentathlon (see the following) are offered at Paralympic competition for athletes with physical, visual and cognitive disabilities. Events include the long jump, triple jump, high jump, shot-put, discus and javelin. The weight of each of the implements is adjusted based on gender and classification (see official IPC rules).

United States Cerebral Palsy Athletic Association

Of all the disability sport organizations, the United States Cerebral Palsy Athletic Association provides services to athletes with more severe disabilities. It is a formidable challenge to provide meaningful athletic competition, and not just token participation requiring little skill or training. To meet this challenge, USCPAA offers seven non-conventional field events. These events are typically not a part of international competition (except the Club throw). Each was designed specifically for either Class I or Class II athletes, with the club throw being offered to Classes II through VI.

Class I Events

The four Class I events are the distance throw, soft discus, precision event, and high toss.

Distance throw: As the name implies, the distance throw involves throwing an implement, the soft shot, as far as possible.

Soft discus: Similar to the conventional discus event, a soft rubber disc is thrown for distance (Figure 40.11).

Precision event: The athlete participating in this event attempts to accumulate the highest possible score by throwing six soft shots at an eight-ringed target placed on the ground.

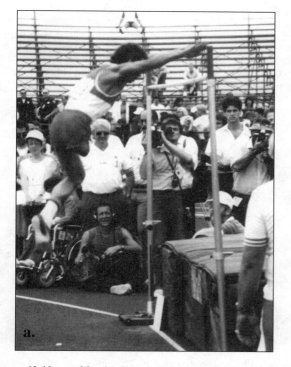
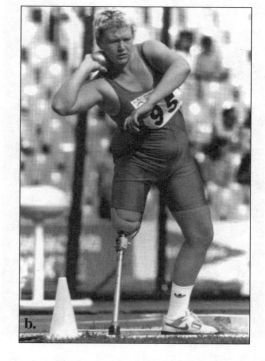

Figure 40.10 a and b. (a) Canadian Arnie Bolt high jumps almost 7 feet on one leg. (b) The shot-put is one of the most popular field events offered by disabled sports organizations. (Courtesy of Specialized Sports Unlimited)

High toss: The high toss involves throwing a soft shot over a progressively higher bar, usually a pole vault bar (Figure 40.12). Competitors are given three attempts at each height with the athlete throwing over the highest height being declared the winner.

Kicking Events

As in Class I events, Class II foot-kicking events which include the thrust kick and the distance kick are unique to cerebral palsy sports. These events were the result of early disability innovators finding suitable field events for athletes with lower extremity dominance.

With the exception of two major rules, the events are very similar. The thrust kick uses a 6-pound medicine ball, while the distance kick uses a 13-inch rubber utility ball. In the thrust kick, the athlete's foot must maintain contact with the ball at all times prior to the thrust, whereas in the distance kick (Figure 40.13) the athlete is given the opportunity to wind up before kicking the ball.

Club Throw

The club throw is used in national and world competition and is typically offered for Classes II through VI Figure 40.14 a and b). It involves the throwing of an Indian Club for distance.

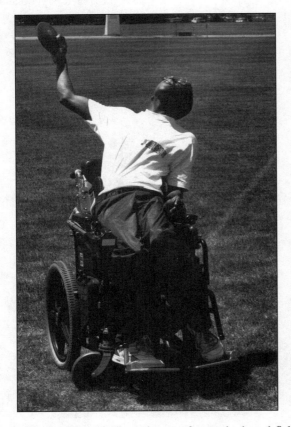

Figure 40.11. The soft discus is one of several adapted field events offered by USCPAA. (Courtesy of Rehabilitation Institute of Chicago's Wirtz Sports Program and Oscar Izquierdo)

Junior Events

To encourage participation by youth, USCPAA includes the softball throw, soft discus, and standing long jump for certain age group competitions as developmental events leading to the standard open division events.

Field Events for Athletes who are Blind

Athletes who are blind compete in the same field events as individuals without visual impairments including shot put, javelin, discus, long jump, and high jump. Various modifications are made for blind athletes who

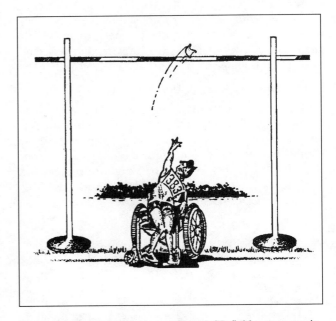

Figure 40.12. The high toss, a Class I CP field event, was introduced in Great Britain in 1984. (Courtesy of Human Kinetics Publishers)

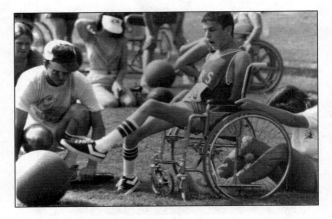

Figure 40.13. The distance kick is one of two field events specifically designed for Class 2 lower cerebral palsy athletes. (Courtesy of Specialized Sports Unlimited)

compete in field events. Visual modification of the existing facility is permitted (i.e. paint, chalk, powder, cones, flags, etc.) for some classifications to increase orientation. Acoustic signals may also be used. High jumpers are allowed to touch the bar before jumping, and some may place tape or cloth on the bar for better sighting purposes. In the long jump, the take off board is extended one meter into the sand. A coach with a bull horn may provide auditory cues to keep the long jumper running straight and to ensure they hit their mark properly (Figure 40.15 a and b and Figure 40.16).

PENTATHLON

Most of the disability sport organizations offer the pentathlon during competitions. The five pentathlon events vary depending on the athlete's disability. Wheelchair athletes compete in a mixture of throwing and track

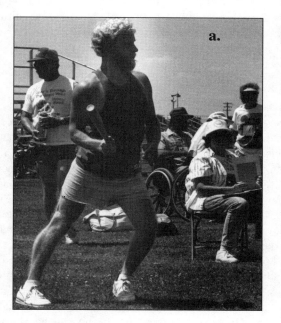
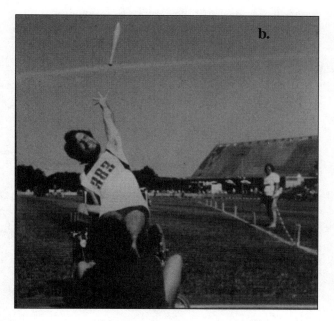

Figure 40.14 a and b. USCPAA offers the club throw as both a wheelchair and ambulatory event. (Courtesy of Specialized Sports Unlimited and USCPAA)

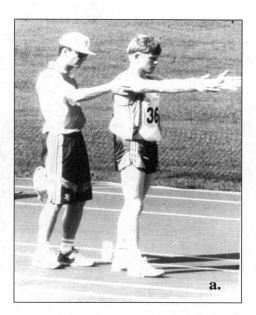
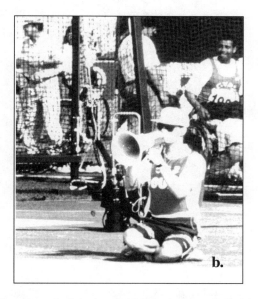

Figure 40.15 a and b. Blind athletes use directional orientation and auditory cues for jumping field events. (Photo by Michael J. Paciorek)

events, while athletes with amputations participate in a mixture of jumping and running events. Special Olympics athletes compete in the 100 meter and 400 meter running races and field events including long jump, shot put and high jump.

SPECIALIZED EQUIPMENT

Many individuals with disabilities need few equipment modifications to begin track and field fitness programs. Individuals who do require some modifications should refer to the Fitness Chapter, and Weight Training

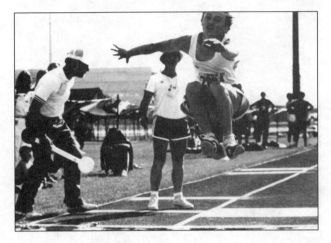

Figure 40.16. A coach provides auditory cues to the long jumper near the take-off board, as an official looks on. (Courtesy of USABA)

Chapter in this book and to the suggestions provided below.

Arm Ergometers

Applicable for wheelchair users, the arm ergometer allows a person with physical disabilities to improve upper body strength, aerobic capacity, and stamina. Various models are available through the manufacturers listed in this section, including table and floor models and models adapted for wheelchair users. The Saratoga Cycle offers a quick-release interchangeable hand grip to suit individuals with varying levels of hand function, while SCI FIT offers several models that use both the upper and lower extremities.

Prosthetic Devices

Until about the late 1980's lower extremity prostheses were built for walking as the primary activity. The increased popularity of sports for individuals with amputations, particularly lower extremity amputations, has inspired the development of technologically advanced prosthetic devices that enable individuals with amputations not only to run, but to compete in track events (Figure 40.17 a and b). Participation by single and bilateral above-the-knee amputees, once regarded as medically impossible, now occurs around the world. The orthotics and prosthetic profession deserves credit for meeting the challenges and in the promotion of athletic competition for athletes with amputations. Running prostheses such as the VA Seattle Foot and Flex-foot are the most popular running choices. By recreating the normal heel-to-toe gate, runners with amputations are able to run with greater mechanical efficiency. Improvements in socket technology have decreased such problems as residual limb movement, excess perspiration and irritation, and rotation of the entire prosthesis while running. Advancements in mechanical knee joints allow individuals with

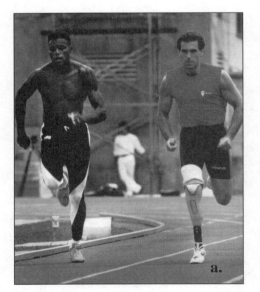

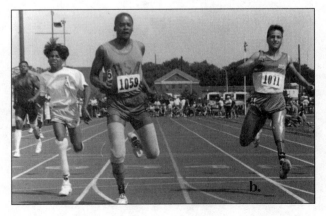

Figure 40.17 a and b. The Flex Foot stores and releases energy, recreating normal heel-to-toe action for lower extremity amputees who participate in rigorous high-energy activities. **(a)** Dennis Ohler, former world record holder, training with Carl Lewis. **(b)** Double below-the-knee and single above-the-knee amputees finishing the 100 meter dash. (Courtesy of Flex Foot, Inc., Oscar Izquierdo and Specialized Sports Unlimited)

above-the-knee amputations to run more efficiently. In all cases, individuals should consult their doctors and prosthetists before beginning a running program.

Throwing Chair

Innovations within field events have traditionally been made in technique. In the high jump it was the introduction of the Fosbery Flop, and in the shot-put it was the use of a discuss spin rather than the customary glide motion. Within wheelchair field events, innovations in throwing techniques have resulted from changes in equipment, specifically the wheelchair. Flexible interpretations of field event rules have allowed the standard wheelchair to be replaced with what is known as a "throwing chair", originally an extremely heavy metal chair that will not tip over (a common problem in typical wheelchairs when throwing) (Figure 40.18 a and b). New throwing chairs are made of PVC and are as varied in type and style as racing chairs (Figure 40.19). If tie downs or heavy chairs are not available, coaches or volunteers must physically support the wheelchair (Figure 40.20). The basic design principle is to provide the athlete with a stable chair-like platform from which to throw while maintaining a sitting position. Handles, foot-rests, and various adaptations are made to each athletes' individual needs. Athletes may use a holding device (grasped with their free hand) to help maintain their balance while throwing. Although most throwing chairs are also tied down, their increased height and design allows for much

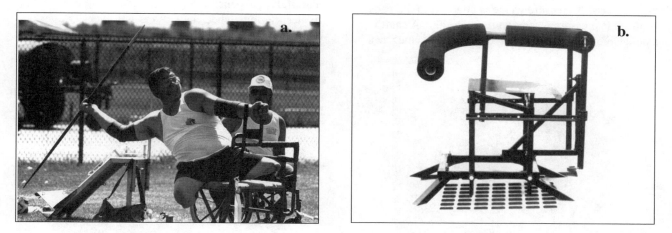

Figure 40.18 a and b. The development of heavy throwing chairs has dramatically changed the nature of wheelchair field events. (Photo by Michael J. Paciorek)

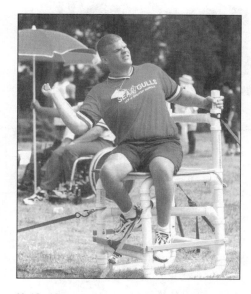

Figure 40.19. Newer versions of throwing chairs are made of PVC pipe making them much lighter and less expensive. (Courtesy of USCPAA's National Sports Festival and Ron Pacchiana)

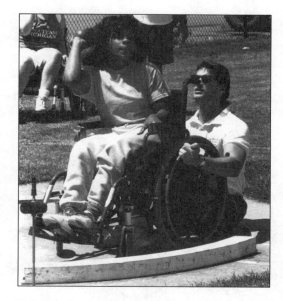

Figure 40.20. When tie-downs are not available, wheelchair stability is often maintained manually. (Courtesy of Rehabilitation Institute of Chicago's Wirtz Sports Program)

more efficient throwing motions, thus better performances. Previous to the development of throwing chair, sport wheelchairs were secured by a variety of tie-down mechanisms, each of which was time-consuming to attach and did not provide sufficient stability (Figure 40.21 a and b).

A technologically advanced tie-down was first used by many athletes at the 1992 Paralympic Games in Barcelona (Figure 40.21 c and d). It enabled them to compete from the comfort of their own wheelchairs, while maintaining the stability found in specialized throwing chairs. The system was developed by Armando Alvarez, Olympic Stadium Competition Director, and industrial engineer Manuel Sanchez Aguilera. It requires four strong suction pads that are used in the transportation of glass. A pressure gauge is attached to the pads to control the pressure when securing the chair. A shaft with a notched bar has been added to these pads, along with a

hook that is rubber-lined to protect the chairs. The process of anchoring chairs that once took 10 to 15 minutes can now be accomplished in under 10 seconds with trained volunteers. The system must be attached to a strong, dry, clean, non-porous (usually a metal base plate) surface to be effective.

Wheelchairs

Nothing has done more during the last 30-35 years to change perceptions of people with disabilities then the development of the racing wheelchair. The site of a racing wheelchair moving at incredible speed as effectively demonstrated the capabilities of individuals with physical disabilities. The racing wheelchair continues to evolve with the use of lightweight but strong metals and other materials, suspension systems, and various types of frames. Serious wheelchair racers will want to consider expensive but essential customized chairs. Figure 40.22

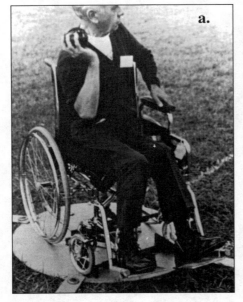

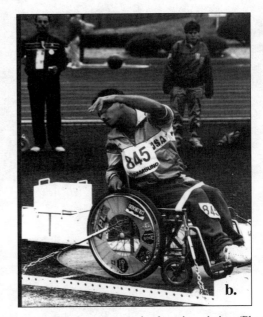

Figure 40.21 a-d. The technology used in wheelchair tie-downs has kept pace with advancements in throwing chairs. (Photo by Michael J. Paciorek)

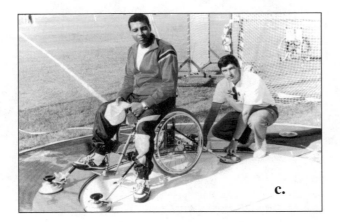

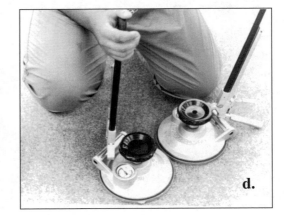

a-f are illustrative of the many advancements in racing wheelchair designs over the past 20 years.

A unique wheelchair race involves Class II athletes with cerebral palsy. These athletes have greater functional ability in their lower limbs. Their method of wheelchair propulsion is with their legs. Class II athletes push backwards. Specially designed racing wheelchairs have been designed for these athletes. Figure 40.23a provides an example of the Class II chair in the late 1980's while Figure 40.23 b and c illustrate state of the art racing wheelchairs for Class II athletes.

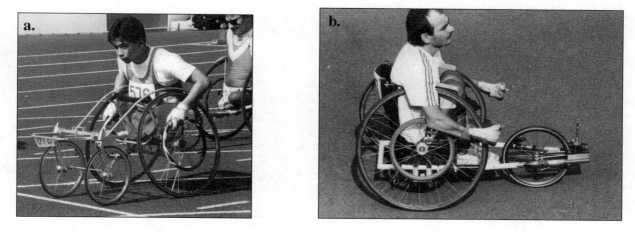

Figure 40.22 a-f. Racing wheelchairs have changed dramatically in the past decade. (Courtesy of Specialized Sports Unlimited and IDEA)

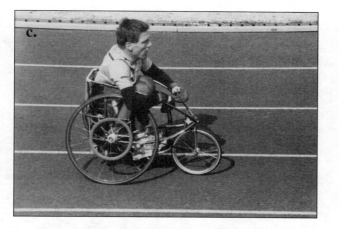

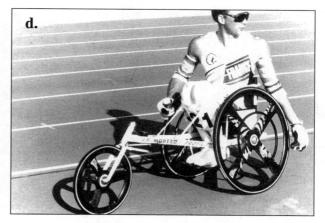

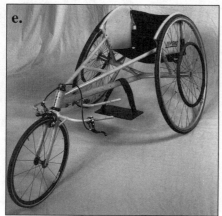

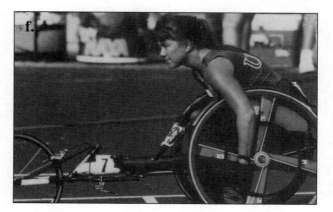

Wheelchair Rollers

Similar to a treadmill for people who are ambulatory, the wheelchair roller is a popular way to continue training indoors during inclement weather (Figure 40.24). It is

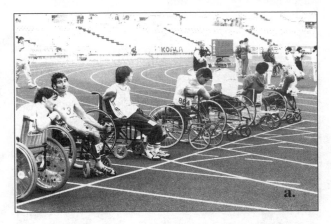

Figure 40.23 a-c. **(a)** Class 2 cerebral palsy athletes use their lower extremities to propel their wheelchairs. **(b)** and **(c)**. The technology used in Class 2 racing wheelchairs has kept pace with that of conventional track chairs. (Courtesy of Specialized Sports Unlimited, USCPAA's National Sports Festival and Ron Pacchiana)

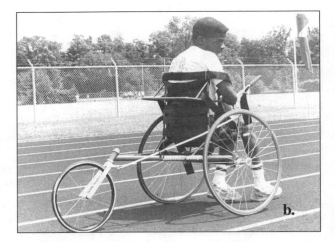

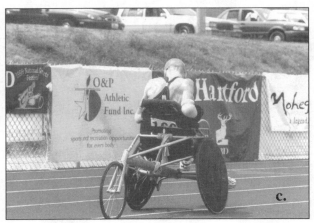

also a valuable tool for a coach who wishes to video tape strokes for biomechanical analysis. The wheelchair is placed securely on top of one or two steel rollers while the individual practices free wheeling and endurance training. For suppliers of ergometers and rollers, see the Fitness Chapter in this book.

EQUIPMENT SUPPLIERS

Prosthetic Suppliers

Most larger communities will have a neighbor hood prosthetist. These local prosthetists will have access to the latest in prosthetic designs for active wear in sport. The following companies are listed as examples of some larger manufacturers.

College Park Industries, Inc.
17505 Helro Drive
Fraser, MI 48026
(800) 728-7950
(800) 294-0067 (fax)
Email: info@college-park.com
Website: http://www.college-park.com/

Flex-Foot, Inc.
27412-A Laguna Hills
Aliso Viejo, CA, 92656
 (800) 233-6263
(949) 362-3883
(949) 362-3888 (fax)
Email: information@flexfoot.com
Website: http://www.flexfoot.com/

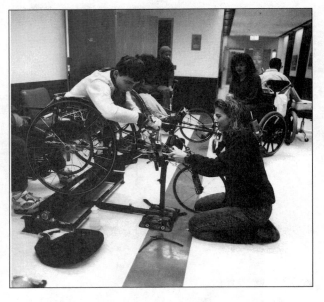

Figure 40.24. Wheelchair rollers allow racers to train year-round. (Courtesy of Rehabilitation Institute of Chicago's Wirtz Sports Program)

Hanger Orthopedic Group
2 Bethesda Metro Center, Suite 1200
Bethesda, MD 20814
(877) 442-6437
(301) 986-0701
(301) 986-0702 (fax)
Website: http://www.hanger.com/

RGP Prosthetic Research Center
6147 University Avenue
San Diego, CA 92115
(800) 545-1932
Website: http://www.rgp.com/

Seattle Orthopedic Group, Inc. (Seattle Foot)
26296 Twelve Trees Lane NW
Building One
Poulsbo, WA. 98370
(800 248-6463
Email: CustSvc@soginc.com
Website: http://www.m-ind.com/

Racing Wheelchairs

Most serious wheelchair racers will want to consider expensive but essential customized chairs. Several manufacturers should be contacted in order to compare information on warranties, guarantees, and cost. Many medical supply companies now routinely carry sport wheelchairs such as Eagle, Quickie, and Top End. *Sports 'n Spokes* magazine conducts a yearly survey of a variety of sport and racing wheelchair companies. This review is based on the response of the companies themselves, but it should provide an example of some of the manufacturers and types of wheelchair designs available. A list of some of the lightweight wheelchair suppliers can be found below but this list is not meant to be inclusive, only representative.

Allegro Home Health Care Supplies
(888) 462-5534
Website: http://www.goallegro.com
Allegro is an online discount source for a variety of wheelchairs.

Care
1877 NE Seventh Avenue
Portland, OR 97212
(800) 443-7091
(503) 287-3957 (fax)
Email: ccs@caremedical.com
Website: http://www.caremedical.com/ccs

Eagle Sportchairs
2351 Parkwood Road
Snellville, GA 30039

(800) 932-9380
(770) 972-0763
(770) 985-4885 (fax)
Email: beweing@bellsouth.net
Website: http://www.harb.net/EagleSportchairs

Invacare Corporation (Action, Top End)
One Invacare Way
P.O. Box 4028
Elyria, OH 44036-2125
440-329-6000
Email: info@invacare.com
Website: http://www.invacare.com

New Hall's Wheels
P.O. Box 380784
Cambridge, MA 02238
(617) 628-7955
(617) 628-6546 (fax)
Email: newhalls@tiac.net
Website: http://www.newhalls.com/

Spinlife.com
(800) 850-0335
Website: http://www.spinlife.com

Spokes N Motion
2225 S Platte River Drive W
Denver, CO 80223
(303) 922-0605
(303) 922-7943 (fax)
Email: info@spokenmotion.com
Website: http://www.spokesnmotion.com/

Sportaid
78 Bay Creek Rd.
Loganville, GA 30252
(800) 743-7203
(770) 554-594 (fax)
Website: http://www.sportaid.com

Sunrise Medical (Quickie)
7477 East Dry Creek Parkway
Longmont, CO 80503
(800) 333-4000
(800) 300-7502 (fax)
Website: http://www.sunrisemedical.com

TiSport
1426 East Third Avenue
Kennewick, WA 99337
(800) 545-2266
(509) 586-6117

Zebra Sport
16014 North 47th Place
Phoenix, AZ 85032
(602) 672-1901
Email: corbin8or@prodigy.net

ADDITIONAL RESOURCES AND WEBSITES

Individuals interested in track and field will find many websites related to their sport. Because people with disabilities are easily included in most running clubs few organizations have been developed specifically for people with disabilities. Because this sport is accessible for those with and without disabilities, most participants will find the following sites satisfactory for gathering information.

Achilles Track Club International (see Road Racing Chapter)
42 West 38th Street
New York, NY 10018
(212) 354-3978
(212) 354-3978
Email: AchillesClub@aol.com
Website: http://www.achillestrackclub.org/

International Amateur Athletic Federation
17 rue Princesse Florestine
BP 359
MC 98007 Monaco Cedex
(377) 93 10 88 88
(377) 93 15 95 15 (fax)
Email: headquarters@iaaf.org
Website: http://www.iaaf.org/

The Running Page
Website: http://www.runningpage.com/
The Running Page is a complete source for information about running on the Web. The Running Page contains information about upcoming races, running clubs, places to run, running related products, magazines, and other information.

United States of America Deaf Track and Field
Website: http://members.tripod.com/~usadtf/

USA Track & Field
P.O. Box 120 (One RCA Dome, Suite 140)
Indianapolis, IN 46206-0120 (46225)
Email: USATFprogs@aol.com
Website: http://www.usatf.org

Wheelchair Racing Resource Page
Email: birzer@execpc.com
Website: http://www.execpc.com/~birzer/
This website provide updated links related to wheelchair road racing including associations, equipment, and race announcements.

Wheelchair Athletics of the USA
Barry Ewing
2351 Parkwood Road
Snellville, GA 30278
(770) 972-0763
(770) 985-4885 (fax)
Email: bewing@beilesouth.net

Chapter 41

Volleyball

SPORT GOVERNING BODIES:
National: USA Volleyball (USAV)
International: Federation Internationale de Volleyball (FIVB)

Official Sport Of: __x__ **DAAA**   _____ **USABA**   _____ **USCPAA**
                            __x__ **DS/USA**   __x__ **USADSF**   _____ **WS/USA**
                            __x__ **SOI**

DISABLED SPORTS ORGANIZATION:
National:
International: World Organization of Volleyball for the Disabled (WOVD)

PRIMARY DISABILITY: Physical and Mental Disabilities

SPORT ORIGIN

Although a sport resembling volleyball may have been played as early as the 16th century, modern volleyball was not introduced until the late 19th century and volleyball for individuals with disabilities was not introduced until the 1950's.

A Paralympic sport since the 1976 games in Toronto, standing volleyball for individuals with disabilities was played many years earlier by amputees. A classification system based on location of amputation was used to equalize competition. By 1984 standing volleyball included individuals from other disability groups.

Originating from a game developed earlier in Germany called *sitzball*, sitting volleyball was developed by the Dutch Sports Committee in 1956 becoming extremely popular world-wide. Sitting volleyball has been played internationally since 1967 and was accepted as an ISOD official sport in 1978, with Paralympic competition beginning in 1980.

USA Volleyball is the national governing body for the sport of volleyball in the United States and is recognized by the Federation International de Volleyball (FIVB) and the United States Olympic Committee (USOC).

SPORT OVERVIEW

Volleyball can be modified in various ways from changing the size of the court and the height of the net, to using various types and sizes of balls. However, most of the disability sport organizations play on regulation sized courts with standard equipment and with few, if any, rule modifications. Individuals with disabilities may play volleyball competitively or for recreational purposes.

World Organization Volleyball for the Disabled

The World Organization Volleyball for Disabled (WOVD) was established in 1992 replacing the ISOD Volleyball Section originally established in 1981. WOVD is the international organization of volleyball for people with disabilities and is affiliated with the International Sports Organization for Disabled (ISOD). WOVD works with the FIVB and other national associations in promoting competition, education, referee training and the development of volleyball for individuals with disabilities throughout the world. Today, more than 38 countries are members of the World Organization Volleyball for the Disabled (WOVB) made of up both sitting and standing volleyball teams.

United States Disabled Volleyball Team (USDVT)

The United States Disabled Volleyball Team (USDVT) was created in 1983 in preparation for the 1984 Paralympics. The USDVT is a national team made up of disabled athletes from all across the United States. Their disabilities range from above and below the knee amputees to above the elbow amputees and congenital limb disabilities. They compete through out the United States against able-body club teams and internationally against disabled national teams from other countries. Disabled Sports USA partners with the USDVT to promote the sport throughout the United States for individuals with disabilities. Two competitive versions of volleyball are available for persons with physical disabilities, standing volleyball and sitting volleyball.

Standing Volleyball

Standing volleyball is played strictly according to FIVB standard international rules by amputees, deaf, mentally impaired, spinal cord-injured and cerebral palsy athletes on an integrated basis. Athletes with amputations may play with or without their prostheses (Figure 41.1 a and b). Advances in both upper and lower extremity prosthesis design have made it easier for single below-the-elbow, single above-the-knee, and below-the-knee amputees to play with their prostheses. Depending on the sense of balance, some above-the-knee amputees will choose to play without a prosthesis, hopping on a single leg.

Sitting Volley

Sitting volleyball is played with six players per team on a smaller court with a lowered net (Figure 41.2). This version of the game enables double leg amputees and individuals with spinal cord-injuries, polio, and various other lower extremity disabilities to play volleyball. The seated game makes the game considerably faster-paced than the standing version. Sitting volleyball is an excellent activity for physical education classes and to foster inclusion of individuals with and without disabilities. Some differences from the standing game include the following:

- The size of the sitting court is reduced to 10m x 6m, compared to the standing volleyball size of 18m x 9m
- The height of the net is lowered to 1.15 m for men and 1.05 m for women
- The player cannot lift up when carrying out an attack-hit, and some part of the body from the buttocks to the shoulders must remain in contact with the floor at all times
- The use of prosthetic or orthopedic devices is not allowed
- Front row players may not block an opponent's service

Deaf Volleyball

Two organizations promote volleyball for individuals who are hearing impaired.

United States Deaf Volleyball Association (USDVA)

The United States Deaf Volleyball Association (USDVA), a governing body of the USA Deaf Sports Federation, is responsible for player development and tournament play. The USADSF and the International Silent Sports Committee (CISS) sanction playing using current USAV or FIVB rules. A red flag is used as a signaling device instead of a whistle.

American Deaf Volleyball Association (ADVA)

The American Deaf Volleyball Association is a volunteer organization which serves a dedicated membership consisting of recreational and competitive volleyball players who are hearing impaired.

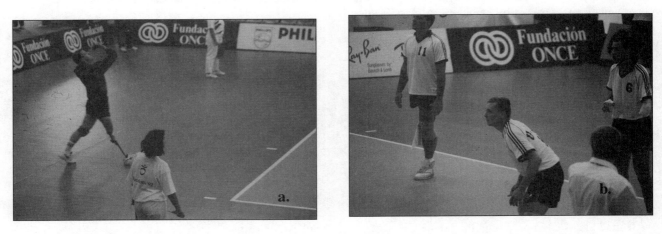

Figure 41.1a and b. Standing volleyball is played with or without prosthesis. (Courtesy of Specialized Sports Unlimited)

Special Olympics

Special Olympics volleyball is offered in every US program and in over 30 countries around the world (Figure 41.3). As in all Special Olympics sports, athletes are grouped in competition divisions according to the athletes' ability level, age and gender.

Volleyball is one of the sports that encourages the development of Special Olympics Officials Program for Athletes®. This program involves interested Special Olympic athletes who want to become certified volleyball officials. These athletes take the same course and meet the same requirements set forth by the United States Volleyball Association for all volleyball officials and are then certified to officiate volleyball competitions.

In addition to the standard competition and Unified Sports® team competition offered, a modified team competition is offered as well. The modified competition is for athletes of lower ability levels and allows for a smaller court with a lower net, and a lighter weight ball. The three-point or five-point serving rule requires an automatic side-out after three or five points have been scored by an individual server. Other events are provided for athletes of lower ability to foster meaningful competition including the individual skills contest, volleyball juggle, volleyball pass, volleyball toss and hit, team skills volleyball. Rules for these events can be found in the official Special Olympics rules book.

The Official Special Olympics Sports Rules govern all Special Olympics volleyball. As an international sports program, Special Olympics has created these rules based upon Federation International de Volleyball (FIVB) and the National Governing Body (NGB) rules for volleyball. FIVB or NGB rules are employed except when they are in conflict with the Official Special Olympics Sports rules. In such cases, the Official Sports Rules apply.

Dwarf Volleyball

The Dwarf Athletic Association of America (DAAA) was the third disability sport organization to offer volleyball as a competitive activity. Competition is conducted according to USVA rules with the lone adaptation being a lower net height.

ADDITIONAL RESOURCES AND WEBSITES

American Deaf Volleyball Association
7582 South Rosemary Circle
Englewood, CO 80112
Attn: Karen Boyd

Disabled Sports USA Volleyball
921 N. Village Lake Dr
Deland, FL32724
904-736-9622 (fax)
Email: seil@totcon.com

Federation Internationale de Volleyball (FIVB)
Avenue de la Gare 12
1000 Lausanne 1
Switzerland

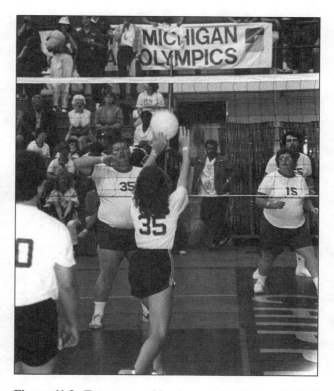

Figure 41.3. Team competition is one of several volleyball events offered by Special Olympics. (Courtesy of Special Olympics Michigan)

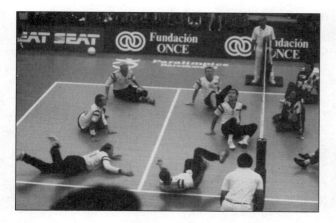

Figure 41.2. Sitting volleyball rules require players to remain seated when making contact with the ball. (Courtesy of Oscar Izquiredo)

(41-21) 345-3535
(41-21) 345-3545
Email: info@mail.fivb.c
Website: www.fivb.ch

United States of America Deaf Volleyball Association
Farley Warshaw (temporary)
(301) 662-9340
Email: farwar@aol.com

USA Volleyball (USAV)
3595 E. Fountain Blvd., Ste. I-2
Colorado Springs, CO 80910-1740
(719) 637-8300
(719) 597-6307 (fax)
(888) 786-5539—Information Line
Email: postmaster@usav.org
Website: www.usavolleyball.org

Volleyball Worldwide
P.O. Box 1872
Cupertino, CA 95015-1872

(408) 358-8622
Email: info@volleyball.org
Website: www.volleyball.org
   An extensive website related to all aspects of volleyball through the world.

World Organization of Volleyball for the Disabled (WOVD)
Klein Heiligland 90
NL-2011 EJ Haarlem
The Netherlands
Email: hqwovd@wovd.com
Website: http://wovd.com

BIBLIOGRAPHY

Official Special Olympics Summer Sports Rules (1996-1999). Special Olympics International: Washington, D.C.

Chapter 42

Water Skiing

SPORT GOVERNING BODIES:
National: USA Water Ski (USAWS)
International: International Water Ski Federation (IWSF)

DISABLED SPORTS ORGANIZATION:
National: Water Skiers with Disabilities Association (USAWS)
International: IWSF World Disabled Council

PRIMARY DISABILITY: All

SPORT OVERVIEW

At first glance, the sport of water skiing may not seem appropriate or possible for many people with disabilities. This is not the case. Advances in equipment technology, instructional techniques and support from national associations have boosted both competitive and recreational water skiing by individuals with physical and mental impairments.

The increased popularity of water skiing has led to the establishment of the annual U.S. National Disabled Water Ski Championship, a sanctioned event of USA Water Ski. Spinal cord-injured, amputee, and blind competitors have participated in consecutive national championships since 1988 (Figure 42.1). The United States was first represented at the World Disabled Ski Championships in 1993, sending 16 competitors from eight states.

A number of private water ski schools exist, providing water ski instruction for individuals with and without disabilities (see Additional Resources). A few of the schools are affiliated with USA Water Ski. The Texas Adaptive Aquatics was founded in 1989 and provides extensive instruction for individuals with mental or physical disabilities. It is one of the premier water ski schools in the country for people with disabilities. Clinics are held nationwide and all disabilities of any age are welcome to come and learn to ski.

A general history of the sport, considerations for increased safety precautions, descriptions of adapted equipment, and an outline for instructional progression are included in this chapter.

SPORT ORIGIN

The invention of water skiing in the United States is credited in 1922 to Ralph Samuelson of Minnesota when he built the first pair of skis and was towed on them behind an outboard-powered boat. The sport became competitive in 1939 with the organization of the American Water Ski Association (now USA Water Ski). Although no formal record exists of when the first person with a disability water skied, it can be assumed this was the case from early on in the history of the sport, although sit skiing was not introduced into the United States until the early 1980's. USA Water Ski is the National Governing Body in the United States and has officially acknowledged adaptive water skiing through the establishment of the Water Skiers with Disabilities Association. USA Water Ski is the proprietor of the U.S. Disabled Water Ski Team and selects the team to represent the United States at the World Championships for the Disabled in addition to sanctioning disabled water ski events. Various ski schools affiliated with USA Water Ski offer instruction for people with disabilities (see Additional Resources).

Internationally the World Disabled Council is affiliated with the International Water Ski Federation. Although people with disabilities have enjoyed the sport for many years, from an organizational standpoint, efforts began in 1986 in Norway to develop a structure to the sport for athletes with disabilities. The initial efforts resulted in the first World Water Ski Tournament being held in England in 1987. By 1992 disabled water skiing had progressed to the point where the International Water Ski Federation gave full council status to the Disabled Council, now having equal status with classic, barefoot, and racing. The tournament evolved until 1993 when the first World Championships were held in France. World championships are now held every other year. Although neither able-bodied nor disabled water-skiing are official Olympic or Paralympic Sports, efforts are being made to change this.

Competitive Water Skiing

Sanctioned water ski competitions generally consist of three events: slalom, trick skiing, and jumping.

Slalom: Sit skiers use an inner course which is a narrow slalom course, vision impaired skiers wake cross, the crosses are counted for 15 seconds, while all other skiers use the standard slalom course of 6 buoys used in traditional competition.

Trick Skiing: In tricks, the contestant performs two, 20-second routines of tricks that each has an assigned point value. The rules are the same as in traditional competition.

Jumping: This event is the same as in able-bodied competitions but skiers with disabilities can choose to have the jump lowered slightly. Here the object is to jump as far as possible without falling.

The sight of a sit-skier jumping off a ramp at 30-35 mph and landing safely is breathtaking. With the exception of the type of skis used, modifications to rules are minimal. Amputee skiers may choose to ski standing up, with or without prosthesis, or to use sit skis.

In some competitions, especially in the United Kingdom, other events may be added such as Wake Crossing and Audio Slalom for the Blind.

DISABLED WATERSKIING CATEGORIES

A variety of techniques and categories for water skiing for people with disabilities have been developed but are still evolving. To date, the following are categories most frequently used.

Sit Skiers: Includes Paraplegics, Quadriplegics, Double Leg Amputees and others who are unable to ski standing. These skis come in a variety of sizes and widths with the wider ski providing greater stability. Narrow skis are used when running the slalom course.

Single Leg Amputees skiing in a standing position, some skiers ski on their one leg, others ski with both legs either on one ski or two while using their prosthesis (Figure 42.2). Those who ski with their prosthesis use a waterproof leg or "ski leg".

Skiers with an arm disability may use one of the many types of harnesses or slings that create a bilateral pull.

Visually Impaired Skiers can use a system of whistle signals to be advised of clear skiing or obstacles. New technology is being developed for competitive blind water skiing (see the following).

Within these four categories, there is further classification to ensure that skiers compete against people with similar abilities. Australia is currently developing a new category that will include people with hemiplegia and arm and leg amputees.

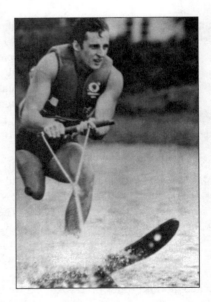

Figure 42.2. Amputees may choose to ski with or without waterproof prostheses. (Courtesy of The British Disabled Water Ski Association)

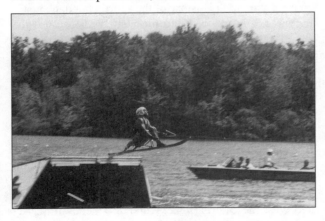

Figure 42.1. The U.S. National Disabled Water Ski Championships include a jumping event. (Photo by Michael J. Paciorek)

Beginners

The Mission Bay Aquatic Center, (1988) undoubtedly one of the leading programs providing aquatic activities for individuals with physical disabilities, offers some suggestions for the beginning water skier (Figure 42.3). Suggestions 1-3 are appropriate for all beginning skiers, while additional suggestions for beginners with specific disabilities are listed separately. Participants should be aware that many ski-areas/lakes are not easily accessed.

1. If an individual questions if water skiing is medically advisable, a physician should be consulted prior to beginning a program.
2. All participants should consider the use of a wet suit to protect the body from extreme heat loss and possible bruises and cuts.
3. Learning progressions should include a complete introduction and fitting to ski equipment while on land.

Beginning Spinal Cord-Injured or Sit Skiers

In addition to the above rules, deep-water practice mounting the ski from the side or rear is encouraged. The skier must find the balance point of the ski, which is very similar to the balance of a chair. A beginning ski (one that is notched at the tip) with a rope attached, will allow the skier greater stability. When using the attached towline, a quick release (trick release) at the boat is mandatory for safety. An assistant (stabilizer person) can ride the tail of the ski until the skier is up and appears to have established balance on the ski. A second boat, or personal watercraft can be used as the pick-up vehicle. Boats with stern mounted platforms make transfers easier. Removable cushions and pads can also be used and are a good idea for any boat. A slower start/pick-up is used when

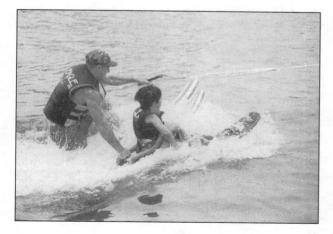

Figure 42.3. It is suggested that an assistant help beginner skiers whenever possible. (Courtesy of *Sports 'n Spokes* 1997 23/7: 59)

driving the boat for a sit-skier. A wider ski will plane more easily out of the water. Ski booms are not to be used if the towline is attached to the ski, but can be used effectively with a short V-line held by the skier.

Beginning Visually Impaired Skiers

The beginning skier with a visual impairment should practice body position on land, emphasizing flexed knees with arms extended. Skiers should touch and examine the rope and ski thoroughly. A communication system between the spotter/driver/skier is essential for safety and success. A loud whistle can be used and is most effective. The following communication system using a whistle has proven successful.

1 short blast: stay behind the boat, i.e., turning, other boat, etc.
2 short blasts: free skiing-skier can cross both sides of the wake safely.
1 long blast: Danger! Let go of the rope. A different whistle pitch can also be used in this situation.

A variety of systems can be used, but the system must be thoroughly known by all involved.

The Mission Bay Aquatic Center offers various other suggestions regarding general safety precautions and individual responsibilities for the skier, boat driver, and accompanying observer in their booklet, *"Water-skiing for the Physically Disabled"*.

Upper Extremity Amputees

Radocy (1987) suggests the following safety suggestions for skiers with upper extremity amputations:

1. Never lock onto a ski rope handle with a terminal device.
2. Never use a terminal device that requires a cable or harness system.
3. Use a ski rope equipped with a single handle.
4. Use a self-suspending, condylar socket that can be twisted free under stress.
5. Use a neoprene arm cover, which will assist in keeping the arm afloat if the arm comes off.
6. As with all skiers, always wear an approved flotation device.

ADAPTED EQUIPMENT

Regardless of the person's disability, there is a variety of water skiing equipment, some standard, some adapted (Figure 42.4), that will assist in the teaching and ongoing enjoyment of water-skiing. Listed below is some of the most popular adapted equipment.

Delgar Sling

A person with a missing or nonfunctional upper extremity will find it easier to ski once he or she has learned to compensate for the uneven pull. For those who have a difficult time adjusting to the uneven pull, the British have developed the Delgar sling, a harness into which the ski handle can fit, creating an even pull bilaterally (Figure 42.5) . If the skier falls, the handle is easily dislodged to prevent injury. Other types of harness systems are available from Achievable Concepts (see Equipment Suppliers).

Dual Ski Rope Handle

For those with visual impairments, the use of a dual ski rope handle with a sighted partner is the best alternative (Figure 42.6).

Ski Trainer

Most water ski shops carry a device called the ski-trainer that incorporates wide tails, flat bottoms, and a training harness to make learning easier (Figure 42.7).

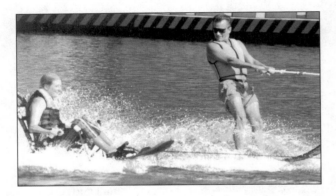

Figure 42.4. Water ski sleds can be custom-made to provide additional support to participants with specific needs. (Courtesy of Roger Randall, Texas Adaptive Aquatics)

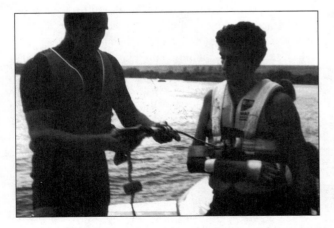

Figure 42.5. The Delgar Sling provides an even pull bilaterally for hemiplegic or upper extremity amputees. (Photo by Michael J. Paciorek)

Ski-Boom

Many ambulatory skiers begin water skiing with the use of a "ski-boom" or "trick bar", consisting of 15-foot bar attached directly to the boat (Figure 42.8). The use of the ski-boom permits the skier to use his or her hands to maintain balance. It also allows side-by-side teaching by enabling an instructor to remain close to the beginning skier (Kegel, 1985).

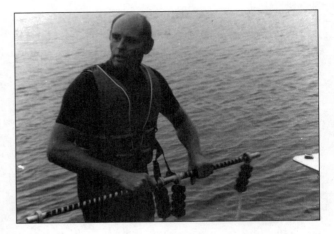

Figure 42.6. A dual ski rope handle used by blind skiers. (Photo by Michael J. Paciorek)

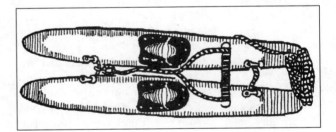

Figure 42.7. Wide tails, flat bottoms, and the use of a training harness are all incorporated in the ski-trainer.

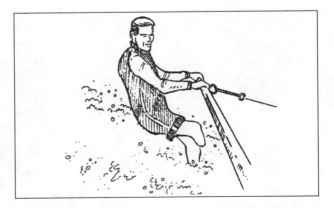

Figure 42.8. Beginning skiers may choose to use a ski-boom.

Sit-Skis

The single most significant factor influencing the participation of water skiers with mobility impairments was the development of the "sit-ski", or adapted water ski. A variety of models and styles exist (Figure 42.9 a-c). Currently, sit-skis are only being manufacturd by Quickie Designs.

Outriggers can also be attached to the main ski with a pair of aluminum bars. The outriggers allow skiers who may not be able to balance a sit ski to enjoy skiing.

The Sit-Ski is a dual ski version of sit-skis that has incorporated a molded seat into its design. Padded metal tubes are formed to provide handles for the skier.

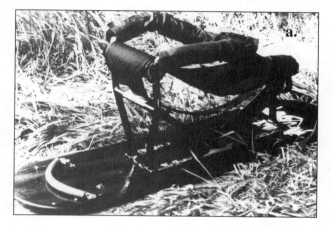

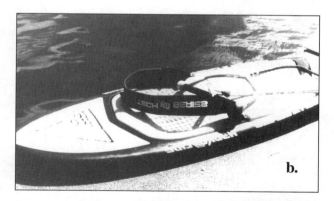

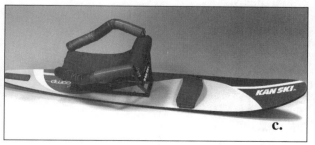

Figure 42.9 a-c. Water ski-skis come in various shapes and styles depending on intended use. (Courtesy of (a) Shadow Water-ski School for the Physically Challenged, (b) Michael J. Paciorek), (c) Kan-Ski Water Ski: Products)

Saucers or Disc-Shaped Equipment

Depending on the person's disability, skiers may find ski discs or saucers easier to use in the beginning stages of water skiing (Figure 42.10). Wider and more stable than conventional skis, saucers can be used in the prone, kneeling or standing position.

ADAPTATION FOR VISUALLY IMPAIRED

The Mark 5 Bat Blaster (Audio Slalom Device)

The new Mark 5 Bat Blaster from the British Disabled Water Ski Association is the ultimate training and competition system for blind and partially sighted water ski slalom. Until now, the most popular of the competition disciplines has been impossible for people with visual impairments. Audio Slalom was specially devised for skiers with visual impairments to accurately simulate the traditional slalom event. Blind and visually impaired skiers no longer needs to see the buoys, but can instead compete by using audible 'buoy' signals. The device attaches directly to the ski boat. The skier receives an audible indication of when to commence turning for the buoy as well as the actual signal when the correct width for the buoy is reached. Medals were awarded to skiers with visual impairments for the first time at the 1999 World Disabled Water Ski Championships in slalom. The device costs about $800. See Equipment Suppliers for ordering information.

EQUIPMENT SUPPLIERS

The Mark 5 Bat Blaster (Audio Slalom Device)

Chris Mairs
Weavers Mill, Avoncliff
Bradford-on-Avon

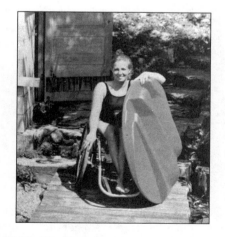

Figure 42.10. The Manta Ray is suitable for both physically disabled and nondisabled, at 20% of the cost of most water skis. (Courtesy of Access to Recreation)

Wiltshire, BA15 2HB
England
+44 1225 868845 (phone and fax)
Email: chris.mairs@virgin.net

Various Sit Ski Models
Achievable Concepts
P.O. Box 361
Moonee Ponds 3039
Victoria, Australia
(61) 3 9752 5958
(61) 3 9754 4798 (fax)
Email: sales@achievableconcepts.com.au
Website: http://www.achievableconcepts.com.au

Advanced Mobility Products Ltd.
Unit # 111-2323 Boundary Rd.,
Vancouver, B.C., V5M 4V8
Canada
(604) 293-0002
(800) 665-4442
(604) 293-0005 (fax)
Email: mobility@mobilityproducts.com
Website: http://www.mobilityproducts.com

ADDITIONAL RESOURCES AND WEBSITES

Water skiers will find many websites related to their sport. Because this sport is accessible for those with and without disabilities, most participants will find the following sites satisfactory for gathering information.

American Disabled Water Skiers
WILLIAM FURBISH
3480 Statfield Drive
Atlanta, GA 30319
(404) 261-9527
(404) 364-9405 (fax)
Email: bfurbish@mindspring.com

British Disabled Water Ski Association
The Tony Edge National Centre
Heron Lake
Wraysbury
Middlesex TW19 6HW
United Kingdom
Website: http://www.bdwsa.org.uk/
Affiliated with the British Water Ski Association, disabled water skiing in Britain appears to be quite advanced. Much information on disabled water-skiing can be found at this site.

International Water Ski Federation (IWSF)
World Disabled Council
C.P. 5537 BO 22
40134 Bologna, Italy
Website: http://www.IWSF.com/
The World Governing Body for Water Skiing includes a World Disabled Council for water skiing.

USAWater Ski
C/o Water Skiers with Disabilities Association
1251 Holy Cow Rd.
Polk City, FL 33868
(863) 324-4341
Website: http://www.usawaterski.org/
USA Water Ski web site is very complete and provides links to many other sites. A listing of many affiliated ski schools are provided as well. A directory of the affiliated ski schools who provide instruction to water skiers with disabilities is provided below. Additionally, the reader may wish to check with the affiliated water ski club in their area for disabled water ski programs.

USA Water Ski Affiliated Ski Schools For Disabled Skiers

The following ski schools have identified instruction for disabled water skiers in their literature:

Aquatic Sports Training
Orlando, FL
(407) 251-9037
(800) 330-8090
(407 399-9242 (fax)
Email: SkiOrlando@aol.com
Website: http://www.LisaStJohn.com/

Kierstead Ski School
Abled-Aquatics
1040 Carlton St.
Melbourne, FL 33803
(407) 259-6737
(407) 255-1654 (fax)
Website: http://www.usawaterski.org/

Cutting Edge Water Ski School
308 Virginia St. #A
El Segundo, CA 90245
(310) 322-3231
Email: waterski@mindspring.com
Website: http://www.waterski-school.com

International Tournament Skiers
Jack Travers
P.O. Box 331

Okahumpka, FL 34762
(352) 429-9027
Email: info@jacktravers.com
Website: http://www.jacktravers.com

Sammy Duvall's Water Sports Centre
4600 World Drive
Lake Buena Vista, FL 32830
(407) 939-0754
(407) 939-0756 (fax)
Email: duvallwatersports@compuserve.com
Website: http://www.duvallsports.com/

Ski-For-All
RR #22
Cambridge, Ontario
Canada N3C 2V4
(519) 638-5403
Email: Ski4all@istar.ca
Website: www.skiforall.on.ca

Other Water Ski Schools and Resources

Abili-ski Adaptive Watersports
950 Avenue K
Seaside, OR 97138
(503) 791-0572
Email: Chris@abili-ski.com
Website: http://abili-ski.com

Mission Bay Aquatic Center/Disabled Water Sports
1001 Santa Clara Point
San Diego, CA 92109
(858) 488-1036
    The Disabled Water Sports Program at the Mission Bay Aquatic Center is devoted to providing accessible water sports (including water skiing) for individuals with disabilities.

National Ability Center
Post Office Box 682799
Park City, Utah 84068
(435) 649-3991 (voice/TDD)
(435) 658-3992 (fax)
Email: nac@xmission.com
Website: http://nationalabilitycenter.org
    The National Ability Center's water-ski program utilizes a variety of specialized and adapted equipment for many types of disabilities.

Texas Adaptive Aquatics
17003 Bentana Court
Houston, TX 77095
Email: neosoft.com/tzadaqua
Website: http://www.neosoft.com/~txadaqua/
    One of the premier water ski programs for individuals with disabilities.

Water Skiers Web
Website: http://www.waterski.net/
    A complete website for the avid water skier. Includes information on clubs, events, boats, ski locations, jobs, links to water ski sites. The ultimate site for the water skier.

Chapter 43

Weight Training

ACTIVITY OVERVIEW

For the purpose of distinction, this text discusses fitness, powerlifting, and weight training as separate chapters. In many ways, and for some athletes, these are closely related. For others, these relationships (especially weight training to fitness) are commonly overlooked.

Weight training has become a very popular and critical method of preparing for athletic competition. Weight training can increase athletic performance and can also be used to improve the health related fitness components of muscular strength and muscular endurance. This is particularly true with respect to the use of weight training within the rehabilitation setting. A great many rehabilitation programs are incorporating specific principles of weight training as a supplement to their therapy programs. It is also very likely that weight training can have a positive effect on self-image.

This chapter is not meant to discuss the physiological aspects of weight training or the issues of specificity, intensity, frequency, or duration. These important considerations should be discussed with a rehabilitation specialist or weight training advisor when setting up a program. It is the intent of this chapter to introduce the reader to various options available to an individual with a disability who might be interested in beginning or revamping a weight training program. Consultation with a physician is always recommended prior to beginning or changing a weight training program.

ACCESSIBLE WEIGHT EQUIPMENT

With the passage of the American's with Disabilities Act (ADA) more private and public fitness clubs and gyms are providing access for people with disabilities, however challenges remain in many other facilities. Those who have crawled in and out of various "monster machines" that exercise a particular muscle group, can easily imagine the difficulty of doing so from a wheelchair. The desire within the disabled population to become physically fit has turned the field of accessible weight training and exercise equipment into a profitable business.

Increases in the number of manufacturers that design and produce equipment for individuals with disabilities have boosted the number of fully accessible programs. Arizona State University's Adaptive Recreation Program, Oregon's Rehabilitation Center's cooperative venture with the Eugene YMCA, the Rehabilitation Institute of Chicago's Center for Health and Fitness, and New Jersey's Kessler Institute for Rehabilitation are a few examples of fitness and weight training programs designed for individuals with disabilities. Specialized equipment ranges from single-station, single exercise units such as the Rickshaw Rehabilitation Exerciser (Figure 43.1) and the Accessible Fitness System's Tricep Extension Unit (Figure 43.2), to the single-station multi-exercise machines such as the Versatrainer (Figure 43.3 a-c) and multi-station, multi-exercise units such as the Freedom machine by Olympic Enterprises (Figure 43.4), the Equalizer that was developed by a person with paraplegia (Figure 43.5 a-d), and the Uppertone Quad Gym designed for wheelchair access by individuals with quadriplegia. The Access Series by Pulse Fitness (Figure 43.6 a and b) is a fully integrated line of strength training equipment targeted to include not only the able bodied, but also the physically challenged. Other machines distributed by other companies (see Equipment Suppliers) make it relatively easy to equip a full-size gym or a basement workout room with just the right equipment.

Although a variety of distributors and examples of machines are listed in this chapter, the authors do not

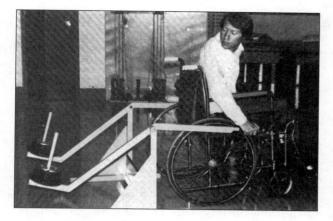

Figure 43.1. The Rickshaw Exerciser.

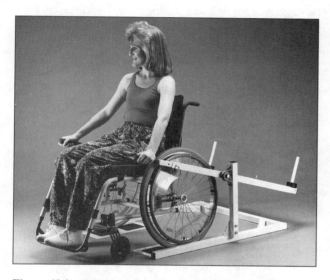

Figure 43.2. The Tricep Extension Unit. (Courtesy of Accessible Fitness Systems)

recommend or endorse any individual company or machine. Interested individuals should investigate options prior to purchase or use.

CONVENTIONAL WEIGHT EQUIPMENT

Depending on the disability, many individuals will be able to use conventional weight training equipment found in many health clubs with little or no adaptations. Radocy (1987) indicates that although lifting is most effectively accomplished while wearing an upper extremity prosthesis, conventional machines such as Nautilus, Hydro-Fitness, and Universal can be used by upper extremity

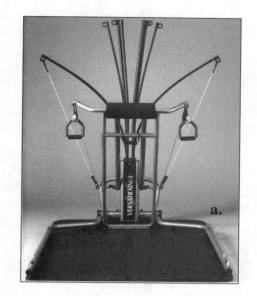

Figure 43.3 a-c. The Versatrainer allows the user to perform a number of different exercises at one station. (Courtesy of Bowflex of America)

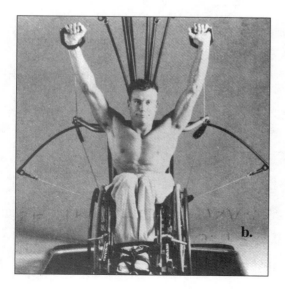

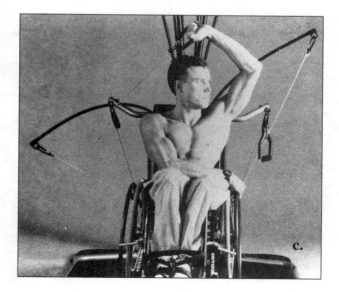

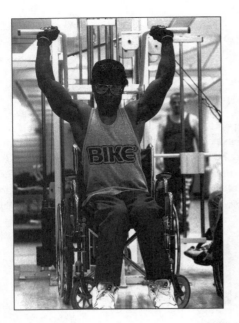

Figure 43.4. The Freedom Machine is a popular single unit, multi-exercise machine. Courtesy of Rehabilitation Institute of Chicago's Center for Health and Fitness and Oscar Izquierdo)

amputees who choose not to wear a prosthesis (Figure 43.7).

The use of these machines is also common among individuals with cerebral palsy and lower limb amputations, in addition to people who are deaf, or who have visual impairments. With the inclusion of powerlifting competition in Special Olympics, and the realization of the benefits of such training, more individuals with mental retardation have become involved as well.

ADAPTED TECHNIQUES

Successful resistance training does not always involve the use of barbells and expensive weight machines. The Rehabilitation Institute of Chicago's Center for Health and Fitness has had great success using standard therapy equipment such as slings and springs (Figure 43.8). The use of wrist cuffs (Figure 43.9 a-d) enable individuals with varying degrees of hand function to perform a number of weight training exercises and leg and wrist weight wraps (Figures 43.10 a-d) provide resistance exercise to a variety of disability groups.

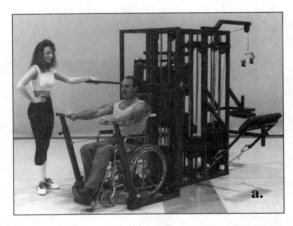

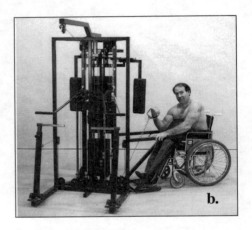

Figure 43.5 a-d. Parts of the Equalizer Series by Helm Distributing, Inc. (Courtesy of Helm Distributing, Inc.)

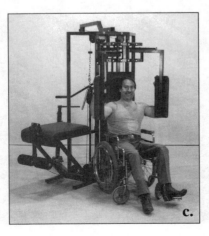

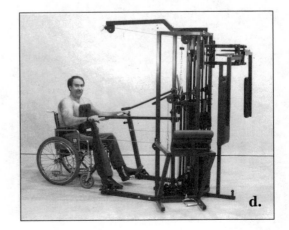

EQUIPMENT SUPPLIERS

The number of reputable weight training equipment suppliers is tremendous. The following is a sample of some of these companies and is not meant to be inclusive.

Accessible Weight Machines

Access To Recreation
8 Sandra Court
Newbury Park CA 91320

(800) 634-4351
(805) 498-7535
(805) 498-8186 (fax)
Email: dkrebs@gte.net
Website: http://www.accesstr.com

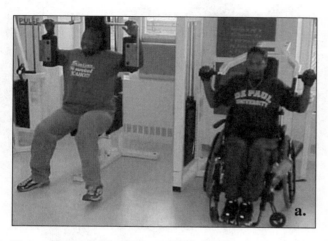

Figure 43.6 a and b. Access machines by Pulse Fitness Systems are specially designed with seats that swing away to allow wheelchair access. (Courtesy of Rehabilitation Institute of Chicago's Center for Health and Fitness)

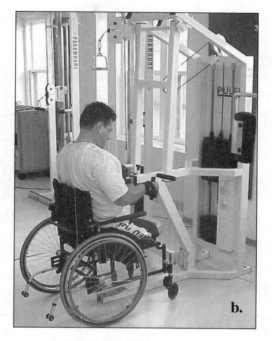

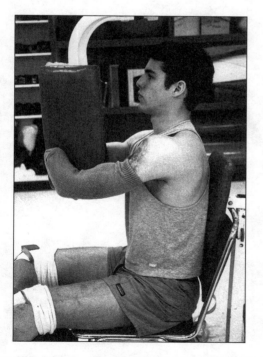

Figure 43.7. Many weight machine exercises can be done correctly and effectively without a prostheses. (Courtesy of Rehabilitation Institute of Chicago's Center for Health and Fitness)

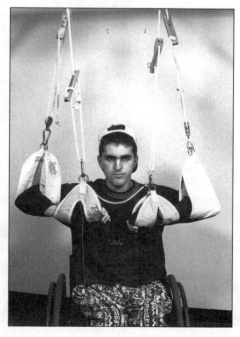

Figure 43.8. The use of slings and springs provides variable resistance with the use of traditional weightlifting equipment. (Courtesy of Rehabilitation Institute of Center for Health and Fitness)

Endorphin Corporation
ProGym CT Cross-Trainer
6901 90th Avenue North
Pinellas Park, Florida 33782
(800) 940-9844
(727) 545-9848
(727) 546-0613 (fax)

Email: endorph@gte.net
Website: http://www.endorphin.net

GPK Inc. (uppertoner)
535 Floyd Smith Drive
El Cajon, CA 92020, USA
(619) 593-7381

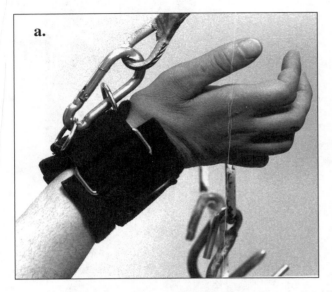

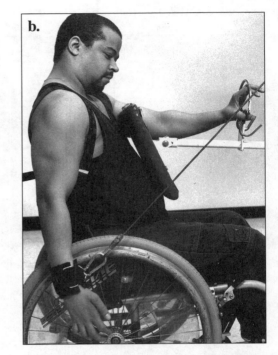

Figure 43.9 a-d. Wrist cuffs enable individuals with various degrees of hand function to perform a number of weight training exercises. (Courtesy of Rehabilitation Institute of Chicago's Center for Health and Fitness and Oscar Izquierdo)

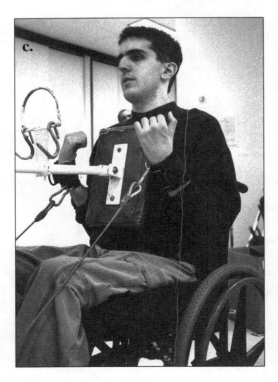

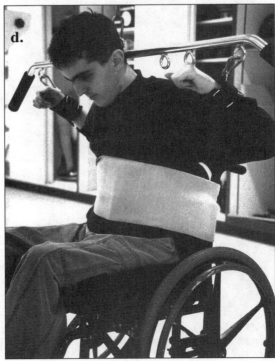

(800) 468-8679
(619) 593-7514 (fax)
Email: info@gpk.com
Website: http://www.gpk.com/
    Products for people with quadriplegia.

Flaghouse Rehab (Power Trainer)
601 Flaghouse Drive
Hasbrouck Heights, NJ 07604-3116
(800) 793-7900
(800) 793-7922 (fax)
Email: sales@flaghouse.com
Website: http://www.flaghouse.com/

Helm Distributing Co.
911 Kings Point Road
Polson, Montana 59860
(406) 883-2147
(406) 883-6207 (fax)
 Email   equalizr@digisys.net
Website: http://www.equalizerexercise.com/

Hoist Systems (Access Trainer)
9990 Empire St., Ste. 130

San Diego, CA 92126
(800) 548-5438
(858) 578-7676
(800) 547-5439 (fax)
Website: http://www.hoistfitness.com

Innovative Medical Inc. (Challenge Circuit)
P.O. Box 4780
Overland Park, KS 66204
(800) 851-1122
(913) 642-5106
(913) 642-9709 (fax)
Email: info@imiquantum.com
Website: http://www.imiquantum.com

Life Extension Systems Inc.
424 Richardson St.
Kalamazoo, MI 49007
(616) 343-4015
(616) 349-3300
Website: http://www.lifeforce1.com

LifeFitness
10601 W. Belmont Ave.

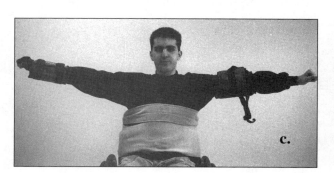
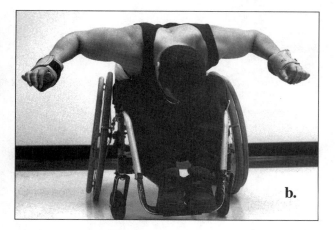
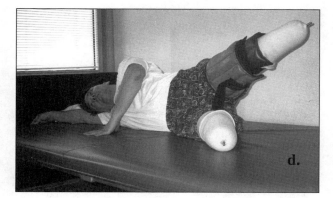

Figure 43.10 a-d. Weight wraps vary from 2 to 20 pounds and can be used for many different types of exercises. (Courtesy of Rehabilitation Institute of Chicago's Center for Health and Fitness)

Franklin Park, IL. 60131
(800) 735-3867
(847) 288-3300
(847) 288-3703
Website: http://www.lifefitness.com/

MedFit Systems
2759 Secret Lake Lane
Fallbrook, CA 92028
(800) 831-7665
Email: medfit@aol.com
Website: http://www.medfitsystems.com

No Boundaries
12882 Valley View Street #5
Garden Grove CA 92845
(800) 926-8637
(714-) 91-5899
(714) 891-0658 (fax)
Website: http://www.powertrainer.com/

Paramount Fitness Corp.
6450 E. Bandini Blvd.
Los Angeles, CA 90040
(800) 721-2121
(323) 724-2000 (fax)
Email: sales@paramountfitness.com
Website: http://www.paramountfitness.com/

Pulse Fitness Systems Inc.
600 Mission Street
Winnipeg, MB, Canada R2J 0A2
(204) 235-0904
(204) 231–1499 (fax)
Email: pulfit@mb.sympatico.ca
Website: http://www.pulfit.com/

SCIFIT, Inc.
5616A. S.122nd E. Ave.
Tulsa, OK 74143
(800) 278-3933
(918) 254-4189 (fax)
Email: scifit@busprod.com
Website: http://www.scifit.com/

Sportime
One Sportime Way
Atlanta, GA 30340
(770) 449-5700
(800) 444-5700
(800) 845-1535 (fax)
Email: customer.service@sportime.com
Website: http://www.sportime.com

Activity Mitts

Access To Recreation
8 Sandra Court
Newbury Park CA 91320
(800) 634-4351
(805) 498-7535
(805) 498-8186 (fax)
Website: http://www.accesstr.com
Email: dkrebs@gte.net

Felco Products Inc.
297 High St.
Dedham, MA 02026
(800) 973-6599

Patton Medical Glove Inc.
P.O. Box 7100
Jacksonville, FL 32210
(904) 388-1182

Arm Ergometers (see Fitness Chapter)

Cuff Weights

Flaghouse Rehab
(see above)

Sammons Preston
AbilityOne Corporation
4 Sammons Court
Bolingbrook, IL 60440
(800) 323-5547
(800) 547-4333 (fax)
Email: sp@sammonspreston.com
Website: http://www.sammonspreston.com/

Power Medicine Ball

M-F Athletic Company
11 Amflex Drive
P.O. Box 8090
Cranston, RI 02920-0090
(800) 556-7464
(800) 682-6950 (fax)
Email: mfathletic@mfathletic.com
Website: http://www.mfathletic.com/

Wheelchair Scale

Flaghouse Rehab
601 Flaghouse Drive
Hasbrouck Heights, NJ 07604-3116
(800) 793-7900
(800) 793-7922 (fax)
Email: sales@flaghouse.com
Website: http://www.flaghouse.com/

Other Resources

Disability Mall
Disability mall is an online resource that features many companies that provide exercise equipment as well as other products for individuals with disabilities
Website: http://www.disabilitymall.com

National Strength and Conditioning Association
1955 N. Union Blvd.
Colorado Springs, CO 80909
(719) 632-6722
(800) 815-6826
(719) 632-6367 (fax)
Email: nsca@nsca-lift.org
Website: http://www.nsca-lift.org/

The North American Academy of Health, Fitness & Rehabilitation Professionals
The Medical Exercise Specialist
(888) 610-0923
Email: medfit2000@aol.com
Website: http://www.medicalexercisespecialist.com
    The *Medical Exercise Specialist* is an excellent publication with articles related to fitness and weight training for people with disabilities.

BIBLIOGRAPHY

American College of Sports Medicine (1997). *Exercise Management for Persons with Chronic Disease and Disabilities*. Champaign, IL:Human Kinetics.

Lockette, K.F. and Keyes, A.M. (1994). *Conditioning with Physical Disabilities*. Champaign, IL: Human Kinetics.

Miller, P. (ed) (1995). *Fitness Programming and Physical Disability*. Champaign, IL: Human Kinetics.

Radocy, B. & Beiswenger, W. (1994). *Pumping Iron with Upper Limb Amputations*. Palaestra (Spring) pp41-46.

Saltin, B., Boushel, R., Secher, N., & Mitchell, J. (2000). *Exercise and Circulation in Healthand Disease*. Champaign, IL: Human Kinetics.

Thompson, B. & Morse, M. (1998) Training Tips: Functional Adaptation. *Sports 'n Spokes 24*(2)38-41.

Wise, J.B. (1996). Weight Training for those with Physical Disabilities at Idaho State University. *Strength and Conditioning 18*(2)67-71.

Chapter 44

Wheelchair Dance Sport

SPORT GOVERNING BODIES:
National: The United States Amateur Ballroom Dancers Association (USABDA)
International: International Dance Sport Federation (IDSF)

DISABLED SPORTS ORGANIZATION:
National:
International: International Paralympic Committee-Wheelchair Dance Sport Committee

PRIMARY DISABILITY: Wheelchair Users

SPORT OVERVIEW

Adapted Physical Educators and Therapeutic Recreation professionals have used wheelchair dance in their programs for decades. Various professional and amateur wheelchair dance companies have also promoted the activity. Many wheelchair dance groups exist that promote everything from line dance to modern dance to ballet (Figure 44.1). The combination of ambulatory and wheelchair dancers performing together has served not only as a wonderful art form, but has helped to dismiss biased attitudes towards the capabilities of individuals with disabilities. The sport or art of dance can be enjoyed on a recreational or competitive basis. On a recreational level, wheelchair dance can be enjoyed in different styles, such as ballroom, ballet, modern, square or folk dance. Wheelchair dancers may dance with other wheelchair users in pairs or groups, with an able–bodied partner, or by themselves.

Only recently has the sport been taken to the next level within the International Paralympic offerings of sports. In international competition, wheelchair dancers perform with an able-bodied partner in Standard dances such as the Quickstep, Slow Foxtrot, Tango, Viennese Waltz, and Waltz; and in Latin American Dances such as Cha-Cha-Cha, Jive, Paso Doble, and the Samba.

SPORT HISTORY

Within the able-bodied community, Dance Sport, better known as Ballroom Dancing, traces its roots to before World War I to Europe, as private competitions emerged in some of the larger cities. More formal competitions did not begin however, until the 1930's. The first formal organization was founded in 1935 as the International Amateur Dancers Federation (FIDA). Interest and membership quickly grew. World War II brought an abrupt halt to the growth of this group and efforts at revival floundered after the war. In 1950, the International Council of Ballroom Dancing (ICBD) was founded in Edinburgh, Scotland, and became the first international professional dance organization. Attempts at cooperation between the amatuer dancers of FIDA and professional dancers of ICBD were in vain. Efforts to revive FIDA were unsuccessful. For all intents and purposes FIDA was an inactive organization for many years prior to formally disbanding in 1964. Due to the inactivity of FIDA, a group of interested amateurs founded the international Council of Amateur Dancers (ICAD) in 1957. The various difficulties that plagued FIDA, now provided ICAD with the same challenges. The squabbles between ICAB and ICAD were finally resolved in 1965 when a joint committee was established to discuss issues related to each group and the bringing together amateur and professional dancers. The time for greater cooperation had arrived. This cooperation lead to a more efficiently run federation and the sport enjoyed greater growth and prosperity. The International Olympic Committee acknowledged the joint operation between ICAB and ICAD in 1990. With this acknowledgement of the IOC in hand, the federation changed its name to The International Dance Sports Federation (IDSF) to identify the group as a true sports organization.

The International Dance Sport Federation (IDSF)

The International Dance Sport Federation (IDSF), is the international governing body for Amateur Dance Sport. The organization was officially welcomed into the International Olympic Committee in 1995. Although Dance Sport is not as yet an Olympic sport, the IDSF continues to work for the inclusion of Dance Sport as a medal sport in the Olympic Games and to promote the sport throughout the world.

The National Dance Council of America (NDCA)

The National Dance Council of America (NDCA) is the official governing body for dancing in the United States. Its purpose is to provide, on a nation-wide basis, a united inter-association agency to represent the interests of those in the dance profession and other dance-related entities and organizations and to act as the agency for cooperation with similar councils in other countries. The United States Amateur Ballroom Dancers Association (USABDA) is a member of the NDCA.

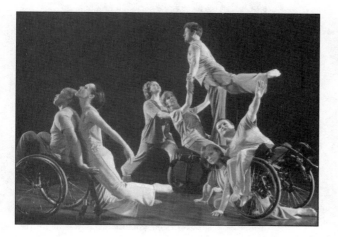

Figure 44.1. Wheelchair dance groups promote a variety of dance forms from line dance to modern dance to ballet. (Photo: Neil Dent; Courtesy of Full Radius Dance)

The United States Amateur Ballroom Dancers Association (USABDA)

The United States Amateur Ballroom Dancers Association (USABDA) functions as the national governing body in the USA for amateur ballroom dancing (also known as Dance Sport). USABDA was established in 1965 to promote the acceptance of ballroom dancing into the Olympic Games. This organization offers programs for competitive, college and social Amateur Ballroom Dancers in the United States.

The United States Dance Sport Council (USDSC) is the division of the United States Amateur Ballroom Dancers Association (USABDA) which is responsible for regulating Amateur Dance Sport competition in the United States. The USDSC is formally recognized by the International Dance Sport Federation (IDSF) as the organization that promotes Dance Sport in the United States.

During the past decade, Dance Sport has undergone unprecedented growth due to the fall of communism in Eastern Europe and the increased popularity of the sport within Asia. Over 60 countries enjoy membership in the IDSF. A complete historical record of Dance Sport can be found on the International Dance Sport Federation web page (see Additional Resources).

Wheelchair Dance Sport

Wheelchair dance has been performed for decades by various groups including the famous Dancing Wheels (formerly the Cleveland Ballet Dancing Wheels). The first international competition in Wheelchair Dance occurred in 1977 in Sweden, with the first World Championships not occurring until 1998 in Japan. Under the leadership of the International Paralympic Wheelchair Dance Sport Committee, the sport became a part of the Winter Paralympic Games sport offerings in 1998.

Wheelchair Dance Sport continues to gain popularity around the world with an estimated 5,500 dancers (4,000 wheelchair users and 1,500 able-bodied partners) participating in recreational and competitive dance. The International Paralympic Committee Wheelchair Dance Sport Committee is continuing to promote the sport to increase the numbers of individuals and countries participating.

At the present time vertical integration of wheelchair dancers does not exist within the International Dance Sport Federation, but both groups remain in close communication. Wheelchair Dance Sport uses rules that compliment the competition rules of the IDSF.

Basic Rules of Wheelchair Dance Sport

- A dance couple must be comprised of a male and a female partner, and one of them must be a wheelchair user with at least a minimal disability that makes walking impossible.
- Athletes with obvious locomotor disabilities in the

lower part of their body such as amputation, paralysis, cerebral palsy, and leg shortening (at least 7 cm) are eligible for competition.

- Athletes are expected to have normal upper body function.
- Athletes are placed in one of 2 functional classes based on their ability to maneuver a wheelchair, rotate their trunk, and arm function.
- In all rounds of International Wheelchair Dance Sport Competitions, the music is played for a minimum of one and a half minutes duration for Waltz, Tango, Slow Foxtrot, Quickstep, Samba, Cha-Cha-Cha, Rumba and Paso Doble. The time for the Viennese Waltz and Jive is one minute. In the qualifying rounds the same music must be played for different heats.
- International Wheelchair Dance Sport Competitions are comprised of at least two qualifying rounds to allow couples the opportunity of dancing twice. The number of rounds is determined by the number of participants.
- At least 50% of participating couples are recalled to the next round excluding the final.
- Winners are selected by a panel of adjudicators from different countries.

DANCE COMPANIES

Wheelchair dance companies exist throughout the country. Two of the more well-known companies include the Dancing Wheels, and Full Radius Dance Company.

Dancing Wheels

The Dancing Wheels, formerly known as the Cleveland Ballet Dancing Wheels is a professional, integrated dance company comprised of dancers with and without disabilities located in Cleveland, Ohio. The Dancing Wheels were created in 1980 by Mary Verdi-Fletcher, as an opportunity for people with disabilities to play a more active role in dance. Having been born with spina bifida, Ms. Fletcher wanted to help change negative perceptions of individuals with disabilities through her art.

In addition to performing various repertory dances, the company educates the audience about disability, choreography, and dance training through interaction and audience participation. These performances are tailored for specific audiences. The company performs hundreds of days per year throughout the world including residency workshops. These residency workshops offer professionals in the fields of dance, theater, rehabilitation, and physical therapy the opportunity to study Dancing Wheels' technique. They can then incorporate these methods into their work within the arts and disabled communities. Students with and without disabilities are of-

fered a full range of technique, composition, improvisation, and repertory. Each residency concludes with a performance by students and company members reflecting the week's work.

Full Radius Dance Company

Full Radius Dance was created in May of 1998, in Atlanta, Georgia, when the professional dance companies Dance Force and E=motion merged. Full Radius Dance is a modern dance company that challenges traditional gender portrayals in mature, choreographically complex works that celebrate technique and physicality. Additionally, the company has a desire to share the talents of dancers who have disabilities with the mainstream audience (Figure 44.2).

Full Radius Dance's focus is on skill and artistry. That some of the dancers use wheelchairs is secondary. The wheelchair may lend additional movement possibilities to the choreography, but is not the focal point of the work. The goal of this company is to neither promote nor diminish the significance of the wheelchair itself, but to focus the attention of the audience on the dance.

EQUIPMENT

The only equipment needed includes an easily maneuverable sports wheelchair and appropriate costuming for the performers.

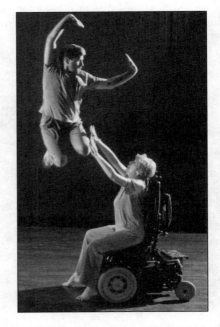

Figure 44.2. The Full Radius Dance Company shares the talents of dancers who have disabilities with the mainstream audience (Photo: Neil Dent; Courtesy of Full Radius Dance)

ADDITIONAL RESOURCES AND WEBSITES

American Dance Therapy Association
2000 Century Plaza, Suite 108
10632 Little Patuxent Parkway
Columbia, MD 21044
(410) 997-4040
(410) 997-4048 (fax)
Email: info@adta.org
Website: http://www.adta.org/

Dancing Wheels
3615 Euclid Avenue
Cleveland, Ohio 44115
(216) 432-0306
(216) 432-0308 (fax)
Email: proflair1@aol.com
Website: http://www.dancingwheels.org

Dancescape's World of Ballroom Dancing and Dance Sport
Website: http://www.dancescape.com

Full Radius Dance Company
Email: dsdance@aol.com
Website: http://www.fullradiusdance.org/

Gallaudet Dance Company
Gallaudet University
Department of Physical Education and Recreation
Washington, D.C.
(202) 651-5493
    A dance company composed of people who are deaf and hearing impaired.

International Dance Sport Federation (IDSF).
Website: http://www.idsf.net

International Paralympic Committee Wheelchair Dance Sport Committee (IPC-WDSC)
Dr. Gertrude Krombholz, Chairperson
Nederlingerstr. 30
80638 Munich, Germany

(49) - 89 - 157 3601
(49) - 89 - 157 3503 (fax)
Email: G.Krombholz@t-online.de
Website:
http://www.paralympic.org/sports/sections/dancing.asp

Light Motion
1520 32nd Avenue South
Seattle, WA 98144
(206) 328-0818

The United States Amateur Ballroom Dancers Association (USABDA)
PO Box 128
New Freedom, PA 17349
(800) 447-9047
(717) 235-4183 (fax)
Email: usabdacent@aol.com
Website: http://www.usabda.org

United States Dancesport Council, (USDSC)
Mr. Gary Stroick, Vice President
3800 France Avenue South
St. Louis Park, MN 55416
(612) 926-7648 (phone/fax)
Email: DanceSportVP.usabda.org

National Dance Council of America (NDCA)
Ballroom Department
Lee Wakefield, Director
P.O. Box 22018
Provo, UT 84602
(801) 378-8381 (phone/fax)
Email: Lee_Wakefield@byu.edu

BIBLIOGRAPHY

Ervin, M. (1998)). Dance, an expression of the soul. *Enable Magazine* 2(1):72-74, 95.

Chapter 45

Wilderness Experiences

SPORT OVERVIEW

Conservation Pledge

I give my pledge to save and faithfully defend from waste the natural resources of my country, its air, soil and minerals, its forests, waters and wildlife.

The ascent to the summit of Mt. Everest by Tom Whittaker in 1998, the first successful attempt by a person with a disability (single leg amputee) to climb the world's tallest mountain, was a terrific athletic accomplishment and provided great evidence that people with disabilities desire to participate in adventure activities. Mark Wellman's (a climber with spinal cord injury) 2 ascents of El Capitan 10 years apart, also were well-documented in the media and brought much attention about the capabilities of individuals with disabilities in tackling even the most challenging adventure activities.

Although most people, with or without disabilities, would probably find the climb of Mt. Everest or El Capitan, to be a bit too challenging, the topic of Wilderness Activities involves a variety of activities and means different things to different people. Some of the traditional wilderness experiences are covered in specific chapters throughout this book. Camping, canoeing, kayaking, skiing, orienteering, mountain climbing, mountain biking, fishing, hunting, rock climbing (Figure 45.1), and white water rafting all involve the great outdoors and can be considered a part of the wilderness experience.

Accessibility to wilderness areas and public lands have been the focus of many individuals and organizations and great growth and improvement in facilities has been seen since the passage of the American's with Disabilities Act (ADA) in 1990. Many outfitting and tour groups now provide wilderness experiences specifically for people with disabilities. Special projects such as the British Columbia Mobility Opportunities Society (see

Additional Resources), established programs such as The Breckenridge Outdoor Education Center (BOEC), Wilderness Inquiry, and special camps such as the Wheelchair Outdoor Adventure Camp in Aspen, Colorado, offer increasing opportunities for people with disabilities to access wilderness activities (Figure 45.2).

The National Park Service (NPS) and U.S. Forest Service are committed to the concept of integrating visitors with disabilities into ongoing opportunities at their sites. Through the technical assistance efforts of its Special Programs and Populations Branch, NPS has helped many national parks to improve the accessibility of their campgrounds. Many public lands and campgrounds now have accessible grounds, bathrooms and campsites.

The Golden Access passport is one such service provided by the NPS. Issued to citizens or U.S. residents who have medical proof of blindness or permanent disabilities, the passport admit the permit holders and accompanying passengers to federally operated properties that charge entrance fees. They are obtained at any federal fee area. The National Parks: Camping Guide is a valuable resource in identifying accessible camping areas (see Additional Resources).

TRAIL ORIENTEERING

Orienteering is the sport of navigation with map and compass and it is an excellent sport for those who enjoy wilderness activities. The object is to run, walk, ski, wheel, or mountain bike to a series of points shown on the map, choosing routes–both on and off trail–that will help you find all the points and get back to the finish in the shortest amount of time. The points on the course are marked with orange and white flags and punches, so the competitor can prove they were there. Each "control" marker is located on a distinct feature, such as a stream junction or the top of a knoll.

Orienteering is a sport for everyone, regardless of age

or experience. The competitive athlete can experience the exhilaration of running through the woods at top speed, while the non-competitive orienteer can enjoy the forest at a more leisurely pace. Most events provide courses for all levels–from beginner to advanced–and the sport has been adapted for small children and wheelchair users in Trail Orienteering.

Trail orienteering is an orienteering discipline centered around map reading in natural terrain. The discipline has been developed to offer everyone, including people with limited mobility, a chance to participate in a meaningful orienteering competition. Manual or power wheelchairs, walking sticks, and assistance with movement are permitted as speed of movement is not part of the competition.

Trail orienteers must identify on the ground control points shown on the map. As this is done from a distance, both able-bodied and participants with disabilities compete on level terms. Proof of correct identification of the control points does not require any manual dexterity, allowing those with severely restricted movement to compete equally. Most trail orienteering events have classes open for everyone.

European Championships in trail orienteering have been organized every year since 1994. Athletes who cannot participate on reasonably equal terms in the sport for able-bodied people because of a functional disadvantage due to a permanent disability are eligible for the event (i.e. the same criterion as for participation in the Paralympics). The first ever World Cup in trail orienteering was held in 1999. Contact the United States Orienteering Federation or the International Orienteering Federation (see Additional Resources) for more information.

WHITEWATER RAFTING

The growth of the whitewater rafting industry has led many outfitters to make it possible for almost anyone to participate safely in some level of whitewater rafting. Oar- guided rafts with lightweight aluminum rowing frames make it possible for disabled individuals, senior citizens, and families with young children to enjoy both singleday and multiday Class I, II and III whitewater trips. On several of the popular river trips of easy and moderate difficulty, it is not at all uncommon to see a person who is paraplegic or quadriplegic, a deaf person, or even a blind person experiencing the unique thrill of whitewater. Please make sure to describe your disability to the outfitter when you make trip reservations. They will help you with equipment and make you comfortable.

It is impossible to do justice to the topic of wilderness activities in a chapter as short as this. The numbers of programs, projects, special camps and activities are overwhelming (Figure 45.3). The purpose of this chapter is to provide the reader with a start to accessing the great outdoors by providing a list of specific major programs and resources throughout the country. This list is not to be considered all-inclusive.

WILDERNESS PROGRAMS AND INITIATIVES

Many local and regional programs exist that offer adventure type activities for children and adults with dis-

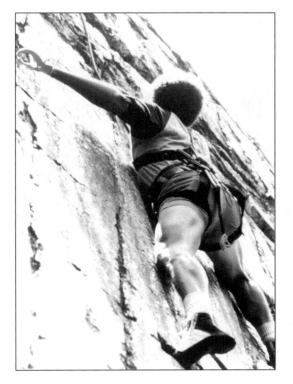

Figure 45.1. Rock climbing is one of many outdoor activities offered by specialty programs to individuals with disabilities. (Courtesy of TRS)

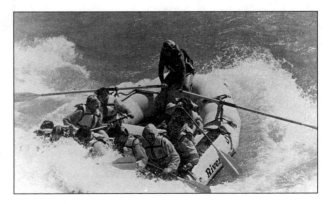

Figure 45.2. Whitewater rafting trips are part of a wide variety of outdoor experiences offered by Wilderness Inquiry. (Courtesy of *Disabled Outdoors*)

abilities. Additionally, specialized camps for specific disabilities or cross-disabilities provide adventure activities for children during the summer season (Figure 45.4). The following resources are some of the major programs and resources available that may be of interest to the reader. Other resources are listed as well under additional resources at the end of the chapter.

American Camping Association

The American Camping Association is a community of camp professionals and is dedicated to enriching the lives of children and adults through the camp experience. Founded in 1910, the American Camping Association (ACA) is the only not-for-profit educational body that accredits all types of camps throughout the United States. The American Camping Association accredits over 2,000 camps. ACA-accredited camps meet up to 300 standards for health, safety, and program quality. The ACA website provides information on locating hundreds of camps for children with specific disabilities and special needs. Of the more than 2,200 ACA-accredited camps, approximately 1,430 are dedicated to meeting the special needs of campers with physical, emotional or mental challenges.

Boy Scouts of America (Scouts With Disabilities and Special Needs)

The Boy Scouts of America represents the introduction of the wilderness and the environment to youth. Since its founding in 1910, the Boy Scouts of America has had fully participating members with physical, mental, and emotional disabilities. Although most of the BSA's efforts have been directed at keeping such boys in the mainstream of Scouting, it has also recognized the special needs of those with severe disabilities. The Boy Scout Handbook has had Braille editions for many years; merit badge pamphlets have been recorded on cassette tapes for blind Scouts; and closed-caption training videos have been produced. In 1965, registration of over-age Scouts who are mentally retarded became possible, a privilege now extended to many people with disabilities. Today, approximately 100,000 Cub Scouts, Boy Scouts, and Venturers with disabilities are registered with the Boy Scouts of America in more than 4,000 units chartered to community organizations.

Breckenridge Outdoor Education Center (BOEC)

Since 1976, the BOEC, located in Breckenridge, Colorado, has offered quality outdoor learning experiences to people of all abilities, including people with disabilities, those with serious illnesses and injuries, and "at-risk" populations. The year-round Wilderness Program focus on abilities, emphasizing fun, challenge by choice, and success. The varied curriculum can include personal development, therapeutic recreation, adventure therapy, disability awareness, teambuilding or natural history. Groups usually combine several of the following activities: rock climbing, canoeing, backpacking & hiking, whitewater

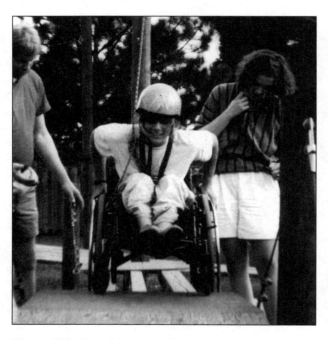

Figure 45.3. Part of the Accessible Challenge Course presents a series of progressive obstacles. (Courtesy of Roland/Diamond Associates, Inc.)

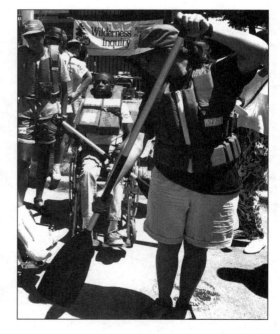

Figure 45.4. Wilderness Inquiry provides in-service clinics in a number of outdoor educational activities including canoeing for persons with disabilities. (Courtesy of Rehabilitation Institute of Chicago's Wirtz Sports Program and Oscar Izquierdo)

rafting, ropes course, initiative games, camping, challenge courses, peak climbs, orienteering, fishing, kayaking, cross country skiing, adaptive skiing, snowshoeing, wilderness first aid, hut skiing, and avalanche awareness.

Casa Colina Center for Rehabilitation: Outdoor Adventures

The Outdoor Adventures Program at Casa Colina is an example of the use of wilderness activities in the rehabilitation process. Many rehabilitation centers have incorporated sports programming as a part of the rehabilitation process. Casa Colina has taken it a step further by incorporating adventure activities. The program is open to all individuals with disabilities throughout the Los Angeles area. It is a unique program to empower people with disabilities by creating opportunities for challenging and exciting experiences in the out-of-doors. Activities include ocean sailing, rock climbing, white-water rafting, snow skiing, horse-packing, water skiing, deep sea fishing, back packing, freshwater fishing, winter camping, dog sledding, sea kayaking, and family camping. This program is open to people of all abilities.

Girl Scouts of America

Similar to the Boy Scouts of America, girls with disabilities have been part of Girl Scouting almost from it's beginning in 1912. The publication of Handicapped Girls & Girl Scouting in 1968 continued the tradition of Girl Scouts' concern for the disabled, begun in 1917, when the first troop of physically disabled girls in the United States was organized. Girls with disabilities join in troop/group activities alongside other girls, and are given the opportunity to participate in the same program. *Focus on Ability: Serving Girls with Special Needs* is the latest resource available from the national office and it offers practical suggestions for leaders, girls, trainers, program staff members, and anyone else looking to include girls with disabilities in Girl Scout activities successfully. This book offers information about specific disabilities, suggestions for inclusion and program adaptations, as well as a lengthy resource list.

National Center on Accessibility

The National Center on Accessibility (NCA) is an organization committed to the full participation in parks, recreation and tourism by people with disabilities. The center provides technical assistance, education and research on accessibility issues to the parks, recreation and tourism industries.

Of interest is *The National Survey on Recreation and the Environment (NSRE)*, the most recent study of outdoor recreation of the US population. The study was prepared for the National Center on Accessibility and was conducted by the US Forest Service from January 1994 through April 1995 and included 17,216 Americans over

the age of 15. Twelve hundred of the respondents identified themselves as having a disability. This report presents summary information on the characteristics, outdoor activity participation, and attitudes of people with disabilities in the NSRE survey. The results of this study are too lengthy for publication here but the full summary may be found at the website: http://www.indiana.edu/~nca/research/nsrekeypoints.htm.

National Sports Center for the Disabled

Founded in 1970, the National Sports Center for the Disabled (NSCD), is a non-profit organization that provides recreation for children and adults with disabilities. Best known for its disabled ski program, the NSCD also offers an extensive summer program of adventure and wilderness activities. Summer recreation opportunities include, hiking, in-line skating, sailing, therapeutic horseback riding, white water rafting, baseball, fishing, rock climbing for the blind, and camping.

Outdoor Buddies, Inc.

Founded in 1984, Outdoor Buddies is a Denver-based non-profit organization, relying on volunteer hunters and anglers who help the mobility disabled and disadvantaged youths enjoy the best of what Colorado's natural resources have to offer. For the mobility disabled, the program gives them a chance to take part in outdoor adventures some thought they'd never be able to do again. Disadvantaged youths, many with troubled home lives or emotional problems, are exposed to alternatives to drugs, alcohol abuse and gangs. Today, Outdoor Buddies hosts a variety of outdoor activities such as hunting, fishing, archery, shooting, camping, canoeing, outdoor survival, and wildlife photography.

Outdoor Explorations (OE)

Outdoor Explorations is an example of the growing number of locally based wilderness programs. Founded in 1990 as a not-for-profit organization, this Boston-based program enables people of all abilities to gain access to opportunities in wilderness experiences such as kayaking, and mountain climbing; and environmental service projects such as urban gardening and trail-building.

From that small venture, OE has grown into a vibrant community of 545 participants annually, involved in a broad array of adventure trips and environmental service projects. It is the only not-for-profit organization in Massachusetts to offer this innovative combination of inclusion, service and learning in the outdoors.

SPLORE—Accessible Outdoor Adventures

SPLORE is a Utah based, not-for-profit organization dedicated to providing life-enhancing wilderness recreation and education to people of all abilities, including people with disabilities and special needs. SPLORE programs lead to increased health, wellness and community integration while promoting environmental stewardship. Year-round activities are offered in four white water rafting, canoeing, rock climbing, and Nordic skiing with additional adventures including kayaking, dog sledding, and fly-fishing.

United States Department of the Interior

The US Department of the Interior is responsible for the running of all public lands and parks in the United States. The Department of the Interior is interested in providing access to America's public lands and resources and is working to assure these opportunities are provided to all Americans. DOI is addressing accessibility issues and is developing a comprehensive strategy to provide persons with disabilities access to all programs, activities, services and facilities consistent with all legal requirements and Departmental policies (Figure 45.5). The US Department of the Interior Coordinating Committee on Accessibility for People with Disabilities is an advisory and proactive working group established to assist the Department in addressing accessibility issues and in developing a comprehensive strategy to provide persons with disabilities access to all programs, activities, services, and facilities consistent with all legal requirements and Departmental policies. This strategy would include the development of processes to more effectively coordinate and guide efforts to provide accessibility to persons with disabilities. See Additional Resources at the end of the chapter.

Wilderness Access Decision Tool

The Wilderness Access Decision Tool is a resource to help managers of the National Wilderness Preservation System (NWPS) make appropriate, objective, and consistent decisions regarding use of the NWPS by persons with disabilities, as defined by the Americans With Disabilities Act of 1990. This tool was developed by Wilderness Inquiry, Inc., under an agreement with the USDA Forest Service and the USDI Bureau of Land Management. It was developed with input from each agency responsible for managing the National Wilderness Preservation System, and is designed to assist wilderness managers regardless of which federal wilderness management agency they work for.

Wilderness Inquiry

Wilderness Inquiry (WI) has been one of the premier programs in the country offering a variety of outdoor adventure activities and trips for people with disabilities. Founded in 1978, Wilderness Inquiry is a non-profit organization that focuses on getting people from all walks of life to personally experience the natural world. In addition to many outdoor adventures, Wilderness Inquiry conducts a variety of activities including community events, research, training, equipment design, trail and facility assessments and policy development, in addition to their multi-day wilderness adventures. However, they are best known for our multi-day adventures that form the core of their programming.

Adventure trips are offered to many wilderness locations throughout the United States, Canada, Central America and Australia. Trips are integrated with people of all abilities and ages. Adventures led by experienced guides include canoeing, kayaking, rafting, skiing, dogsledding, horsepacking, backpacking, and camping to mention a few.

Wilderness on Wheels Foundation

Wilderness On Wheels Foundation was established as a not-for-profit corporation in March of 1986 to provide access for disabled persons to the natural outdoor environment. W.O.W. is supported entirely by donations and has no paid administrative staff.

Through the hard work of volunteers W.O.W. had constructed a model wilderness-access facility. To date, over 100,000 hours have been invested in the project by some 3,000 volunteers. The facility includes campsites, cabins, and a 8-foot wide boardwalk that is just over a mile long. The ultimate goal is complete the boardwalk that starts at 9,100 feet so it reaches the top of a 12,300 foot mountain.

W.O.W. has provided advice and counsel to entities nationwide including the U.S. Forest Service and the National Park Service. See Additional Resources for reservation information.

EQUIPMENT

As with many other activities the use of adaptive equipment varies with each individual and most people

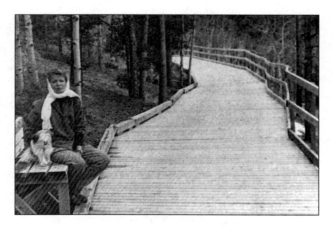

Figure 45.5. Access to the great outdoors is being made possible by more state and federal projects that provide funds for accessible trail systems. (Courtesy of Disabled Outdoors Magazine)

with disabilities will not need any assistive device when participating (Figure 45.6). According to the 1995 National Survey on Recreation and the Environment (NSRE), about 30% of individuals with disabilities indicated they use some type of assistive device when participating in outdoor recreation. Mobility aids such as wheelchairs, walkers, and canes are used to the greatest extent followed by the use of support persons.

Access to wilderness areas by individuals with mobility impairments is a serious concern but one that is easily solved. Depending on the situation, motorized or non-motorized equipment may provide a solution. Local laws pertaining to the use of motorized vehicles by individuals with physical disabilities should be consulted. The use of all terrain vehicles may provide the answer. See chapters on All-Terrain Vehicles, Boating, Hunting, and Fishing for specific adaptive equipment.

ADDITIONAL RESOURCES AND WEBSITES

"Access Challenge Project"
BC Mobility Opportunities Society
Box 27, Plaza of Nations, Suite A-304
770 Pacific Blvd. South
Vancouver, BC V6B 5E7 Canada
(604) 688-6464
(604) 688-6463 (fax)
Email: bcmos@reachdisability.org
Website: http://www.reachdisability.org/bcmos

Adaptive Adventures
P.O. Box 2245
Evergreen, CO 80439
(303) 679-2770
Website: http://www.adaptiveadventures.org

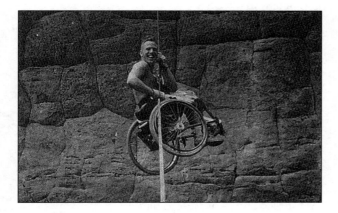

Figure 45.6. Climbing continues to grow in popularity as more programs provide the opportunity to individuals with disabilities. (Courtesy of *Sports 'n Spokes* 1998 24/1: 30)

Adaptive Adventures plans a variety of winter and summer activities for people with disabilities. Some activities offered include camping, kayaking, sailing, mountain biking, skiing, snowmobiling and hut trips.

Adaptive Sports Center
Crested Butte, CO
(907) 349-2296
Email: ascl@rmi.net
Website: http://www.adaptivesports.org
This program provides year-round outdoor recreational experiences for people with disabilities.

The Adaptive Adventure Sports Coalition
833 Eastwind Drive
Westerville, OH 43081
(614) 823-7156
(614) 823-7152 (fax)
Email: TAASC1@aol.com

Adventure Within Inc.
1250 South Odgen
Denver, CO 80210
(303) 744-8813
The purpose of Adventures Within is to provide outdoor experience and confidence-building challenges for individuals with multiple sclerosis.

Alaska Welcomes You
Accessible Alaska Adventures
P.O. Box 91333
Anchorage, AK 99509-1333
(800) 349-6301 (voice/tty)
(907) 344-3259 (fax)
Email: awy@compuserve.com
Website: http://www.accessiblealaska.com

Alternate Mobility Adventure Seekers
Boise State University
Physical Education Department
1910 University Drive
Boise, Idaho 83725
(800) 824-7017

America Outdoors Information Services
Outdoor Management Network Inc.
4607 NE Cedar Creek Rd.
Woodland, WA 98674
(360) 225-5000
Email: omni@americaoutdoors.com
Website: http://www.americaoutdoors.com/
America Outdoors is an outdoor information center and gathering area for outdoor recreationists and for those who enjoy the great outdoors. America Outdoors offers numerous resources.

American Camping Association, Inc.
5000 State Road 67 North
Martinsville, Indiana 46151
(765) 342-8456
(765) 342-2065 (fax)
Website: http://www.acacamps.org/

American Hiking Society
1422 Fenwick Lane
Silver Spring, MD 20910
(301) 565-6704
(301) 565-6714 (Fax)
Email: AmHiker@aol.com
Website: http://www.americanhiking.org/
    American Hiking is a national organization dedicated
to serving hikers and protecting the nation's hiking trails.
From the halls of Congress to the backcountry, AHS
speaks up for America's hikers and the trails they love.

American Whitewater Affiliation
1430 Fenwick Lane
Silver Spring, MD 20910
(301) 589-9453
Website: http://www.awa.org
National organization of whitewater boating enthusiasts.

Boy Scouts of America (Scouts With Disabilities and
Special Needs)
1325 West Walnut Hill Lane
P.O. Box 152079
Irving, TX 75015-2079.
(214) 580-2423
(214) 580-2502
Website: http://www.bsa.scouting.org/

Breckenridge Outdoor Education Center Wilderness program
PO Box 697
Breckenridge, CO 80424
(800) 383-BOEC(2632)
(970) 453-6422
(970) 453-4676 (fax)
Email: boec@boec.org
Website: http://www.boec.org/

Casa Colina Centers for Rehabilitation
Outdoor Adventures Program
2850 N. Garey Avenue
PO Box 6001
Pomona, CA 91769-6001
(909) 596 7733
(909) 593 0153 (fax)
Email: rehab@casacolina.org
Website:
           http://www.casacolina.org/community/index.htm

Common Ground Outdoor Adventures
Whittier Community Center
290 N. 400 E
Logan, UT 84321
(435) 713-0288
Email: cground@cache.net
Website: http://www.cache.net/~cground

Corporative Wilderness Handicapped Outdoor Group
(C.W. HOG)
P.O. Box 8128
Idaho State University
Pocatello, Idaho 83209
(208) 236-3912
Email: http://branjeft@isu.edu
            and www.isu.edu/cwhog/

Courage Center
3915 Golden Valley Road
Minneapolis, MN 55422
(763) 520-0520
(888) 8INTAKE
(763) 520-0577 (fax)
Email: jenim@courage.org
Website: http://www.courage.org/
    Residential camp for children. A variety of outdoor
and educational activities are planned to enhance learning and improve socialization skills. Arts and crafts and
nature study are emphasized, and adventure activities include canoeing, paddle boating, swimming and other outdoor sports. This program is designed to be both fun and
educational for each participant.

Department of the Interior
Coordinating Committee on Accessibility for People
with Disabilities
Website: http://www.pn.usbr.gov/doiacc/

Girl Scouts of the USA
420 5th Avenue
New York, New York 10018-2798
(800) GSUSA 4 U
Email: misc@girlscouts.org
            (see website for specific department)
Website: http://www.gsusa.org/

Great Outdoors Recreation Pages (GORP)
    GORP is the largest and most extensive website for
planning outdoor and adventure activities. This site provides much information on outdoor resources and accessibility for people with disabilities.
Website: http://www.gorp.com/

International Orienteering Federation
Website: http://www.orienteering.org/

National Center on Accessibility
5020 State Road 67 North
Martinsville, Indiana 46151
(765) 349-9240 (voice/TTY)
(765) 342-6658 (fax)
Email: nca@indiana.edu
Website: http://www.indiana.edu/~nca/

National Forest Recreation
Website: http://www.fs.fed.us/recreation

National Park Service
1849 C Street NW
Washington, DC 20240
(202) 208-6843
Website: http://www.nps.gov/

National Sports Center for the Disabled (NSCD)
P.O. Box 1290
Winter Park, CO 80482
(970) 726-1540
(970) 726-4112 (fax)
Website: http://www.nscd.org

Outdoor Buddies, Inc.
P.O. Box 37283
Denver CO 80237
(303) 771-8216
(303) 771-9002 (fax)
Email: outbud@aol.com.
Website: http://www.outdoorbuddies.com/

Outdoor Explorations
98 Winchester Street
Medford, MA 02155
(781) 395-4999
(781) 395-4183 (fax)
(781) 395-4184 (TTY)
Email: Information@outdoorexp.org
Website: http://www.outdoorexp.org/

Outdoor Recreation Coalition of America (ORCA)
2475 Broadway, Suite 100
Boulder, CO 80304
(303) 444-3353
(303) 444-3284
Email: info@orca.org
Website: http://www.orca.org/

ORCA is the trade association for the outdoor recreation industry. They advocate for various federal policies and issues related to outdoor recreation.

Recreation.Gov
Website: http://www.recreation.gov/

Recreation.Gov is a partnership among federal land management agencies aimed at providing a single, easy-to-use web site with information about all federal recreation areas. The site allows you to search for recreation areas by state, by recreational activity, by agency, or by map.

National Sports Center for the Disabled
P.O. Box 1290
Winter Park, CO 80482
(970) 726-1540
(970) 726-4112 (fax)
Email: info@nscd.org
Website: http://www.nscd.org

Turning P.O.I.N.T. (Paraplegics on Independent Nature Trips)
4144 North Central Expressway, Suite 130
Dallas, TX 75204
(214) 827-7404
(214) 827-6468 (fax)
Email: pointntl@aol.com
Website: http://www.turningpoint1.com

SPLORE
27 West 3300 South
Salt Lake City, Utah 84115
(801) 484-4128
(801) 484-4177 (fax)
Email: info@splore.org
Website: http://www.splore.org

SPLORE's mission is to provide life-enhancing wilderness recreation and education to people of all abilities, including people with disabilities and special needs. SPLORE programs lead to increased health, wellness and community integration while promoting environmental stewardship.

United States Adaptive Recreation Center
P.O. Box 2897
Big Bear Lake, CA 92315
(909) 584-0243
Website: http://www.usarc.org

United States Orienteering Federation
P.O.Box 1444
Forest Park, GA 30298
(404) 363 2110
(404) 363 2110 (fax)
Email: rshannonhouse@mindspring.com
Website: http://www.us.orienteering.org/

Wheelchair Outdoor Adventure Camp (Challenge Aspen)
(800) 530-3901
(970) 923-0578

This camp held at various ties each year offers indoor and outdoor climbing activities, off-road wheelchair adventure and white water rafting.

Wheelin Sportsmen of America
5459 Troy Highway
Montgomery, AL 3616-5143
888-832-6967
334-286-8446
Fax: 334-286-8447
Website: http://www.wheelin-sportsmen.org

Wilderness Inquiry
808 14th Ave SE
Minneapolis, MN 55414
(612) 676-9400
(800) 728-0719
(612) 676-9401 (fax)
Email: info@wildernessinquiry.org
Website: http://www.wildernessinquiry.org/

Wilderness On Wheels Foundation
3131 Vaughn Way, Suite 305
Aurora, CO 80014
(303) 751.3959
Email: wow@ecentral.com
Website: http://www.wildernessonwheels.org/

World T.E.A.M. Sports
2108 South Boulevard, Suite 101
Charlotte, NC 28203
(704) 370-6070
(704) 370-7750
Website: http://www.worldteamsports.org

Videos

"Beyond the Barriers"
No Limits
11983 Snowpeak Way
Truckee, CA 96161
(800) 742-0248
Email: info@nolimitstahoe.com
Website: http://www.nolimitstahoe.com
Features the adventures of Mark Wellman and others with physical disabilities as they climb, surf, sail and dive.

BIBLIOGRAPHY

Blazing Trails (1999). *Sports 'n Spokes, 25*(8)34-37.
Cordova, J. & Jones, T. (2000). Cool Running. *Paraplegia News, 54*(9)14-17.
Rogers, D. (2000). To The Top: Future Challenge Courses Offer Access for Persons with Disabilities. *Park & Recreation, 35*(3)76-85.
Sadowsky, D. (1998). No Limits: Adventure Skills Workshop. *Sports 'n Spokes, 24*(5)20-23.
Wellman, M. (1999). Risky Business. *Sports 'n Spokes, 25*(7)9-11.

Chapter 46

Wrestling

SPORT GOVERNING BODIES:
National: USA Wrestling (USAW)
International: Federation of Associated Wrestling Styles (FILA)

Official Sport Of:	_____DAAA	_x_USABA	_____USCPAA
	_____DS/USA	_x_USADSF	_____WS/USA
	_*_SOI		

*prohibited

DISABLED SPORTS ORGANIZATION:
National:
International:

PRIMARY DISABILITY: Blind and Visually Impaired, Deaf and Hearing Impaired

SPORT OVERVIEW

For many years, wrestling has enabled individuals with certain disabilities to compete on an equal basis with their nondisabled peers. Scrapbooks from across the country are filled with stories about high school and college athletes with disabilities participating and succeeding in wrestling, in inclusive (nondisabled vs. disabled) and disabled only (blind and deaf) competition. For this reason, wrestling may be seen as an excellent activity to foster inclusion in physical education classes at the secondary level.

Only two disabled sports organizations, the United States Association for Blind Athletes and the USA Deaf Sports Federation (United States Deaf Wrestling Association), offer wrestling as an official sport. Many athletes from each organization wrestle in high school and college against nondisabled opponents.

Competition is usually conducted in free-style wrestling, however Greco-Roman wrestling has been used at various demonstration events (Figure 46.1).

Wrestling was a promising sport in Special Olympics until it was prohibited by the organization in the mid 1980's. It was determined that this sport and others do not meet SOI's minimum health or safety standards and may expose Special Olympics athletes to unreasonable risks to their health and safety.

SPORT ORIGIN

Wrestling maintains a modest history in sports for people with disabilities. Wrestling for people with visual impairments is sanctioned as an official sport through the International Blind Sports Association (IBSA), but is not an official sport in Paralympic Games even though it was included in the 1984 Paralympic Games. Although many countries have shown some interest in developing this sport, presently only the United States, Canada and Iran have well-established programs due the exposure of the sport in physical education classes.

Wrestling is included as an official sport in the Summer World Games for the Deaf.

RULE ADAPTATIONS

Both the USABA and the USADSF use the official rules of USA Wrestling, the national governing body of wrestling in the United States. One reason for the success of wrestling as an inclusionary sport in physical education classes and other events, is the lack of rule modifications or adapted equipment needed to participate. Generally the rules for individuals who are blind or deaf are identical to those who can see or hear. Although some blind wrestlers choose to participate without modifications, one major adaptation for blind wrestlers is the touch start (Figure 46.2). It is required that the two competitors maintain contact with each other throughout the competition. To begin the match, both competitors assume a standing position and overlap hands. Physical contact must be maintained through the match between the two wrestlers. Once contact is broken, the match will be stopped until contact is reestablished.

For individuals who are deaf, the use of visual or tactile cues by referees seem to be the only modification required.

EQUIPMENT

Equipment used in wrestling is similar for those with or without disabilities and includes items such as uniforms, shoes, mouth guards, and head protection. Information on hundreds of athletic equipment suppliers can be found on the Athletic Business Buyers Guide at <www.athleticbusiness.com>.

EQUIPMENT SUPPLIERS

Helmets

Cliff Keen Athletic
1235 Rosewood
Ann Arbor, MI 48106
(734) 769-9555
(734) 769-0412 (fax)
(800) 992-0799
Email: info@cliffkeen.com

Throw Dummies

Marty Gilman Inc.
30 Gilman Road
Gilman, CT 06336
(800) 243-0398
(860) 889-7334
(860) 823-1859 (fax)
Email: gilmangear@aol.com

Uniforms

Betlin Inc.
1445 Marion Road
Columbus, OH 43207
(614) 443-0248
(614) 443-4658 (fax)
(800) 923-8546
Email: info@betlin.com

Champion Products Inc.
475 Corporate Square Drive
P.O. Box 1550
Winston Salem, NC 27102
(910) 519-6658
(910) 519-7908 (fax)

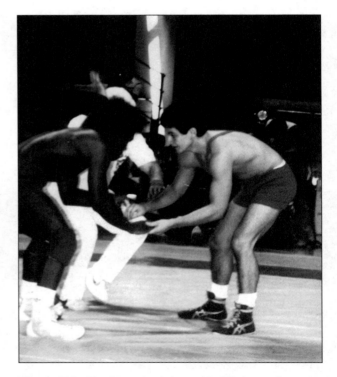

Figure 46.2. The finger touch is used in blind wrestling competition as a starting position at the beginning of each match, and each time the wrestlers are separated. (Courtesy of Specialized Sports Unlimited)

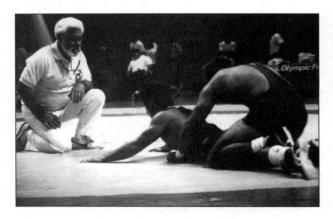

Figure 46.1. Demonstration wrestling event for blind athletes at the United States Olympic Festival. (Courtesy of Specialized Sports Unlimited)

Martin Sales Inc.
P.O. Box 16801
Stamford, CT 06905
(203) 323-5555
(203) 323-0188 (fax)
(888) 441-5090
Email: d.and.j.martin@worldnet.att.net

Protectors, Mouth & Teeth

Everlast
750 E. 132nd St.
Bronx, NY 10454
(718) 993-0100
(718) 665-4116 (fax)

ADDITIONAL RESOURCES AND WEBSITES

Wrestlers will find many websites related to their sport. Because this sport is accessible for those with and without disabilities, most participants will find the following sites satisfactory for gathering information.

Canadian Amateur Wrestling Association
1600 James Naismith Drive, #505
Gloucester, Ontario K1B 5N4
Canada
(613) 748-5686
(613) 748-5756 (fax)
Website: http://www.wrestling.ca/home.html

Intermat Wrestling
Website: http://www.Intermatwrestle.com
This site provides the ultimate amateur wrestling resource.

International Blind Sports Association IBSA)
Website: http://www.ibsa.es

International Federation of Associated Wrestling Styles (FILA)
Avenue Juste-Olivier 17
CH-1006 Lausanne, Switzerland
 (41-21) 312-8426
 (41-21) 323-6073 (fax)
Website: http://www.fila-wrestling.org
This site offers the most comprehensive listing of wrestling related links.

USA Wrestling
6155 Lehman Drive
Colorado Springs, CO 80918
(719) 598-8181
(719) 598-9440 (fax)
Email: usaw@concentric.net
Website: http://www.usawrestling.org
The home page of the National Governing Body for wrestling.

United States Deaf Wrestling Association
Maurice Abenchuchan
(904) 797-5695
(904) 823-4203 (fax)
Email: abenchm@mail.fim.edu

Appendix A
Sport Organizations and Resources

Aquatics

Federation Internationale de Natation Amateur (FINA)
Ave. de Beaumont 9
1012 Lausanne, Switzerland
Website: http://www.fina.org

US Aquatic Association of the Deaf (USAAD)
Carrie Miller, Director
6808 40th Ave NE
Seattle, WA 98115
(206) 616-6143 (TTY)
Email: cmiller@ocean.washington.edu
Email: USAAD@hotmail.com
Website: http://members.tripod.com/USAAD/

US Wheelchair Swimming
C/o Liz DeFrancesco
5730 Chambertin Drive
San Jose, CA 95118
(408) 267-0200
(408) 2672834 (fax)

USA Swimming
One Olympic Plaza
Colorado Springs, CO 80909
(719) 578-4578
Email: ussinfo@usa-swimming.org
Website: http://www.usa-swimming.org/

United States Masters Swimming
P.O. Box 185
Londonderry NH 03053-0185
(603) 537-0203
(603) 537-0204 (fax)
Email: usms@usms.org.
Website: http://www.usms.org/

Archery

International Archery Federation (FITA)
Avenue de Cour 135
1007 Lausanne, Switzerland
41-21-614-3050

41-21-614-3055 (fax)
Email: fita@worldcom.ch
Website: http://www.archery.org

National Archery Association
One Olympic Plaza
Colorado Springs, CO 80909-5778
(719) 578-4576
(719) 632-4733 (fax)
Email: info@usarchery.org
Website: http://www.USArchery.org

National Archery Assn.- Wheelchair Archers USA
Lyn Rourke
528 N. Bauman Street
Indianapolis, IN 46214
317-244-2377
Email: LMR1970@aol.com

National Field Archery Association
31407 Outer I-10
Redlands, CA 92372
(909) 794-2133
(800) 811-2331
(909) 794-8512 (fax)
Website: http://www.nfaa-archery.org/

Physically Challenged Bowhunters of America (PCBA)
Karen Vought
RD#1, Box 470
New Alexandria, PA 15670-9240
(724) 668-7439
Email: mkvought@westol.com
Website: http://www.bowhunting.net/pcba/

United Foundation For Disabled Archers (UFFDA)
Dan Hendricks
P.O. Box 250,
29th Ave
Glenwood, MN 65334
(320) 634-3660
Email: dhendricks@hunting.net
Website: http://www.hunting.net/uffda/

Basketball

Canadian Wheelchair Basketball Association
1600 James Naismith Dr.
Gloucester, Ontario
K1B 5N4 Canada
(613) 841-1824
(613) 841-5151 (fax)
Email: cwba@cwba.ca
Website: http://www.cwba.ca/

International Basketball Federation (FIBA)
P O Box 70 06 07, D-81306
MÜNCHEN, Germany
Tel:+49 89 7481 580 Fax:+49 89 7481 5833
Email: secretariat@office.fiba.com
Website: http://www.fiba.com/

International Wheelchair Basketball Federation (IWBF)
Robert J Szyman, Secretary General
5142 Ville Maria Lane
Hazelwood, MO 63042–1646
(314) 209 9006
(314) 739 6688 (fax)
Email: iwbfsecgen@aol.com
Website: http://www.iwbf.org/

National Wheelchair Basketball Association
Charlotte Institute of Rehabilitation
c/o Adaptive Sports/Adventures
1100 Blythe Blvd.
Charlotte, NC 28203
(704) 355-1064
(704) 466-4999 (fax)
Website: http://www.nwba.org/

Beep Baseball

National Beep Baseball Association
Email: Beepball@nancecomputerservices.com
               or info@nbba.org
Website: http://www.nancecomputerservices.com
               or http:://www.nbba.org

Michael Garrett, NBBA President
4427 Knottynold
Houston, TX 77053

Jeanette Bigger
Secretary, NBBA
2231 West First Street,
Topeka, Kansas 66606

Boating
Kayaking And Canoeing

America Canoe Association
7432 Alban Station Blvd, Suite B-232

Springfield, Virginia 22150
(703) 451-0141
(703) 451-2245 (fax)
Website: http://www-acanet.org

Canadian Recreational Canoeing Association
P.O. Box 398
446 Main St.
West Merrickville, ON
Canada, KDG 1NO
(888) 252-6292
Website: http://www.crca.ca

Federation Internationale de Canoe (FIC)
Dozsa Gyorgy ut 1-3
1143 Budapest, Hungary
Email: icf_hq_budapest@mail.datanet.hu
Website: http://www.datanet.hu/icf_hq/

USA Canoe/Kayak (USACK)
P.O. Box 789 (421 Old Military Rd.)
Lake Placid, NY 12946
Email: USCKT@aol.com
Website: http://www.usacanoekayak.org

United States Canoe Association (USCA)
606 Ross Street
Middletown, OH 45044-5062
(513) 422-3739 (phone/fax)
Email: uscamack@aol.com
Website: http://usca-canoe-kayak.org/

Sailing

Blind Sailing International (BSI)
c/o The Carroll Center for the Blind
770 Centre Street
Newton, MA
(617) 969-6200
Website: http://www.blindsailing.org/

International Foundation for Disabled Sailors (IFDS)
Website: http://ifds.org/

International Sailing Federation (ISAF)
Ariadne House, Town Quay
Southhampton
SO14 2AQ, United Kingdom
Email: sail@isaf.co.uk
Website: http://www.sailing.org

ISAF Disabled Sailing information.
Website: http://sailing.org/disabled/

United States Sailing (USS)
Website: http://www.ussailing.org/

United States Sailing Association Sailors with Special Needs (USSA-SWSN)
Website: http://www.ussailing.org/swsn

Boccia

International Bocce Association
187 Proctor Boulevard
Utica, New York 13501
(315) 733-9611
Website: http://www.borg.com/~iba/index.html

U.S. Bocce Federation
920 Harbor Drive
Martinez, CA 94553
(510) 229-2157

World Bocce Association
1098 West Irving Park Road
Bensenville, IL 60106
(630) 860-2623
(630) 595-2541 (fax)
Email: Mr. Bocce@worldbocce.org
Website: http://www.worldbocce.org/USA/

Bowling

American Blind Bowling Association (ABBA)
315 N. Main
Houston, PA 15342
(724) 745-5986

American Bowling Congress (ABC)
5301 S. 76th St.
Greendale, WI 53129-1127
(414) 421-6400
(414) 421-1194 (fax)
Email: sjames@bowl.com
Website: http://www.bowl.com

American Wheelchair Bowling Association (AWBA)
6264 N. Andrews Ave.
Ft. Lauderdale, FL 33309
(954) 491-2886 (phone/fax)
Website: http://www.amwheelchairbowl.qpg.com/
   or http://members.aol.com/bowlerweb/awba.htm

Federation Internationale des Quilleurs (FIQ)
1631 Mesa Ave., Suite A
Colorado Springs, CO 80906
Email: bowling@fiq.org
Website: www.fiq.org

The National Bowling Association Inc.
National Office Headquarters
377 Park Avenue, South, 7th Floor
New York, New York 10016

(212) 689-8308/8309
(212) 725-5063 (fax)
Website: http://www.trbainc.org

United States Deaf Bowling Federation (USDBF)
Connie Marchione, Liaison and Coach
8071 Cherrystone Avenue
Panorama City, CA 91402-5414
(818) 785-1478 (TTY)
(818) 785-1478 (fax)
Website   http://hometown.aol.com/kchodak/myhome-page/profile.html

USA Bowling
5301 South 76th Street
Greendale, WI 53129-0500
E-mail: cpon@bowl.com
Website: http://www.bowl.com

Women's International Bowling Congress (WIBC)
5301 S. 76th St.
Greendale, WI 53129-1191
(414) 421-9000
(414) 421-4420 (fax)
Email: ssavet@bowl.com
Website: http://www.bowl.com

Young American Bowling Alliance (YABA)
5301 S. 76th St.
Greendale, WI 53129-1192
(414) 421-4700
(414) 421-1301 (fax)
Email: jjocha@bowl.com
Website: http://www.bowl.com

Cycling

International Cycling Union (UCI)
Casa Postale 84 (37 Route de Chavannes)
1000 Lausanne 23, Switzerland (1007)
Email: Admin@uci.ch
Website: http://www.uci.ch

The Tandem Club of America (TCA)
Website: http://www.tandemclub.org

United States Handcycling Federation
(831) 457-7747 (for general information)
C/0 Wheelchair Sport USA
3395 E. Fountain Blvd., L-1
Colorado Springs, CO 80910
(719) 574-1150 (for membership information)
(719) 574-9840 (fax)
Email: info@ushf.org
Website: http://www.ushf.org

USA Cycling
One Olympic Plaza
Colorado Springs, Co 80909-5775
(719) 578-4581
(719) 578-4596 (fax)
Email: usac@usacycling.org
Website: http:// www.usacycling.org

United States Deaf Cycling Association (USDCA)
C/0 USA Deaf Sports Federation
3607 Washington Blvd., Suite 4
Ogden, UT 84403-1737
(801) 393-7916 Office
   (TTY: use your state relay service)
(801) 393-2263 (fax)
Email: usadsf@aol.com
Website: http://www.usadsf.org
Website:
   http://home.earthlink.net/~skedsmo/usdca.htm
   (for USDCA)

Equestrian

American Competition Opportunities for Riders With
Disabilities (ACORD) Inc.
5303 Felter Road
San Jose, CA 95132
(408) 261-2015
(408) 261-9438 (fax)

American Horse Shows Association Inc.
4047 Iron Works Parkway
Lexington, Kentucky 40511
(606) 258-2472
(606) 231-6662 (fax)
Website: http://www.ahsa.org

American Quarter Horse Association (AQHA)
P.O. Box 200.
Amarillo, TX 79168
(806) 376-4811
Website: http://www.aqha.org

Federation Equestre Internationale (FEI)
Avenue Mon-Repos 24
P.O. Box 157
1000 Lausanne 5
Switzerland
(41) 21 310 47 47
(41) 21 310 47 60 (fax)
Website: http://www.horsesport.org

International Paralympic Committee
Equestrian Chairperson
Mrs. Jonquil Solt
Blackdown Farm

Leamington Spa
Warwickshire, CV32 6QS
United Kingdom
44-1926-422-522
44-1926-450-996 (fax)

North American Riding for the Handicapped Association
P.O. Box 33150
Denver, CO 80233
(800) 369-RIDE (7433)
(303) 452-1212
(303) 252-4610 (fax)
(303) 457-8496 (Fax-on-Demand)
Email: Narha@narha.org
Website: http://www.narha.org

Fencing

Canadian Fencing Federation
1600 Prom. James Naismith Drive
Gloucester, ON K1B 5N4
(613) 748-5633
(613) 748-5742 (fax)
Website: http://www.fencing.ca

Federation International d'Escrime (FIE)
Avenue Mon Repos 24
Case Postale 2743
1002 Lausanne, Switzerland
(41-21) 320-3115
(41-21) 320-3116 (fax)
Website: http://www.fie.ch

International Wheelchair Fencing Committee:
Alberto Martinez Vassallo, President
Somatenes 3
08950 Esplugas (Barcelona)
Spain
34-3-4736083 (tel/fax)

United States Fencing Association (USFA)
One Olympic Plaza
Colorado Springs, CO 80909-5774
(719) 578-4511
(719) 632-5737 (fax)
Email: usfencing@aol.com
Website: http://www.usfa.org

USFA National Wheelchair Fencing Coach:
Leszek Stawicki
1609 Ellwood Avenue, #C4
Louisville, KY 40204
(502) 568-6781

Chairman, USFA Wheelchair Fencing Committee:
Marcella Denton

4009 Woodgate Lane
Louisville, KY 40220
(502) 582-5734 (Day)
(502) 491-6883 (Evening)
Email: Marcella.M.Denton@lrl02.usace.army.mil

Wheelchair Sports-USA
US Fencing—Disabled Committee
Bill Murphy
306 Candler Street
Atlanta, GA 30307
404-523-7421
Email: wtmaw@atl.mindspring.com

Fishing

Buckmasters Online
Website: http://buckmasters.rivals.com/

Fishing Has No Boundaries, Inc.
P.O. Box 175
Hayward, WI 54843
(800) 243-3462
(715) 634-3185
Email: info@fhnbinc.org
Website: http://www.fhnbinc.org/

PVA National Bass Trail
Website: http://www.pva.org/basstrail/index.htm

Project Access
Website: http://www.projectaccess.com/

The U.S. Fish and Wildlife Service
Department of the Interior
1849 C Street NW
Washington DC 20240
Email: Contact@fws.gov
              (see FAQ before using email)
Website: http://www.fws.gov/

Fitness Programming

The Aerobics and Fitness Association of America
15250 Ventura Blvd., Suite 200
Sherman Oaks, CA, 91403-3297
(877) 968-2639
(818) 788-6301 (fax)
Website: http://www.afaa.com

American College of Sports Medicine (ACSM)
401 W. Michigan St., Indianapolis, IN 46202-3233
(317) 637-9200
(317) 634-7817 (fax)
Website: http://www.acsm.org/

American Council on Exercise
5820 Oberlin Drive, Suite 102
San Diego, CA 92121-3787
(858) 535-8227
(858) 535-1778 (fax)
Website: http://www.acefitness.org/

American Running Association (ARA)
4405 East West Highway, Suite 405
Bethesda, MD 20814
(301) 913-9517
(800) 776-2732
(301) 913-9520 (fax)
Email: run@americanrunning.org
Website: http://www.americanrunning.org/

Disabled Sports USA (Fitness Department)
451 Hungerford Drive Suite 100
Rockville, MD 20850
 (301) 217-0968 (fax)
(301) 217-0963 (TTY)
(301) 217-9839
Email: programs@dsusa.org
Website: http://www.dsusa.org/

Healthy People 2010
Website: http://www.health.gov/healthypeople/
     This website provided information on all the goals
and objectives of Healthy People 2010.

National Strength and Conditioning Association
1955 N. Union Blvd.
Colorado Springs, CO 80909
(719) 632-6722
(800) 815-6826
(719) 632-6367 (fax)
Email: nsca@nsca-lift.org
Website: http://www.nsca-lift.org/

Football

Santa Barbara Parks and Recreation Department
620 Laguna Street, PO Box 1990
Santa Barbara, CA 93102-1990
(805) 564-5418
Website:
     http://ci.santa-barbara.ca.us/departments/
parks_and_recreation/recreation

Developmental & Adapted Programs (Blisterbowl)
Cabrillo Bathhouse
1118 East Cabrillo Boulevard
Santa Barbara, CA 93103
(805) 564-5421

United States Flag Football Federation
USA Deaf Sports Federation
3607 Washington Blvd. #4
Ogden, UT 84403-1737
(801) 393-7916 (TTY)
(801) 393-2263 (fax)
Email: HomeOffice@USADSF.Org
Website: http://www.USADSF.org

Universal Wheelchair Football Association
John Kraimer
Disability Services
University of Cincinnati- Raymond Walthers College
9555 Plainfield Road
Cincinnati, OH 45236-1096.
(513) 792-8625
(513) 792-8624 (fax)
(513)743-8300 (TTY)
Email: john.kraimer@uc.edu

Warm Spring Sports (Spoke Bender Bowl)
5101 Medical Drive
San Antonio, Texas 78229
(210) 592-5358
Email: sports@warmsprings.org
Website: http://www.warmsprings.org

Goalball

USABA
Women's Head Goalball Coach Men's Head Goalball
Coach
Ken Armbruster (719) 550-1120   Tom Parrigin (904)
824-0260

Goalball New Zealand
Website:
    http://www.blindsport.org.nz/pagegoalball.html

IBSA Goalball Site:
Website: http://www.ibsa.es/sports/goalball.html

Michigan Association for Competitive Goalball Homepage
Website: http://www.bestmidi.com/goalball/

Golf

Association of Disabled American Golfers
PO Box 2647
Littleton, CO 80161-2647
(303) 922-5228
Email: adag@usga.org
Website: http://www.adag.org

Eastern Amputee Golf Association (EAGA)
2015 Amherst Dr.
Bethlehem, PA 18015-5606
(888) 868-0992
(610) 867-9295 (fax)
Email: info@eaga.org
Website: http://www. EAGA.org/

The First Tee
170 Highway A1A North
Ponte Vedra Beach, FL 32082
(904)940-4300
(904)280-9019 (fax)
Website: http://www.thefirsttee.com/

Fore All!
PO Box 2456
Kensington, MD 20891-2456
(301) 881-1818
(301) 881-2828 (fax)
Email: fore_all@juno.com
Website: http://www.foreall.org

Fore Hope, Inc.
c/o Darby Dan Farm
925 Darby Creek Drive
Galloway, Ohio 43119
(614) 870-7299
(614) 870-7245 (fax)
Email: fore.hope@gateway.net

Get A Grip
552 W. Berridge Lane
Phoenix, AZ 85013
(602) 728-0218
Email: GetaGripRw@aol.com
Website: http://www.getagripgolf.com
                Video: Adaptive Golf and the Therapist

HandiGolf Foundation
c/o Andrew Greasley
Stone Cottage, Lanton Road
Stratton Audley, Oxen
England OX6 9BW
Tel: 01869 277369

International Blind Golf Association
Derrick Sheridan - President
25 Langhams Way, Wargrave, Berks,
RG10 8AX, England
Email: Derrick@Sheridan25.freeserve.co.uk
Website:
    http://www.blindgolf.com/International/about_us.htm

National Amputee Golf Association (NAGA)
Dan Cox, Executive Director
P.O.Box 23285
Milwaukee, WI 53223-0285
(800) 633-NAGA
(414) 376-1268 (fax)
Email: info@nagagolf.org
Website: http://www.nagagolf.org

National Center on Accessibility
Gary Robb, Director
5040 State Road 6/ N.
Martinville, IN 46151
(765) 349-9240
(765) 349-1086 (fax)
Email: nca@indiana.edu
Website: http://www.indiana.edu/~nca

National Golf Foundation
1150 U.S. Highway One
Jupiter, FL 33477
(800) 733-6006
Website: http://www.ngf.org/

Physically Challenged Golfers Association, Inc.
Brian Magna, Exec. Dir.
Avondale Medical Center
34 Dale Rd—Suite 001
Avon, CT 06001
(860) 676-2035
(860) 676-2041
Email: pcga@townusa.com
Website: http://www.townusa.com/pcga/index.html

The Professional Golfers' Association of America (PGA)
100 Avenue of the Champions
P.O. Box 109601
Palm Beach Gardens, FL 33410-9601
(407) 624-8400
(407) 624-8439 (fax)
Website: http://www.PGA.com/

United States Blind Golf Association (USBGA)
Bob Andrews, President
3094 Shamrock St. North
Tallahassee, FL 32308-2735
(850) 893-4511 (tel./fax)
Email: USBGA@blindgolf.com
Website: http://www.blindgolf.com

United States Golf Association (USGA)
P.O. Box 708

Far Hills, NJ 07931
(908) 234-2300
(908) 234-9687 (fax)
Email: usga@usga.org
Website: http://www.usga.org/

Walking Impaired Golfers of America
Fred L. Montgomery, Director
PO Box 1058
Los Altos, CA 94022
(877) 480-9442
Email: wiga@mindspring.com
Website: http://www.wiga.org

Western Amputee Golf Association (WAGA)
5980 Sun Valley Way
Sacramento, CA 95823
(800) 592-WAGA
Website: http://www.wagatales@aol.com

Hockey

Electric Wheelchair Hockey

Canadian Electric Wheelchair Hockey Association (CEWHA)
Email: info@wheelchairhockey.com
Website: http://www.wheelchairhockey.com

United States Electric Wheelchair Hockey Association (U.S.EWHA)
7216 39th Ave. No.
Minneapolis, MN 55427
(612) 535-4736
Email: hockey@usewha.org
Website: http://www.usewha.org/

Floor Hockey

Special Olympics
1325 G Street, NW, Suite 500
Washington, DC 20005-3104
(202) 628-3630
(202) 824-0200 (fax)
Email: SOImail@aol.com
Website: www.specialolympics.org

Hearing Impaired Hockey

American Hearing Impaired Hockey Association
1143 West Lake Street
Chicago, IL 60607
(312) 829-2250

Sled Hockey

International Paralympic. Committee Sledge Hockey Page
Website:
http://www.paralympic.org/sports/sections/sledge-hockey.asp

Ottawa-Carleton Sledge Hockey & Ice Picking Association
46 Nestow Dr.
Nepean, Ontario
K2G 3X8, Canada

Sledge Hockey of Canada
P.O. Box 20063
Ottawa, Ontario
K1N 5W0 Canada
(888) 857-8555
(613) 723-5799
(613) 226-2050 (fax)
Email: shoc@shoc.ca
Website: http:// www.shoc.ca/

United States Sled Hockey Association
21 Summerwood Court
Buffalo, NY 14223
(716) 876) 7390
Email: Info@sledhockey.org
Website: http://www.sledhockey.org/

Visually Impaired Hockey

Western Association of Persons with Vision Impairment (WAPVI)
The Vancouver Blind Hockey Program
110 - 5055 Joyce St.
Vancouver, B.C.
V5R 4G7 Canada
Email: office@wapvi.bc.ca
Website: http://www.wapvi.bc.ca

Wheelchair Hockey

Disabled Athletes Floor Hockey League
Southeast Association for Special Parks & Recreation
6000 S. Main St.
Downers Grove, IL 60516

Michigan Wheelchair Hockey League
Email: andyice@aol.com
Website: http://www.scorezone.com/wchl/

Sports on Wheels
1591 South Sinclair St.
Anaheim, CA 92806
(714) 939-8727
(714) 978-2891 (fax)

Other

International Ice Hockey Federation
Parkring 11
8002 Zurich
Switzerland
+41-1-289 86 00
+41-1-289 86 22 (fax)
Email: iihf@iihf.com
Website: http://www.iihf.com/

USA Hockey
1775 Bob Johnson Drive
Colorado Springs, CO 80906-4090
(719) 576-USAH
(719) 538-1160 (fax)
Website: http://www.usahockey.com/

Hunting

Bowhunting Net
Website: http://www.bowhunting.net/

Buckmasters On-Line
David Sullivan
Director, Disabled Sportsman Resources
11802 Creighton Avenue
Northport, Alabama 35475
Email: dsullivan@buckmasters.com
Website: http://buckmasters.rivals.com/

Outdoor Buddies, Inc.
PO Box 37283
Denver, Colorado 80273
(303) 771-8216
Email: outbud@juno.com
Website: http://www.outbud.freeservers.com/

Capable Partners
P.O. Box 28543
St. Paul, MN 55128
(612) 542-8156
Email: comunications@capablepartners.org

Buckmasters Quadriplegic Hunters Association (BQHA)
Jeff Lucas
P.O. Box 117
Hyde Park, NY 12538
(914) 229-4131
Email: lucan1776@aol.com
Website: http://residents.bowhunting.net/Disabled-Hunters/

Disabled Hunters of North America Inc. (DHNA)
Email: normdhna@charter.net
Website: http://www.dhna.org

National Rifle Association (NRA)
NRA Disabled Shooting Services
C/o David Baskin
11250 Waples Mill Road
Fairfax, VA 22030
703-267-1495
703-267-3941 (fax)
Website: http://www.nra.org/
              http://www.nrahq.org/shooting/disabled/asp

North American Bowhunter
P.O. Box 251
Glenwood, MN 56334
(320) 634-3660
Email: dhendricks@hunting.net
Website: http://www.hunting.net/nab/

Physically Challenged Bowhunters of America (PCBA)
Karen Vought
RD#1, Box 470
New Alexandria, PA 15670-9240
(724) 668-7439
Email: mkvought@westol.com
Website: http://www.bowpcba-inc.org

Todd Albaugh's Handicapped Hunting Resource Guide
Website: http://www.ismi.net/handicapinfo/

United Foundation For Disabled Archers (UFFDA)
Dan Hendricks
P.O. Box 250,
29th Ave
Glenwood, MN 65334
(320) 634-3660
Email: dhendricks@hunting.net
Website: http://www.hunting.net/uffda/

Wheelin' Sportsmen Of America, Inc.
5510 Wares Ferry Rd., Suite G
Montgomery, AL 36117
(888) 832-6967
(334) 395-6300
(334) 395-6311 (fax)
Email: mail@wheelin-sportsmen.org
Website: http://www.wheelin-sportsmen.org/

Ice Skating/Picking

Amateur Speedskating Union National Office:
1033 Shady Lane, Glen Ellyn, IL 60137
(630) 790-3230
(630) 790-3235 (fax)
Email: ASUYates@aol.com
Website: http://speedskating.org/

International Skating Union (ISU)
Chemin de Primerose 2

CH 1007 Lausanne, Switzerland
(+41) 21 612 66 66
(+41) 21 612 66 77 (fax)
Email: info@isu.ch
Website: http://www.isu.org/

Ottawa-Carleton Sledge Hockey & Ice Picking Association
46 Nestow Dr.
Nepean, Ontario
K2G 3X8, Canada

Skating Association for the Blind and Handicapped, Inc. (SABAH)
120 East and West Road
West Seneca, NY 14224
(716) 675-7222
Email: sabah@sabahinc.org
Website: http://www.sabahinc.org/

United States Figure Skating Association
20 First Street
Colorado Springs, CO 80906-3697
(719) 635-5200
(719) 635-9548 (fax)
Email: usfsa@usfsa.org
Website: http://www.usfsa.org

United States Figure Skating Association
Special Olympic Committee
Website:
    http://hometown.aol.com/socommittee/index.htm

United States Speed Skating Association
P.O. Box 450639
Westlake, OH 44145
(440) 899-0128
Email: usskate@ix.netcom.com
Website: http://www.usspeedskating.org

Lawn Bowling

American Lawn Bowls Association
Email: woodyo@aol.com
Website: http://www.bowlsamerica.org/

Bowls Canada Boulingrin
1600 James Naismith Drive
Gloucester, Ontario
K1B 5N4 Canada
Phone: (613) 748-5643
Fax: (613) 748-5796
Email: office@bowlscanada.com
Website: http://www.bowlscanada.com/

International Paralympic Committee Lawn Bowl Section
Chairperson
Bob Tinker
2a First Avenue
Forestville 5035, Australia
+ 618 829 38139 (tel/fax)

Lawn Bowls International
Website: http://www.lawnbowls.com.au

Ontario Lawn Bowls Association
1185 Eglinton Avenue East
Suite 205
North York, Ontario M3C 3C6
(416) 426-7161
Email: olba@interlog.com
Website: http://www.interlog.com/~olba/index.html

World Bowls Board (WBB)
Secretary/Treasurer: David W Johnson.
Lyndhurst Road
Worthing, West Sussex
BN11 2AZ, England
National (01903) 820222
International +44 903 820222
International +44 903 820444

Martial Arts

Federation Mondaile de Karate (FMK/WKF)
122 Rue de la Tombe Issoire
75014 Paris, France
Email: support@wkf.net
Website: http://www.wkf.net

International Judo Federation (IJF)
101-1, Ulchi-Ro, 21st Floor Doosan Bldg., I-KA
Chung-Ku, Seoul, Korea
(82+2) 3398 1017
Email: yspark@ijf.org
Website: http:// www.ijf.org

International Disabled Self-Defense Association (IDSA)
22-C New Leicester Hwy., #259
Asheville, North Carolina 28806
(828)683-5528
(828)683-4691 (fax)
Email: info@defenseability.com
Website: http://www.defenseability.com/

Kenpo Karate: Wheelchair Self-defense Studio
562 Monterey Blvd.
San Francisco, CA 94127
(415) 586-8566

Martial Arts for the Handicapable, Inc.
22 Knight Rd.
Harrisburg, Pa. 17111
(717) 583-2150
Email: Yudncha@aol.com
Website: http://mahinc.net/

National Handicapable Martial Arts Association (NHMAA)
C/o D. Richard Eunice
112 East Gay Street
Lancaster, SC 29270
(803) 286-5155

Ron Scanlon's Kung Fu San Soo Academy
12740 Culver Blvd, Unit E.
Marina Del Rey, CA 90066
(310) 305-4144
Website: http://home.sprynet.com/~syzygy/Ron.htm

U.S. Taekwondo Union
One Olympic Plaza, Suite 405
Colorado Springs, CO 80909-5792
(719) 578-4632
(719) 578-4642
Email: USTUTKD1@aol.com
Website: http://www.ustu.org

USA Judo
One Olympic Plaza
Colorado Springs, CO 80909
Email: usjudoexdr@aol.com
Website: www.usjudo.org

USA National Karate-do Federation
P.O. Box 77083 Seattle, WA 98177-7083
(206) 440-8386
(206) 367-7557 (fax)
Email: karate@usankf.org
Website: http://www.usankf.org/

United States Judo Association
21 North Union Blvd.
Colorado Springs, CO USA 80909
(719) 633-7750
(719) 633-4041 (fax)

United States Judo Federation
P. O. Box 338
Ontario, OR 97914
(541) 889-8753
(541) 889-5836 (fax)
Email: natofc@usjf.com

United States Martial Arts Association
8011 Mariposa Avenue
Citrus Heights, CA 95610
(916) 727-1486
(916) 727-7236 (fax)
Email: psp4@flash.net
Website: http://www.mararts.org/

World Taekwondo Federation (WTF)
635 Yuksam-Dong, Kangnam-ku
Seoul 135-081 Korea
Email: wft@unitel.co.kr

Multisport

(US Based)

America's Athletes with Disabilities
Website: http://www.americasathletes.org

Disabled Sports, USA (DS-USA)
451 Hungerford Dr., Suite 100
Rockville, MD 20805
(301) 217-9838
(301) 217-0968 (FAX)
Email: information@dsusa.org
Website: http://www.dsusa.org/~dsusa/dsusa.html

Dwarf Athletic Association of America (DAAA)
418 Willow Way
Lewisville, TX 75067
(972) 317-8299
(972) 317-8299 (FAX)
Email: daaa@flash.net
Website: http://www.daaa.org/

Special Olympics, Inc. (SOI)
1325 G Street, NW, Suite 500
Washington, DC 20005-3104
(202) 628-3630
(202) 824-0200 (FAX)
Email: SOImail@aol.com
Website: http://www.specialolympics.org

United States Association for Blind Athletes (USABA)
33 North Institute Street
Colorado Springs, CO 80903
(719) 630-0422
(719) 630-0616 (FAX)
Email: usaba@usa.net
Website: http://www.usaba.org/

United States Cerebral Palsy Athletic Association
(USCPAA)

25 West Independence Way
Kingston, RI 02881
(401) 848-2460
(401) 848-5280 (FAX)
Email: uscpaa@mail.bbsnet.com
Website: http://www.uscpaa.org

USA Deaf Sports Federation (USADSF)
3607 Washington Blvd., Suite 4
Ogden, UT 84403-1737
(801) 393-7916 Office (tty: use your state relay service)
(801) 393-2263 (FAX)
Email: usadsf@aol.com
Website: http://www.usadsf.org

The United States Olympic Committee (USOC)
Disabled Sports Services Dept.
One Olympic Plaza
Colorado Springs, CO 80909-5760
(719) 578-4958 or 4818
(719) 578-4976 (FAX)
(719) 447-8773 (TTY)
Email: mark.shepherd@usoc.org
Website: http://www.usoc.com/

Wheelchair Sports USA (WS/USA)
3395 E. Fountain Blvd., L-1
Colorado Springs, CO 80910
(719) 574-1150
(719) 574-9840 (FAX)
Email: wsusa@aol.com
Website: http://www.wsusa.org/

(International Based)

Cerebral Palsy International Sports and Recreation
Association (CP-ISRA)
Secretariat CP-ISRA
Trudie Rombouts
P.O. Box 16
6666 ZG HETEREN, The Netherlands
Email: cpisra_nl@hotmail.com
Website: http://www.cpisra.org/

International Committee on Silent Sports (CISS)
814 Thayer Avenue, Suite #350
Silver Spring, Maryland 20910 USA
Email: info@ciss.org
Website: http://www.ciss.org/

International Blind Sports Association (IBSA)
Email: ibsa@ibsa.es
Website: http://www.ibsa.es/ibsa/ibsa.html

International Paralympic Committee (IPC)
Email: info@paralympic.org
Website: http://www.paralympic.org

International Stoke Mandeville Wheelchair Sports
Federation (ISMWSF)
Head Office
Olympic Village, Guttmann Road
Aylesbury
Bucks HP219PP, United Kingdom
Email: info@wsw.org.uk
Website: http://www.wsw.org.uk/

Powerlifting

International Powerlifting Federation
Email: mike@ipf.com
Website: http://www.powerlifting-ipf.com

International Weightlifting Federation (IWF)
Hold u.1
1374 Budapest, P.O.Box 614 Hungary
Email: iwf@iwf.net
Website: http://www.iwf.net

USA Powerlifting Disabled Athletes Committee
Fran Haley
12101 Reagan St.
Los Alamitos, CA 90720
(562) 596-6866

USA Weightlifting
One Olympic Plaza
Colorado Springs, CO 80909-5764
Email: usaw@worldnet.att.net
Website: http://www.usaweightlifting.org

USCPAA Sport Technical Officer (Powerlifting)
Michael McDevitt
8420 West Chester Pike
Upper Darby, PA 19082
(610) 356-1910
Website: http://www.uscpaa.org/

US Wheelchair Weightlifting Federation
Bill Hens (Director)
39 Michael Place
Levittown, PA 19057
(215) 945-1964
(215) 946-2574 (fax)
Website: http://www.wsusa.org/weightrule.htm (rules)

Quad Rugby

International Wheelchair Rugby Federation
Pawel Zbieranowski
67 Riverside Blvd.
Thornhill Ontario L4J 1H8 Canada
(905) 886-1252 (res)
(416) 396-6765 (bus)
(416) 396-6770 (fax)

Canadian Wheelchair Rugby Association
Marco DisPaltro – Chairman
1155 Monte Ste-Therese, # C
Bellefeuille, QC
J0R 1A0, Canada
(514) 585-5300
(514) 585-5300 (fax)

United States Quad Rugby Association
Kevin Orr
101 Park Place Circle
Alabaster, Alabama 35007
(205) 868-2281
(205) 868-2283 (fax)
Email: supersports@mindspring.com
Website: http://www.quadrugby.com

Racquetball

United States Racquetball Association
1685 West Uintah
Colorado Springs, CO 80904-2921
(719) 635-5396
(719) 635-0685 (fax)
Email: usragen@webaccess.net
Website: http://www.usra.org

International Racquetball Federation (IRF)
1685 West Uintah
Colorado Springs, CO 80904-2921
(719) 635-5396
(719) 635-0685 (fax)
Website:
   http://www.worldsport.com/worldsport/sports/rac-
quetball/home.html

Morris Adams, USRA Commissioner for Wheelchair
8644 Portola Circle, #12-A
Huntington Beach, CA 92645
714/969-5786 (H)

Road Racing

Achilles Track Club International
42 West 38th Street

New York, NY 10018
(212) 354-3978
(212) 354-3978
Email: AchillesClub@aol.com
Website: http://www.achillestrackclub.org/

All American Trail Running Association
PO Box 9175
Colorado Springs, CO 80932

American Ultrarunning Association (AUA)
Email: aua@americanultra.org

Challenge Alaska
Midnite Sun Ultra Challenge
P.O. Box 110065
Anchorage, AK 99511
(907) 344-7399
(907) 344-7349
Email: challenge@artic.net

International Amateur Athletic Federation
17 rue Princesse Florestine
BP 359
MC 98007 Monaco Cedex
(377) 93 10 88 88
(377) 93 15 95 15 (fax)
Email: headquarters@iaaf.org
Website: http://www.iaaf.org/

Road Runners Club of America (RRCA)
1150 South Washington, Suite 250
Alexandria, VA 22314
(703) 836-0558
(703) 836-4430 (fax)
Email: execdir@rrca.org
Website: http://www.rrca.org/

United States of America Deaf Track and Field
Website: http://members.tripod.com/~usadtf/

USA Track & Field
P.O. Box 120 (One RCA Dome, Suite 140)
Indianapolis, IN 46206-0120 (46225)
Email: USATFprogs@aol.com
Website: http://www.usatf.org
Website: http://www.usaldr.org/
               (USATF Road Running Information Center)

Wheelchair Racing Resource Page
Email: birzer@execpc.com
Website: http://www.execpc.com/~birzer/

Wheelchair Athletics of the USA
Barry Ewing
2351 Parkwood Road
Snellville, GA 30278
(770) 972-0763
(770) 985-4885 (fax)
Email: bewing@beilesouth.net

Roller Skating

Federation Internationale de Roller-Skating (FIRS)
Rambla Cataluna 80, piso 1
08008 Barcelona, Spain
Email: firs@idgrup.ibernet.com
Website: http://www.rollersport.org

Roller Skating Association International
6905 Corporate Drive
Indianapolis, IN 46278
(317) 347-2626
(317) 347-2636 (fax)
Website: http://www.rollerskating.org/

USA Roller Skating
P.O. Box 6579 (4730 South Street)
Lincoln, NE 68506
E-mail: usacrs@usacrs.com
Website: http://www.usarollerskating.com/

Special Olympics Director of Roller Skating
1325 G Street, NW, Suite 500
Washington, DC 20005-3104
(202) 628-3630
(202) 824-0200 (fax)
Email: SOImail@aol.com
Website: www.specialolympics.org

Scuba Diving

American Association of Challenged Divers
John Ellerbrock
P.O. Box 8862
Sparren Way
San Diego, CA 92129
(619) 538-3483
Email: pinnacle@cts.com

Divers Unlimbited
724 Loranne Ave. #1100
Pomona CA, 91767
(909) 623-2412 (voice/fax))
Email: Info@DiversUnlimbited.org
Website: http://www.diversunlimbited.org/

Diving Medicine Online
Diving With Disabilities
Website: http://www.gulftel.com/~scubadoc/

Eels on Wheels Adaptive Scuba Club
4020 Travis Country Circle
Austin, TX 78735
(512) 892-0863
Email: tskelley@sig.net
Website: http://www.eels.org/

Handicapped Scuba Association International (HSAI)
1104 El Prado
San Clemente, CA 92672
(949) 498-6128 (voice/fax)
Website: http://hsascuba.com

International Association for Handicapped Divers (IAHD)
Vargmötesvagen 4, SE- 186 30
Vallentuna, SWEDEN
Email: info@iahd.org
Website: http://www.iahd.org/

Moray Wheels
P.O. Box 1660 GMF
Boston, MA 02205
Email: Info@MorayWheels.org
Website: http://www.moraywheels.org/

National Association of Underwater Instructors (NAUI)
9942 Currie Davis Drive, Suite H
Tampa, FL 33619-2667
(800) 553-6284
(813) 628-6284.
Email: nauihq@nauiww.org
Website: http://www.naui.org/index-top.html

National Instructors Association for Divers with Disabilities (NIADD)
P.O. Box 112223
Campbell, CA 95011-2223
(408) 379-6536 or
(408) 244-4433
(408) 244- 8652 (fax)
Email: degnan@degnandivers.com

Open Waters Program
Alpha One
127 Main Street
South Portland, ME 04106
(207) 767-2189 (voice or TTY)
(800) 640-7200 (voice or TTY)

(207) 799-8346 (fax)
Email: info@alpha-one.org or Owscuba@aol.com
Website: http://www.alpha-one.org/

Professional Association of Diving Instructors (PADI)
30151 Tomas Street
Rancho Santa Margarita, CA 92688-2125
(800) 729-7234
(949) 858-7234
(949) 858-7264 (fax)
Website: http://www.padi.com/

Shooting

Amateur Trapshooting Association of America
601 W. National Road
Vandalia, Ohio 45377
(937) 898-4638
(937) 898-5472 (fax)
Email: Shootata@bright.net
Website: http://www.shootata.com/

International Shooting Committee for the Disabled (ISCD)
Email: wvl@bigfoot.com
Website: http://members.tripod.com/ShootISCD/

International Shooting Sport Federation (ISSF)
Bavariaring 21
D-80336 München, Germany
49-89-5443550
49-89-54435544 (fax)
Email: issfmunich@compuserve.com
Website: http://www.issf-shooting.org

National Wheelchair Shooting Federation
C/o David Baskin
NRA Disabled Shooting Services
11250 Waples Mill Road
Fairfax, VA 22030
703-267-1495
703-267-3941 (fax)
Website: http://www.nra.org/

Paralyzed Veterans of America (PVA) National Trapshoot Circuit
Paralyzed Veterans of America
80l 18th Street, NW
Washington, DC 20006 USA
(202) 872-1300
(800) 424-8200
Email: info@pva.org
Website:
http://www.pva.org/sports/trapshoot/trapoverview.htm

Single Action Shooting Society (TASS)
23255 La Palma Avenue
Yorba Linda, California 92887
(714) 694-1800;
(714) 694-1815 (fax)
Email: sasseot@aol.com
Website: http://www.sassnet.com

USA Shooting
One Olympic Plaza
Colorado Springs, CO 80909-5762
(719) 578-4670
Email: Admin.Info@usashooting.org
Website: http://www.usashooting.com

Showdown

British Columbia Blind Sports and Recreation Association
317-1367 West Broadway
Vancouver, British Columbia
Canada V6H 4A9
(604) 325-8638
(604) 325-1638 (fax)

IBSA Showdown Sub-committee
(604) 325-8638
(604) 325-1638 (fax)
Email: bcbs@express.ca

IBSA Showndown Site:
Website: http://www.ibsa.es/sports/showdown.html

IBSA Showdown Table Construction site:
Website: http://www.ibsa.es/sports/planos.html

Skiing

American Blind Skiing Foundation (ABSF)
227 East North Avenue
Elmhurst IL 60126
Email: ABSF@bigfoot.com
Website: http://www.absf.org/

Canadian Association for Disabled Skiing
P.O. Box 307
Kimberly, B.C. V1A 2Y9
(250) 427-7712
(250) 427-7715 (fax)
Email: info@disabledskiing.ca
Website: http://www.disabledskiing.ca/

Disabled Sports USA

The following website has a complete list of DSUSA chapters
Website: http://www.dsusa.org/chapter-state.htm

International Paralympic Committee
Website: http://www.paralympic.org
              For a complete set of rules.

Extreme Adaptive Sports
    This monoski and adaptive sport resource provides links and reviews of ski manufacturers
Website: http://www.sitski.com/

International Ski Federation (FIS)
Blochstrasse 2
3653 Oberhofen/Thunersee, Switzerland
Email: webmaster@fisski.ch
Website: http://www.fis-ski.com/home/default.sps

National Ability Center
P.O. Box 682799
Park City, UT 84068
(435) 649-3991
Website: http://www.nationalabilitycenter.org/

National Sports Center for the Disabled
P.O. Box 1290
Winter Park, CO 80482
(970) 726-1540
(970) 726-4112
Email: info@nscd.org
Website: http://www.nscd.org/

Ski Central
Website: http://skicentral.com/adaptive.html

Special Olympics Director of Alpine and Nordic Skiing
1325 G Street, NW, Suite 500
Washington, DC 20005-3104
(202) 628-3630
(202) 824-0200 (fax)
Email: SOImail@aol.com
Website: http://www.specialolympics.org

The U.S. Deaf Ski & Snowboarding Association (US-DSSA)
C/o U.S. Deaf Sports Federation
Website: http://www.usdssa.org/

U.S. Ski and Snowboard Association
Box 100
1500 Kearns Blvd.
Park City, UT 84060

(435) 649-9090
(435) 649-3613 (fax)
Email: special2@ussa.org
Website: http://www.usskiteam.com

United States Ski and Snowboard Association: Disabled Home Page
Linda Johnson
Prog. Mgr./Team Mgr.
(435) 647-2055
Email: ljohnson@ussa.org
Website: http://www.usskiteam.com/disabled/dis-abled.htm

Skydiving

Fédération Aéronautique Internationale (FAI)
Avenue Mon Repos 24
CH-1005 Lausanne, Switzerland
Phone: +41 21 345 1070
Fax: +41 21 345 1077
Email: info@fai.org
Website: http://www.fai.org/

Landings: Skydiving links
Website:
http://www.landings.com/_landings/pages/skydiving.html

Pieces of Eight Amputee Skydiving Team
Mike DiMenichi
13700 Alton #154
Irvine, CA 92718

United States Parachute Association (USPA)
1440 Duke St.
Alexandria, VA 22314
703-836-3495
703-836-2843 (fax)
Email: USPA@USPA.org
Website: http://www.USPA.org/

Soccer

American Amputee Soccer Association
Website: http://www.ampsoccer.org

Federation Internationale de Football Association (FIFA)
Case Postale 85 (Hitzigweg 11)
8030 Zurich, Switzerland
(41-1) 384-9595
(41-1) 384-9696 (fax)
website: http://www.fifa.com

International Amputee Football Federation
Website: http://www.ampsoccer.org/iaff/index.htm
     Full set of rules and field dimensions are available on this web site.

International Paralympic Committee 7-A-Side Soccer Rules
Website:
http://www.paralympic.org/ipc/handbook/section4/chapter13/content.htm

International Blind Sports Association
Website: http://www.ibsa.es/ibsa/ibsa.html

United States of America Deaf Soccer Association
Farley Warshaw (temporary)
(301) 662-9340
(301) 662-1371 (fax)
Email: farwar@aol.com

United States Amputee Soccer Association
% Disabled Sports USA – Northwest
117 E. Louisa St., #202
Seattle, WA 98102
(260) 467-5157
Email: USAsteam@dsusa.org

United States Soccer Federation
U.S. Soccer House
1801-1811 South Prairie Avenue
Chicago, IL 60616
(312) 808-1300
(312) 808-9566 (fax)
Email: socfed@aol.com
Website: http://www.us-soccer.com

US Youth Soccer Association
899 Presidential Drive, Suite 117
Richardson, TX 75081
(800) 4-Soccer
Website: http://www.youthsoccer.org

Softball

Amateur Softball Association (USA Softball)
2801 N.E. 50th Street
Oklahoma City, OK 73111-7203
Email: info@softball.org
Website: http:www.usasoftball.com/
            (national team information only)
Website: http://www.softball.org/

International Softball Federation

1900 S. Park Road
Plant City, FL 33566-8113 USA
(813) 707 7204
(813) 707 7209 (fax)
Email: isfsoftball@ci.plant-city.fl.us
Website:
http://www.worldsport.com/worldsport/sports/softball/home.html

Little League Baseball
Website: http://www.littleleague.org/
Challenger Division
Website:
    http://www.littleleague.org/divisions/chall.htm

National Softball Association of the Deaf (NSAD)
USA Deaf Sports Federation
3607 Washington Blvd., Suite 4
Ogden, UT 84403-1737
(801) 393-7916 Office (TTY: use your state relay service)
(801) 393-2263 (fax)
Email: Officers@NSAD
Website: http://www.nsad.org/

National Wheelchair Softball Association
1616 Todd Court
Hastings, MN 55033
Website: http://www.wheelchairsoftball.com/

Table Tennis

American Wheelchair Table Tennis Association (AWTTA)
Attn: Jennifer Johnson
23 Parker Street
Port Chester, NY 10573
(914) 937-3932

International Table Tennis Federation (ITTF)
53, London Road
St. Leonards-on-Sea, East Sussex
TN37 6AY, Great Britain
Email: http://www@ittf.com
Website: http://www.ittf.com

International Table Tennis Committee for the Disabled
Website: http://www.tabletennis.org/ittc/
    This website provides extensive information on players rankings, profiles, rules, competition updates, and links

USA Table Tennis (USATT)

USATT Disabled Athletes & Tournaments Committee
One Olympic Plaza
Colorado Springs, CO 80909-5769
(719) 578-4583
(719) 632-6071 (fax)
Email: usatt@iex.net
Website: http://www.usatt.org/

Team Handball

International Handball Federation
Case Postale 312 (Lange Gasse 10)
4020 Basel, Switzerland (4052)
(41-61) 272-1300
(41-61) 272-1344 (fax)
Email: IHF@magnet.ch
Website: http://www.worldsport.com/sports/handball/home.html

Special Olympics Director of Team Handball
1325 G Street, N.W., Suite 500
Washington, DC 20005
(202) 628-3630
(202) 824-0200 (fax)
Email: SOImail@aol.com
Website: http://www.specialolympics.org

United States Deaf Team Handball Association
Gene Duve
(510) 862-2907
Email: geneduve@aol.com

USA Team Handball
1903 Powers Ferry Rd., Suite 230
Atlanta, Ga. 30339
(770) 956-7660
(770) 956-7976 (fax)
(888) Play-THB
Email: info@usateamhandball.org
Website: http://www.usateamhandball.org

Tennis

Wheelchair Tennis Department
C/o International Tennis Federation
Bank Lane, Roehampton
London SW15 5XZ, United Kingdom
(011) 44-181-878-6464
(011) 44-181-392-4745 (fax)
Email: ITF@ITFTennis.com
Website: http://www.itftennis.com

United States Tennis Association
70 West Red Oak Lane
White Plains, NY 10604-3602

(800) 990-8782
(914) 696-7008 (fax)
Website: http://www.usta.com
    http://www.usta.com/usatennis/wheelchair/index.html

Track & Field

Achilles Track Club International (see Road Racing Chapter)
42 West 38th Street
New York, NY 10018
(212) 354-3978
(212) 354-3978
Email: AchillesClub@aol.com
Website: http://www.achillestrackclub.org/

International Amateur Athletic Federation
17 rue Princesse Florestine
BP 359
MC 98007 Monaco Cedex
(377) 93 10 88 88
(377) 93 15 95 15 (fax)
Email: headquarters@iaaf.org
Website: http://www.iaaf.org/

United States of America Deaf Track and Field
Website: http://members.tripod.com/~usadtf/

USA Track & Field
P.O. Box 120 (One RCA Dome, Suite 140)
Indianapolis, IN 46206-0120 (46225)
Email: USATFprogs@aol.com
Website: http://www.usatf.org

Wheelchair Racing Resource Page
Email: birzer@execpc.com
Website: http://www.execpc.com/~birzer/

Wheelchair Athletics of the USA
Barry Ewing
2351 Parkwood Road
Snellville, GA 30278
(770) 972-0763
(770) 985-4885 (fax)
Email: bewing@beilesouth.net

Volleyball

American Deaf Volleyball Association
7582 South Rosemary Circle
Englewood, CO 80112
Attn: Karen Boyd

Disabled Sports USA Volleyball

921 N. Village Lake Dr
Deland, FL32724
904-736-9622 (fax)
Email: seil@totcon.com

Federation Internationale de Volleyball (FIVB)
Avenue de la Gare 12
1000 Lausanne 1
Switzerland
(41-21) 345-3535
(41-21) 345-3545
Email: info@mail.fivb.ch
Website: http://www.fivb.ch

United States of America Deaf Volleyball Association
Farley Warshaw (temporary)
(301) 662-9340
Email: farwar@aol.com

USA Volleyball (USAV)
3595 E. Fountain Blvd., Ste. I-2
Colorado Springs, CO 80910-1740
(719) 637-8300
(719) 597-6307 (fax)
(888) 786-5539—Information Line
Email: postmaster@usav.org
Website: www.usavolleyball.org

World Organization Volleyball Disabled (WOVD)
Klein Heiligland 90
NL-2011 EJ Haarlem
The Netherlands
Email: hqwovd@wovd.com
Website: http://www.wovd.com

Water Skiing

British Disabled Water Ski Association
The Tony Edge National Centre
Heron Lake
Wraysbury
Middlesex TW19 6HW
United Kingdom
Website: http://www.bdwsa.org.uk/

International Water Ski Federation (IWSF)
World Disabled Council
C.P. 5537 BO 22
40134 Bologna, Italy
Website: http://www.IWSF.com/
    The World Governing Body for Water Skiing includes a World Disabled Council for water skiing.

USAWater Ski
C/o Water Skiers with Disabilities Association
1251 Holy Cow Rd.
Polk City, FL 33868
(863) 324-4341

Mission Bay Aquatic Center/Disabled Water Sports
1001 Santa Clara Point
San Diego, CA 92109
(619) 488-1036

National Ability Center
Post Office Box 682799
Park City, Utah 84068
(435) 649-3991 (voice/TTY)
(435) 658-3992 (fax)
Email: nac@xmission.com
Website: http://nationalabilitycenter.org

Texas Adaptive Aquatics
17003 Bentana Court
Houston, TX 77095
(713) 462-0016
Email: neosoft.com/tzadaqua
Website: http://www.neosoft.com/~txadaqua/

Wheelchair Dance Sport

American Dance Therapy Association
2000 Century Plaza, Suite 108
10632 Little Patuxent Parkway
Columbia, MD 21044
(410) 997-4040
(410) 997-4048 (fax)
Email: info@adta.org
Website: http://www.adta.org/

Dancing Wheels
3615 Euclid Avenue
Cleveland, Ohio 44115
(216) 432-0306
(216) 432-0308 (fax)
Email: proflair1@aol.com
Website: http://www.dancingwheels.org

Dancescape's World of Ballroom Dancing and Dance Sport
Website: http://www.dancescape.com

Full Radius Dance Company
Email: dsdance@aol.com
Website: http://www.fullradiusdance.org/

Gallaudet Dance Company
Gallaudet University

Department of Physical Education and Recreation
Washington, D.C.
(202) 651-5493

International Dance Sport Federation (IDSF).
Website: http://www.idsf.net

International Paralympic Committee Wheelchair Dance Sport Committee (IPC-WDSC)
Dr. Gertrude Krombholz, Chairperson
Nederlingerstr. 30
80638 Munich, Germany
(49)–89–157 3601
(49)–89–157 3503 (fax)
Email: G.Krombholz@t-online.de
Website:
   http://www.paralympic.org/sports/sections/dancing.asp

Light Motion
1520 32nd Avenue South
Seattle, WA 98144
(206) 328-0818

The United States Amateur Ballroom Dancers Association (USABDA)
PO Box 128
New Freedom, PA 17349
(800) 447-9047
(717) 235-4183 (fax)
Email: usabdacent@aol.com
Website: http://www.usabda.org

United States Dancesport Council, (USDSC)
Mr. Gary Stroick, Vice President
3800 France Avenue South
St. Louis Park, MN 55416
(612) 926-7648 (phone/fax)
Email: DanceSportVP.usabda.org

National Dance Council of America (NDCA)
Ballroom Department
Lee Wakefield, Director
P.O. Box 22018
Provo, UT 84602
(801) 378-8381 (phone/fax)
Email: Lee_Wakefield@byu.edu

Weight Training

National Strength and Conditioning Association
1955 N. Union Blvd.
Colorado Springs, CO 80909
(719) 632-6722
(800) 815-6826
(719) 632-6367 (fax)

Email: nsca@nsca-lift.org
Website: http://www.nsca-lift.org/

The North American Academy of Health, Fitness & Rehabilitation Professionals
The Medical Exercise Specialist
(888) 610-0923
Email: medfit2000@aol.com
Website: http://www.medicalexercisespecialist.com

Wilderness Experiences

"Access Challenge Project"
BC Mobility Opportunities Society
Box 27, Plaza of Nations, Suite A-304
770 Pacific Blvd. South
Vancouver, BC V6B 5E7 Canada
(604) 688-6464
(604) 688-6463 (fax)
Email: bcmos@reachdisability.org
Website: http://www.reachdisability.org/bcmos

Adaptive Adventures
P.O. Box 2245
Evergreen, CO 80439
(303) 679-2770
Website: http://www.adaptiveadventures.org

Adaptive Sports Center
Crested Butte, CO
(907) 349-2296
Email: ascl@rmi.net
Website: http://www.adaptivesports.org

American Camping Association, Inc.
5000 State Road 67 North
Martinsville, Indiana 46151
(765) 342-8456
(765) 342-2065 (fax)
Website: http://www.acacamps.org/

American Hiking Society
1422 Fenwick Lane
Silver Spring, MD 20910
(301) 565-6704
(301) 565-6714 (fax)
Email: AmHiker@aol.com
Website: http://www.americanhiking.org/

American Whitewater Affiliation
1430 Fenwick Lane
Silver Spring, MD 20910
(301) 589-9453
Website: http://www.awa.org
    National organization of whitewater boating enthusiasts.

Boy Scouts of America (Scouts With Disabilities and Special Needs)
1325 West Walnut Hill Lane
P.O. Box 152079
Irving, TX 75015-2079.
(214) 580-2423
(214) 580-2502
Website: http://www.bsa.scouting.org/

Breckenridge Outdoor Education Center Wilderness program
PO Box 697
Breckenridge, CO 80424
(800) 383-BOEC(2632)
(970) 453-6422
(970) 453-4676 (fax)
Email: boec@boec.org
Website: http://www.boec.org/

Courage Center
3915 Golden Valley Road
Minneapolis, MN 55422
(763) 520-0520
(888) 8INTAKE
(763) 520-0577 (fax)
Email: jenim@courage.org
Website: http://www.courage.org/

Department of the Interior
Coordinating Committee on Accessibility for People with Disabilities
Website: http://www.pn.usbr.gov/doiacc/

Great Outdoors Recreation Pages (GORP)
Website: http://www.gorp.com/

International Orienteering Federation
Website: http://www.orienteering.org/

National Center on Accessibility
5020 State Road 67 North
Martinsville, Indiana 46151
(765) 349-9240 (voice/TTY)
(765) 342-6658 (fax)
Email: nca@indiana.edu
Website: http://www.indiana.edu/~nca/

National Park Service
1849 C Street NW
Washington, DC 20240
(202) 208-6843
Website: http://www.nps.gov/

Outdoor Buddies, Inc.
P.O. Box 37283

Denver CO 80237
(303) 771-8216
(303) 771-9002 (fax)
Email: outbud@aol.com.
Website: http://www.outdoorbuddies.com/

National Sports Center for the Disabled
P.O. Box 1290
Winter Park, CO 80482
(970) 726-1540
(970) 726-4112 (fax)
Email: info@nscd.org
Website: http://www.nscd.org

Turning P.O.I.N.T. (Paraplegics on Independent Nature
Trips)
4144 North Central Expressway, Suite 130
Dallas, TX 75204
(214) 827-7404
(214) 827-6468 (fax)
Website: http://www.turningpoint1.com

SPLORE
27 West 3300 South
Salt Lake City, Utah 84115
(801) 484-4128
(801) 484-4177 (fax)
Email: info@splore.org
Website: http://www.splore.org

United States Orienteering Federation
P.O.Box 1444
Forest Park, GA 30298
(404) 363 2110
(404) 363 2110 (fax)
Email: rshannonhouse@mindspring.com
Website: http://www.us.orienteering.org/

Wilderness Inquiry
808 14th Ave SE
Minneapolis, MN 55414
(612) 676-9400
(800) 728-0719
(612) 676-9401 (fax)
Email: info@wildernessinquiry.org
Website: http://www.wildernessinquiry.org/

Wheelchair Outdoor Adventure Camp (Challenge Aspen)
(800) 530-3901
(970) 923-0578

Wilderness On Wheels Foundation
3131 Vaughn Way, Suite 305
Aurora, CO 80014
(303) 751-3959
Email: wow@ecentral.com
Website: http://www.wildernessonwheels.org/

Wrestling

Canadian Amateur Wrestling Association
1600 James Naismith Drive, #505
Gloucester, Ontario K1B 5N4
Canada
(613) 748-5686
(613) 748-5756 (fax)
Website: http://www.wrestling.ca/home.html

Intermat Wrestling
Website: http://www.Intermatwrestle.com
     This site provides the ultimate amateur wrestling re-
source.

International Blind Sports Association IBSA)
Website: http://www..es/sports/wrestling.html
                 http://www.ibsa.es/sports/wrestling.html

International Federation of Associated Wrestling Styles
(FILA)
Avenue Juste-Olivier 17
CH-1006 Lausanne, Switzerland
 (41-21) 312-8426
 (41-21) 323-6073 (FAX)
Website: http://www.fila-wrestling.org

USA Wrestling
6155 Lehman Drive
Colorado Springs, CO 80918
(719) 598-8181
(719) 598-9440 (fax)
Email: usaw@concentric.net
Website: http://www.usawrestling.org

United States Deaf Wrestling Association
Maurice Abenchuchan
(904) 797-5695
(904) 823-4203 (fax)
Email: abenchm@mail.fim.edu

Appendix B

Sport Wheelchair Suppliers

Allnight Wheelchairs
7730-238th Place SW
Edmonds, WA 98026
(425) 774-9802
Email: customcmpt@aol.com
    Sport Chairs For: basketball, hockey, tennis, rugby

Colours By Permobile
1591 South Sinclair Street, Unit 1
Anaheim, CA 92806
(800) 892-8998
(714) 978-2891 (fax)
Email: amalebox@aol.com
    Sport Chairs For: basketball, hockey, rugby, tennis

Eagle Sportchairs
2351 Parkwood Road
Snellville, GA 30039
(800) 932-9380
(700 972-0763 (fax)
Email: bewing@harb.net
    Sport Chairs For: all sport, all terrain, basketball, racing, rugby, tennis

Everest & Jennings
3601 Rider Trail South
Earth City, MO 63045
(800) 235-4661
(512) 7038 (fax)

Invacare Corporation
One Invacare Way
Elyria, OH 44036
(800) 333-6900

New Hall's Wheels
P.O. Box 380784
Cambridge, MA 02238
(800) 628-7956
(617) 628-6546 (FAX)
Website: http://www.NEWHALLS@tiac.com
    Sport Chairs For: basketball, racing, tennis

Otto Back Rehab
3000 Xenium Lane

Minneapolis, MN 55441
(800) 328-4058
(612) 553-9464 (fax)

Per4Max Medical
2550 114th Street, Suite 180
Grand Prarie, TX 75050
(972) 641-6773
(972) 623-0585 (fax)
    Sport Chairs For: all sport, basketball, racing, rugby, tennis

SPORTAID/MEDAID
(800) 743-7203
(770) 554-5385 (fax)
Email: info@Sportaid.com
Website: http://www.sportaid.com
    Largest wheelchair supply mail order company

Sunrise Medical
7477 East Dry Creek Parkway
Longmont, CO 80503
(800) 333-4000
(800) 300-7502 (fax)
Website: http://www.sunrisemedical.com
    Sport Chairs For: basketball, rugby

Top End
4501 63rd Circle North
Pinellas Park, FL 33781
(800) 532-8677
(7727) 522-1007 (fax)
Website: http://www.invacare.com
    Sport Chairs For: basketball, racing, rugby, tennis

Appendix C
Sports Offered By Disability Sport Organizations

	DAAA	DS/USA	SOI	USABA	USADSF	USCPAA	WS-USA
Alpine Skiing	x	x	x	x	x		
Archery		x					x
Badminton	x		*		x		
Baseball					x		
Basketball	x		x		x		x
Boccia	x		*			x	
Bowling			x		x	x	
Cross Country						x	
Cycling	x	x	x	x	x	x	
Equestrian	x		x			x	
Fencing							x
Figure Skating		x					
Floor Hockey		x					
Goalball				x			
Golf			x		x		
Gymnastics			x				
Ice Hockey					x		
Judo				x			
Lawn Bowling		x					
Nordic Skiing		x	x	x	x		x
Powerlifting	x			x			x
Quad Rugby						x	x
Racquetball							x
Roller Skating			x				
Sailing		x	*				
Shooting							x
Sled Hockey						x	
Snowboarding					x		
Soccer	x		x		x	x	
Soccer (Wheelchair)					x		
Softball			x		x		
Speed Skating			x				
Swimming	x	x	x	x	x	x	x
Table Tennis	x	x	x	*	x		x
Team Handball					*		x
Tennis		x		x		1	
Track & Field	x	x	x	x	x	x	x
Volleyball-stand	x		x		x		x
Volleyball (sit)		x					
Water Skiing							x
Wrestling				x			x

*Nationally Popular Sport
WS-USA: Sport Federations
USADSF: Sport Federations
1:          Potential Member

Appendix D

Special Olympics United States Chapters

Below is the list of Special Olympics United States Chapters at the time this book went to print. The reader should be aware that names and addresses have a habit of frequent change. A current list of these associations may be found on the Special Olympics website: <http://www.specialolympics.org/program_locations/program_locations_frame.html>

Special Olympics Alabama
880 South Court Street
Montgomery, AL 36104
(334) 242-3383
(334) 262-9794 (fax)
Email: Also@juno.com

Special Olympics Alaska
4055 Arctic Warrior Drive
Elemendorf Air Force Base AFB, AK 99506
(907) 753-2182
(907) 753-2192 (fax)
Email: info@specialolympicsalaska.org
Website: http://www.specialolympicsalaska.org

Special Olympics Arizona
3816 N. 7th Street
Phoenix, AZ 85014-5004
(602) 230-1200
(602) 230-1110 (fax)
Email: spolympaz@aol.com
Website: http://www.specialolympicsarizona.org

Special Olympics Arkansas
2115 Main St.
North Little Rock, AR 72114
(800) 722 9063
(501) 771-0222
(501) 771-1020 (fax)
Email: arkso@juno.com

Special Olympics Southern California
6071 Bristol Parkway, Suite 100
Culver City, CA 90230-6601
(310) 215-8380
(310) 215-8388 (fax)
Email: sosc@sosc.org
Website: http://www.sosc.org/

Special Olympics Northern California
3480 Buskirk Avenue, Suite 340
Pleasant Hill, CA 94523
(925) 944-8801
(925) 944-8803 (fax)
Email: rick@sonc.org
Website: http://www.sonc.org/

Special Olympics Colorado
410 17th Street, Suite 200
Denver, CO 80202
(303) 592-1361
(303) 592-1364 (fax)
Email: pl@specialolympicsco.org
Website: http://specialolympicsco.org

Special Olympics Connecticut
2666 State Street, Suite 1
Hamden, CT 06517-2232
(203) 230-1201
(203) 230-1202 (fax)
Email: mailbox@soct.org
Website: http://www.soct.org/

Special Olympics Delaware
University of Delaware
619 South College Ave.
Newark, DE 19716-1901
(302) 831-4653
(302) 831-3483 (fax)
Email: agrunert@udel.edu
Website: http://www.sode.org

Special Olympics District of Columbia
300 Eye Street, N.E. Suite 102
Washington, DC 20002
(202) 544-7770
(202) 546-8249 (fax)
Email: wdcso@aol.com

Special Olympics Florida
8 Broadway, Suite D
Kissimmee, FL 34741
(407) 870-2292
(407) 870-9810 (fax)

Email: sofl1@aol.com
Website: http://www.sofl.org

Special Olympics Georgia
3772 Pleasantdale Road, Suite 195
Atlanta, GA 30340
(770) 414-9390
(770) 414-9389 (fax)
Email: georgia.milton-sheats@specialolympicsga.org

Special Olympics Hawaii
P.O. Box 3295
Honolulu, HI 96801
(808) 531-1888
(808) 528-0881 (fax)
Email: nbottelo@aol.com
Website: http://www.specialolympicshawaii.com/

Special Olympics Idaho
8426 Fairview Avenue
Boise, ID 83704
(208) 323-0482
(208) 323-0486 (fax)
Email: iso@micron.net
Website: http://www.idso.org

Special Olympics Illinois
605 East Willow Street
Normal, IL 61761
(309) 888-2551
(309) 888-2570 (fax)
Email: soill@aol.com
Website: http://www.soill.org

Special Olympics Indiana
5648 West 74th Street
Indianapolis, IN 46278-1752
(317) 328-2000
(317) 328-2018 (fax)
Email: info@specialolympicsindiana.org
Website: http://www.specialolympicsindiana.org

Special Olympics Iowa
3737 Woodland Avenue, Suite 325
West Des Moines, IA 50266
(515) 267-0131
(515) 267-0232 (fax)
Email: soiowa@soiowa.org
Website: http://www.soiowa.org

Special Olympics Kansas
5280 Foxridge Drive
Mission, KS 66202-1567
(913) 236-9290

(913) 236-9771 (fax)
Email: kso@ksso.org
Website: http://www.ksso.org

Special Olympics Kentucky
105 Lakeview Court
Frankfort, KY 40601-8749
(502) 695-8222
(502) 695-0496 (fax)
Email: dkercher@soky.org
Website: http://www.soky.org

Special Olympics Louisiana
200 Southwest. Railroad Ave
Hammond, LA 70403
(504) 345-6644
(504) 345-6649 (fax)
Email: emmanuelbourgeois@hotmail.com
Website: http://www.laso.org

Special Olympics Maine
125 John Roberts Road, Suite 19
South Portland, ME 04106
(207) 879-0489
(207) 879-0672 (fax)
Email: SOMEemail@aol.com
Website: http://www.specialolympicsmaine.org

Special Olympics Maryland
8300 Guilford Road, Suite A
Columbia, MD 21046
(410) 290-7611 3007
(410) 381-4483 (fax)
Email: pkrebs@somd.org
Website: http://www.somd.org/

Special Olympics Massachusetts
P.O. Box 303
Hathorne, MA 01937
(978) 774-1501
(978) 750-4686 (fax)
Email: ceo@specialolympicsma.org

Special Olympics Michigan
East Campus Drive, Central Michigan University
Mt. Pleasant, MI 48859
(517) 774-3911
(517) 774-3034 (fax)
Email: lois.r.t.arnold@cmich.edu
Website: http://www.somi.org

Special Olympics Minnesota
400 South Fourth Street , Suite 915
Minneapolis, MN 55415-1423

(612) 333-0999 11
(612) 333-8782 (fax)
Email: somn@somn.org
website: http://www.somn.org/

Special Olympics Mississippi
15 Olympic Way
Madison, MS 39110
(601) 856-7748
(601) 856-8132 (fax)
Email: SpOlyMiss@aol.com

Special Olympics Missouri
520 Dix Road, Suite C
Jefferson City, MO 65109
(573) 635-1660
(573) 635-8233 (fax)
Email: hq@somo.org
Website: http://www.somo.org

Special Olympics Montana
P.O. Box 3507
3117 5th Avenue North
Great Falls, MT 59403-3507
(406) 268-6759
(406) 454-9043 (fax)
Email: info@specialolympicsmt.org
Website: http://www.specialolympicsmt.org

Special Olympics Nebraska
8801 F St.
P.O. Box 27085
Omaha, NE 68127
(402) 331-5545
(402) 331-5964 (fax)
Email: sone@radiks.net
Website: http://www.sone.org/

Special Olympics Nevada
624 S. 4th Street, Suite B,
Las Vegas, NV 89101
(702) 474-0690
(702) 474-0694 (fax)
Email: sparks1son@aol.com
Website: http://www.nvso.org

Special Olympics New Hampshire
650 Elm Street, Suite 101
Manchester, NH 03101
(603) 624-1250
(603) 624-4911 (fax)
Email: sonewh@aol.com
Website: http://www.sonh.org/

Special Olympics New Jersey
Princeton Forrestal Village
201 Rockingham Row
Princeton, NJ 08540
(609) 734-8400
(609) 734-0911 (fax)
Email: mse@njso.org
Website: http://www.sonj.org

Special Olympics New Mexico
6600 Palomas N.E., Suite 207
Albuquerque, NM 87109
(505) 856-0342
(505) 856-0346 (fax)
Email: sonmrandy@aol.com

Special Olympics New York
504 Balltown Road
Schenectady, NY 12304-2290
(518) 388-0790F
(518) 388-0795 (fax)
Email: njohnson@nyso.org
Website: http://www.specialolympicsnewyork.org

Special Olympics North Carolina
P.O. Box 25968
Raleigh, NC 27611-5968
(919) 719-SONC (7662)
(919) 719-7663 (fax)
Email: kfishburne@sonc.net
Website: http://www.sonc.net/

Special Olympics North Dakota
2616 South 26th Street
Grand Forks, ND 58201
(701) 746-0331
(701) 772-1265 (fax)
Email: gfndso@corpcomm.net

Special Olympics Ohio
3303 Winchester Pike
Columbus, OH 43232
(614) 239-7050
(614) 239-1873 (fax)
Email: rwrsooh@aol.com

Special Olympics Oklahoma
6835 South Canton Avenue
Tulsa, OK 74136-3433
(918) 481-1234
(918) 496-1515 (fax)
Email: info@sook.org
Website: http://www.sook.org/

Special Olympics Oregon
3325 NW Yeon Ave.
Portland, OR 97210-1525

(503) 248-0600
(800) 452-6079
(503) 248-0603 (fax)
Email: soor@soor.org
Website: http://www.soor.org

Special Olympics Pennsylvania
124 Washington Sq.
2570 Blvd. of the Generals
Norristown, PA 19403
(800) 235-9058
(610) 630-9456 (fax)
Email: jschoeniger@paso.org
Website: http://www.paso.org/

Special Olympics Rhode Island
33 College Hill Road, Suite 31
Warwick, RI 02886
(401) 823-7411
(401) 823-7415 (fax)
Email: mmcgovsori@aol.com

Special Olympics South Carolina
Dutch Plaza
810 Dutch Square Blvd., Suite 204
Columbia, SC 29210
(803) 772-1555 ext. 2925
(800) 765 7276
(803) 772-0094 (fax)
Email: bcoats@so-sc.org
Website: http://www.so-sc.org

Special Olympics South Dakota
305 West 39th Street
Sioux Falls, SD 57105
(605) 331-4117
(605) 331-4328 (fax)
Email: sosdak@aol.com
Website: http://www.sosd.org

Special Olympics Tennessee
1900 12th Avenue South
Nashville, TN 37203
(615) 327-1465
(800) 288-5225
(615) 343-9473 (fax)
Email: Absotn@aol.com
Website: http://www.specialolympics-tn.org

Special Olympics Texas
11442 North Interstate 35
Austin, TX 78753
(512) 835-9873
(512) 835-7756 (fax)
Email: info@sotx.org
Website: http://www.sotx.org/

Special Olympics Utah
4 Triad Center, Suite 105
Salt Lake City, UT 84180
(801) 363-1111 121
(801) 363-1524 (fax)
Email: utsoinfo@utso.org
Website: http://www.utso.org

Special Olympics Vermont
368 Avenue D, Suite 30
Williston, VT 05495
(802) 863-5222
(802) 863-3911 (fax)
Email: mderda@vtso.org
Website: http://www.vtso.org/

Special Olympics Virginia
3212 Skipwith Road, Suite 100
Richmond, VA 23294

(804) 346-5544
(800) 932-GOLD
(804) 346-9633 (fax)
Email: spolva@aol.com
Website: http://www.specialolympicsva.com

Special Olympics Washington
2150 North 107th Avenue, Suite 220
Seattle, WA 98133
(206) 362-4949 ext. 219 210
(206) 361-8158 (fax)
Email: dsiebert@sowa.org
Website: http://www.sowa.org

Special Olympics West Virginia
914 Market Street, Suite 201
Parkersburg, WV 26101
(304) 422-1868
(800) 926 1616
(304) 428-8395 (fax)

Special Olympics Wisconsin
5900 Monona Drive, Suite 301
Madison, WI 53716
(608) 222-1324

(608) 222-3578 (fax)
Email: wisoinfo@wiso.org
Website: http://www.wiso.org/

Special Olympics Wyoming
735 English Drive,

Casper, WY 82601
(307) 235-3062
(307) 235-3063 (fax)
Email: sow@caspers.net

Appendix E
USA Deaf Sports Federation National Sports Organizations and International Affiliations

Below is the list of USA Deaf Sports Federation (National Sports Organizations) at the time this book went to print. The reader should be aware that names and addresses USA Deaf Sports Federation website: < http://www.usadsf.org>

USA Deaf Sports Federation (National Sports Organizations)

United States Aquatic Association of the Deaf
Caroline A. Miller
(206) 543-0275
Email: cmiller@ocean.washington.edu

United States of America Deaf Track and Field
Thomas E. Withrow
(301) 464-1284
Email: tewithrow@aol.com

United States Deaf Badminton Association
Kenneth Eurek
(719) 475-0693
Email: ped10@aol.com

United States of America Deaf Baseball
Jeff Salit
(202) 708-3577
Email: jeffsalit@aol.com

United States of America Deaf Basketball
Bennie Maucere, Comm.
(818) 789-2087
Email: usadb@jps.net

United States Deaf Bowling Federation
Connie Marchione
(818) 785-1478

United States Deaf Cycling Association
Bobby Skedsmo
(510) 471-6064
Email: skedsmo@earthlink.net

United States Flag Football of the Deaf
John Schlutz
(716) 825-2305
Email: usffdjcs@webtv.com

United States Deaf Golf Foundation
James Hynes
(301) 464-9581
Email: jhynesjr@aol.com

American Hearing Impaired Hockey Association
Stan Mikita
(312) 829-2098

United States Deaf Skiers and Snowboarders Association
Robert Lewis
(512) 328-6457
Email: razlewis@texas.net

United States of America Deaf Soccer Association
Farley Warshaw (temporary)
(301) 662-1371
Email: farwar@aol.com

National Softball Association of the Deaf
Vance Rewolinski, Comm.
(512) 444-6983
Email: vbut@texas.net
United States Deaf Table Tennis Association
Emanuel Golden
(904) 794-0458

United States Deaf Team Handball Association
Gene Duve
(510) 862-2907
Email: geneduve@aol.com

United States Deaf Tennis Association
Jamie McElfresh
(954) 349-0662
Email: jamtennis@aol.com

United States of America Deaf Volleyball Association
Farley Warshaw (temporary)
(301) 662-1371
Email: farwar@aol.com

United States Deaf Wrestling Association
Maurice Abenchuchan
(904) 823-4203
Email: abenchm@mail.fim.edu

Appendix F
Wheelchair Sports—USA National Governing Bodies and Regional Sport Organizations

Below is the list of Wheelchair Sport USA National Governing Bodies and regional Sport Organizations at the time this book went to print. The reader should be aware that names and addresses have a habit of frequent change. A current list of these associations may be found on the Wheelchair Sports USA website <http://www.wsusa.org/directory.htm>

Wheelchair Sports USA National Governing Bodies

American Amateur Racquetball Association—Wheelchair
Luke St. Onge, Executive Director
1685 West Uintah
Colorado Springs, CO 80904
(719) 635-6395
(719) 638-0585 (fax)

American Disabled Water Skiers
William Furbish
3480 Statfield Drive
Atlanta, GA 30319
(404) 261-9527
(404) 364-9405 (fax)
Email: bfurbish@mindspring.com

American Sled Hockey Association
Rich DeGlopper
21 Summerwood Court
Buffalo, NY 14223
(716) 874-8411 ext. 7328
(716) 874-8518
Email: rich_deglopper@admgat.kenton.k12.ny.us

American Wheelchair Table Tennis Association
Jennifer Johnson
23 Parker Street
Port Chester, NY 10573
(914) 937-3932

National Wheelchair Basketball Association
Roger A.Davis Sr., Commisioner
710 Queensbury Loop
Winter Garden FL 34787
(407) 654-4215
(407) 654-6682

OR

David Kiley
1100 Blythe Blvd.
Charlotte, NC 28203
(704) 355-1064
Email: nwba@carolines.org

Wheelchair Track and Field USA
Barry Ewing
2351 Parkwood Road
Snellville, GA 30278
(770) 972-0763
(770) 985-4885 (fax)
Email: bewing@beilesouth.net

National Wheelchair Shooting Federation
David Baskin
NRA Disabled Shooting Services
11250 Waples Mill Road
Fairfax, VA 22030
(703) 267-1495
(703) 267-3941 (fax)

US Handcycling Association
Ian Lawless
115 Du Four St.
Santa Cruz, Ca 95060
(831) 457-7747

US Quad Rugby Association
Ed Suhr
3340 SE Morrison
Portland, OR 97214

(503) 238-1324 (phone/fax)
Email: esuhr@aol.com

US Wheelchair Swimming
Liz DeFrancesco
5730 Chambertin Drive
San Jose, CA 95118
(408) 267-0200
(408) 267-2834 fax

US Wheelchair Weightlifting Federation
Bill Hens
39 Michael Place
Levittown, PA 19057
(215) 945-1964
(215) 946-2574 (fax)

Wheelchair Archers, USA
Lyn Rourke
528 N. Bauman Street
Indianapolis, IN 46214
(317) 244-2377
Email: LMR1970@aol.com

Wheelchair Athletics of the USA
Barry Ewing
2351 Parkwood Road
Snellville, GA 30278
(770) 972-0763
(770) 985-4885 (fax)
Email: bewing@harb.net

Wheelchair Fencing
Mario Rodriguez
2023 Steber
Houston, TX
(713) 946-1780
Email: usfencer@hotmail.com

Wheelchair Sports USA Regional Sports Organizations

Appalachian Wheelchair Athletic Association
Gerry Herman
22 Mitchell Drive
Abingdon, MD 21009
(410) 669-2015 ext 16
(410) 669-7215 (fax)
Email: gherman@abs.net

Dixie Wheelchair Athletic Association
Laverne Achenbach
3230 Skyland Drive SW
Snellville, GA 30278
(770) 978-8183

Far West Wheelchair Athletic Association
Lauri Yarwasky
5730 Chambertin
San Jose, CA 95118
(408) 267-0200
(408) 267-0200
(408) 267-2834 (fax)

Great Lakes Adaptive Athletic Association
Cindy Housner
P.O. Box 5333
Vernon Hills, IL 60051
(547) 249-8655

Wheelchair Sports, Hawaii
Jeff Sampaga
95-1086 Lalai Street
Honolulu, HI 96789
(808) 943-1250

Michigan Wheelchair Athletic Association
Diane Winterstein
14410 Vale Court
Sterling Heights, MI 48312
(810) 977-6123 ext 217
(810) 977-6239 (fax)

Mid-Atlantic Wheelchair Athletic Association
Stephen Bridge
Box 103, WWRC
Fishersville, VA 22939
(540) 332-7184
(540) 332-7394 (fax)

New England Wheelchair Athletic Association
Dick Crisafulli
MA Hospital School
3 Randolph Street
Canton, MA 02021
(617) 828-2440 ext. 388
(617) 821-4086 (fax)

North Central Wheelchair Athletic Association
Tobe Broadrick
Courage Center
3915 Golden Valley Road
Golden Valley, MN 55422
(612) 520-0479
(612) 520-0577 (fax)

Northwest Wheelchair Athletic Association
Joe Todisco
PO Box 1596

Big Timber, MT 59011
(406) 932-5237 (phone/fax)

Rocky Mountain Wheelchair Athletic Association
Mary Carpenter
1080 South Independence Court
Lakewood, CO 80226
(303) 985-7525
(303) 985-0090 (fax)
Email: mcarpent@jeffco.k12.co.us

Southeastern Wheelchair Athletic Association
Lana Witiak
Rt. 25 Box 346N
Fayettvile, NC 28306
(910) 323-9010 ext. 334

Southwest Wheelchair Athletic Association
Jerry Terry
705 West Ave. B Suite 300
Garland, TX 75040
(972) 494-3160
(972) 494-0150
Email: jtswaa@aol.com

Tri-State Wheelchair Athletic Association
Ralph Armento
45 Richford Road
Kendall Park, NJ 08824
(732) 422-9094
(732) 422-4546
Email: ralpharm@aol.com

Michael J. Paciorek, Ph.D.

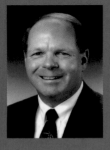

Michael J. Paciorek, Ph.D. is a professor and Physical Education Program Coordinator in the Department of Health, Physical Education, Recreation and Dance at Eastern Michigan University, with specialties in adapted physical education and motor development. He received his B.S. in Physical Education from St. Bonaventure University, his M.A. in adapted physical education from The George Washington University, and his Ph.D. from Peabody College of Vanderbilt University. He has taught adapted physical education in the Norfolk, VA City Schools and been involved in sports for individuals with disabilities for the past 25 years. He has served as a volunteer, coach, and member of the Board of Directors for Special Olympics Michigan and is Past President of the Michigan Association for Health, Physical Education, Recreation and Dance . He is a member of the Adapted Physical Activity Council (APAC) of AAHPERD and the National Consortium on Physical Education and Recreation for Individuals with Disabilities (NCPERID). He was an Assistant Coordinator of disabled athlete participation at the 1990 and 1991 United State Olympic Festivals, and was a staff member on the 1992 United States Disabled Sports Team at the Barcelona Paralympic games.

Jeffery A. Jones, M.P.E.

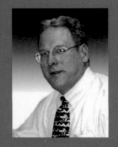

Jeffery A. Jones, M.P.E. received his B.S. in Physical Education from Southern Connecticut State College and his M.P.E. in Adapted Physical Education from Springfield College, and has done post-graduate work in Therapeutic Recreation at Wayne State University.

He has been working in the field of sports and recreation for individuals with disabilities for more than 20 years. His direct coaching experience in disability sports includes track & field, soccer, wheelchair team handball, cycling, quad rugby and sled hockey. He has been a member of the coaching or administrative staff of six United States Cerebral Palsy Sports Teams, including the teams that competed in the 1988,1992 & 1996 Paralympic Games. Jones is also the editor of a 1988 publication titled Training Guide to Cerebral Palsy Sports and the co-author of the 1994 and 1989 publication titled Sports and Recreation for the Disabled .

His disability sports work includes a consulting practice in sports and recreation (Specialized Sports Unlimited) and organization of more than 50 regional or national sports competitions, including the 1985 National Cerebral Palsy-Les Autres Games, the 1986 International Dwarf Games, and the 1992 National Women's Wheelchair Basketball Tournament, 2000 National Wheelchair Softball Tournament. He was the Assistant Coordinator of disabled athlete participation for the United States Olympic Festival from 1987 to 1991. He also served as President of the U.S. Cerebral Palsy Athletic Association from 1994 through the end of 2000.

He is currently the Director of Rehabilitation Institute of Chicago's Center for Health and Fitness and the Wirtz Sports Program, one of the largest disability sports and recreation program in the United States. Currently, the program offers 18 sports and recreation activities and is involved in several fitness/exercise related research projects. His wife, Marybeth, shares his passion for disability sports and works in a community-based Special Recreation Association. His children, Kristyn and Benjamin, are avid sports fans, youth sports participants and frequent volunteers in Dad's programs.